PRAISE FOR
THE ENVIRONMENTAL AND GENETIC CAUSES OF AUTISM

"With nearly one in fifty US children being diagnosed with autism, *The Environmental and Genetic Causes of Autism* could not come soon enough. The information in this book needs to be read by all medical students, physicians, and parents. I highly recommend this book."

—Dr. David Brownstein, MD, medical director,
Center for Holistic Medicine

"Dr. Lyons-Weiler is an inspired American scientist. . . . I can say without reservation that this learned person has the ethics of a true teacher, the type idealized from the roots of Western Civilization. He analyzes scientific data for the sake of improving the human condition without monetary influence. . . . His work is encyclopedic."

—Dr. Edward "Ted" Fogarty, MD, chair, Department of Radiology,
University of North Dakota School of Medicine and Health Sciences

"With over one million new cases per year, a current incidence of one in 45–68 children, and a projected incidence of one in two children within two decades, autism is more than an epidemic—it is a national crisis. At this rate, our entire nation will either be autistic or caring for someone who is. While nearly all efforts and public pronouncements are about management and care, very few are exploring cause. We hear from the medical community that autism is a tragic but inevitable outcome of genetic roulette. Dr. Lyons-Weiler, an impeccably credentialed biologist . . . clearly explains the environmental causes of this terrible spectrum of disorders. In so doing, he provides much-needed hope for its prevention and cure. If you are a parent, health professional, or scientist, this is an essential book to read."

—Michael Gaeta, DAc, MS, CDN, clinician and educator

"This book is a Bible for anyone who wants to understand the deep science behind the autism epidemic in America. Dr. Lyons-Weiler shows us convincingly that autism is not a mysterious disease with no known cause and no known treatment: it is the expected outcome when you expose a child with a certain genetic makeup to multiple neurotoxins simultaneously."

—Dr. Stephanie Seneff, senior research scientist
at the Massachusetts Institute of Technology (MIT)

"[Dr. James Lyons-Weiler's new book is a call to action] for the pediatric community to 'awaken from its dogmatic slumber.' . . . Until our understanding of [autism spectrum disorders] (and their environmental, genetic, and immunological underpinnings) is secure, we must all be willing to evolve as practitioners and scientists and, thusly, light our own candles in the darkness, lest we fall into an abyss."

—Dr. Anthony Kovatch, MD, pediatrician, Pediatric Alliance

"Lyons-Weiler has done us all an immense service by putting together this well-documented and highly informative overview of autism. Those who are really seeking answers and a way forward will welcome this book. Those whose interests are threatened will not. Indeed, Lyons-Weiler will be able to measure just how much he has stung big pharma by the number of pharma-paid negative reviews in the media, and by the troll attacks, and the denunciations by the CDC. He should wear all these as a badge of [honor] for ultimately the truth will come out. This book will help the truth emerge."

—Christopher A. Shaw, PhD,
author of *Neural Dynamics of Neurological Disease*

The Environmental and Genetic Causes of Autism

THE ENVIRONMENTAL AND GENETIC CAUSES OF AUTISM

JAMES LYONS-WEILER, PhD

Skyhorse Publishing

Skyhorse Publishing books may be purchased in bulk at special discounts for sales promotion, corporate gifts, fund-raising, or educational purposes. Special editions can also be created to specifications. For details, contact the Special Sales Department, Skyhorse Publishing, 307 West 36th Street, 11th Floor, New York, NY 10018 or info@skyhorse-publishing.com.

Skyhorse® and Skyhorse Publishing® are registered trademarks of Skyhorse Publishing, Inc.®, a Delaware corporation.

Visit our website at www.skyhorsepublishing.com.

10 9 8 7 6 5 4 3 2

Library of Congress Cataloging-in-Publication Data is available on file.

Cover design by Rain Saukas

Print ISBN: 978-1-5107-1086-3
Ebook ISBN: 978-1-5107-1087-0

Printed in the United States of America

DEDICATION

This book is dedicated to six groups of people.

The first group are the tens of thousands of patients who have participated in the studies that generated the discoveries presented in this book. The second group are scientists whose hundreds of thousands of person-hours have contributed to a magnificent body of knowledge that has not been given its proper consideration in the formulation of public policy on vaccines. The third group are the brave pediatricians willing to examine deeply the issues with mercury and aluminum and other neurotoxins in vaccines. The fourth group are the many foundations that fund autism research, to whom we all owe an immense debt of gratitude for their wisdom, foresight, and generosity that allow us to pursue the research that generates knowledge. The fifth group are the parents of children and adults with autism, who know all too well that

> *Grief is not just the prerogative of those who have recently lost a loved one; it is also a constant companion for the spouse watching his or her life partner gradually succumb to a life-threatening or debilitating illness. Grief is woven in the days of anxious parents as they watch their ill or disabled child struggle and fail to keep up with healthy siblings and peers. . . . So grief is part and parcel of many illness experiences, whether that illness ultimately leads to death or not. If you allow yourself to love, then at some point in time you will probably need to figure out how to grieve.* (Michele Reiss, PhD, "Lessons in Loss and Living")

Finally, and most important, the sixth and final group this book is dedicated to are all the children injured by vaccines, who are dramatically undercounted in the Vaccine Adverse Event Reporting System (VAERS), including those who developed autism as a consequence of the US Centers for Disease Control and Prevention (CDC) vaccine policy, which has been formulated with a full dose of willful, egregious, and intolerable ignorance of the published studies that appear on the pages of this book.

I would like to thank the many people who have made this book possible, including first and foremost Grace Ruggirello Innes and my sons, Ben and Zach, for their sacrifices during the months of work on this project. I am indebted to Louis Conte and Tony Lyons, for being courageous enough to have me take on this project, and to Louis in particular for much-needed encouragement and support. To many informal reviewers for your improvements and additions, including Tim Lundeen, Josh Mazen, Dan, Alex Snelgrove, and Bernadette Pajer. I thank Grace, Dan, Stephanie Seneff, James Grunvig, Bernadette Pajer, and Gary Null for various references and sources of useful information. I thank Robert F. Kennedy Jr. for setting the example in the importance of bringing the science forward. I thank all of the autism research foundations that have supported the various aspects of the mountain of evidence brought forward here. I thank the Simons Foundation Autism Research Initiative (SFARI) for curating their SFARI Gene Database and for making it available to the public. I thank Bonnie Auyeung for granting an interview and wish her the very best of luck in conducting research on improving mood and sociality in ASD. I thank Mary Holland and Louis Conte for inspiration.

I thank Russell Blaylock for being an early, clear voice on the importance of focusing on glutamate signaling of chronic microglial activation as one of the more important factors in the processes that are involved in autism. I thank all of the researchers whose work I cite, as well as all of those whose work I did not cite, for their contributions toward understanding the causes of autism.

I thank Brian Hooker for his stalwart bravery in bringing forward the truth about the deficient and corrupt manner of doing vaccine safety research by the CDC. I thank Congressman Bill Posey for excellent stewardship of public trust for being the conscience of the House of Representatives in amplifying the message. I thank William Thompson, wherever you are. This book would not exist were it not for your forthrightness and honesty in sharing with Brian Hooker and with all of us the scientific treachery that exists within the CDC. And I thank Dr. Andrew Wakefield and Del Bigtree for their central roles in bringing about the change our society so desperately needs.

I congratulate all of the thousands of scientists who work in autism research on a fantastic job at unraveling the molecular basis of autism. If we push together for change, your work will impact public health policy and no longer be trivialized. I would like to extend my most sincere gratitude to Jonathan Mitchell and to Richard Âû, each for his bravery in sharing his uniquely personal experiences with the world. Reader, you must read Richard's blog; it is a clear voice on who autistics are and their experience.

And to Anne Dachel, whose willingness to connect those from different walks in a journey to help others suffer less, I offer a hearty thank-you and a commendation of your incredible passion for educating others on the injustices that have led to this pandemic. I am proud to know you.

"If the effects of genetic variation can vary depending on characteristics of the environment, then what are environments doing to genes to alter their impact?"

—Champagne and Mashoodh

"Autistic individuals show signs of neuroinflammation, altered inflammatory responses and immune abnormalities throughout life."

—Lucchina and Depino

"Together, these findings indicate that the immune system is a point of convergence for multiple ASD-related genetic and environmental risk factors."

—Estes and McAllister

"I wonder is there a particular health outcome that is related to aluminum salts that may have anything that we are looking at today."

—Dr. Tom Sinks, Associate Director for Science at the National Center for Environmental Health at the CDC and the Acting Division Director for Division of Birth Defects, Developmental Disabilities and Health, Simpsonwood Meeting, June 2000

"I believe in evidence. I believe in observation, measurement and reasoning, confirmed by independent observers. I'll believe anything, no matter how wild and ridiculous, if there is evidence for it. The wilder and more ridiculous something is, however, the firmer and more solid the evidence will have to be."

—Isaac Asimov

"I will burn you at the stake of science!"

—No One, Ever. Until Now.

CONTENTS

FOREWORD

Autism spectrum disorder (ASD) has grown tremendously in prevalence over the past several decades. While thirty years ago this disorder was considered rare, it now has become very common, affecting about 2 percent of children. This is more than many childhood diseases for which campaigns have been launched to eradicate and find cures for them. For example, in the United States, cancer and diabetes affect about 0.02 percent and 0.2 percent of children and adolescents, respectively. Thus, ASD is, at this time, about ten to one hundred times more prevalent than these important childhood diseases, yet its cause remains elusive, effective treatments are lacking, and limited research dollars are dedicated to solving these problems. The National Institutes of Health has dedicated institutes to research the causes and treatments for diabetes and cancer, but it has yet to dedicate an institute for combating ASD or even find a solid home for this disorder.

So why has ASD fallen through the cracks? One of the reasons is that it is a complicated disorder that has been approached using traditional paradigms for studying and treating medical and psychiatric disorders. It has thus far apparently defied these approaches. For decades, standard approaches have been used to investigate ASD, but few have substantially improved our understanding of the causes or treatments for ASD, and approaches that have provided some insight have provided only preliminary information.

One of the major approaches to understanding disease in the modern era is genetic research. Substantial funding has gone into building technology and knowledge focusing on genetics. Near the end of the last century, these efforts were celebrated when it was announced that we had successfully sequenced (read) the complete human genetic code. Now we are able to sequence (read) the important parts of any patients' genome (so-called whole exome sequencing) within a week or two (or even days if it is urgent). Yet this massive amount of information has not provided the tremendous insight that was promised. Why is this? The promise of genetic sequencing relied on several assumptions that have ended up not to be as solid as previously believed. ASD is a prime example of this.

First, many diseases found to have a strong genetic basis are found to have an error in the code for one of the twenty-four thousand genes on our twenty-three pairs of chromosomes. Now it is being realized that many diseases are not that simple. Like eye color, which is determined by multiple genes, it may be that some medical diseases may involve multiple genes that have no particular obvious relationship to each other or the disease itself. Given the large number of genes in our body, this becomes a large and complicated puzzle.

Second, not all changes in the genetic code cause the development of disease by themselves; they may simply be risk factors that require another causal factor. Without identifying such factors, it is difficult to identify the changes in the genetic code that lead to disease. Also, many of these genetic changes are what we call polymorphism, indicating that they are relatively common changes in the genetic code that are possessed by many people without disease.

Third, even with genetic disorders that are very closely linked to ASD, the association with ASD is not one-to-one. For example, Fragile X is the most common single-gene disorder associated with ASD, supposedly accounting for up to 5 percent of ASD cases. However, only 30 percent of cases of children with Fragile X have ASD. This theme is true for many other genetic disorders closely associated with ASD. Thus, there must be some additional factor that causes ASD in these genetic disorders.

Fourth, there is good evidence than many diseases, like ASD, involve disruption of mitochondrial function. The mitochondrion is the only other part of the cell besides the cell nucleus (where the chromosomes reside) that carries genetic information. Mitochondria are exclusively inherited from the mother, so the inheritance of genes in the mitochondria is different from other genes in the cell, but the effects of mitochondrial dysfunction can be profound.

Fifth, we are learning that genes are regulated through complicated molecular mechanisms. Some of these epigenetic processes rely on metabolic processes called methylation, which is known to be disrupted in ASD. Epigenetic processes are responsible for turning genes on or off, regardless of whether there are errors in their genetic code. Thus, standard methods for sequencing the genetic code to search for dysfunctional genes will not easily pick up genes that are silenced because of epigenetic processes.

Sixth, like many developmental disorders, the errors in the genetic code identified in many children with ASD appear as what is called de novo, meaning that they are new mutations not found in the genetic code of the parents. Thus, these mutations arose during formation of the egg or sperm or shortly after the egg and sperm combined to form the zygote. These de novo mutations are usually caused by errors induced into the genetic code mostly by negative environmental influences. So even when genetic mutations are found to cause ASD, the ultimate culprit may not be genetic; in fact, it might be environmental.

Finally, one of the reasons that ASD research focuses on genetics is that it has high heritability. For example, siblings are more likely to have ASD if their sibling has ASD. This idea that ASD runs in families suggests, at the surface, that the disorder must be inherited from a gene defect. But when we step back and consider other possibilities, we can see that, besides sharing part of the genetic code, siblings also share the most important environmental influence of their development, the same womb.

An increasing number of studies have confirmed that the environment has a large influence on the cause of ASD. The definition of environment is very broad. Many people immediately think of environmental toxicants as negative environmental influences, but the environment is much broader and includes diet, medications, infections, parenting, and so on. Perhaps the most influential environment an individual will experience is during development in the mother's uterus.

The maternal environment has only been recently recognized. One of the most important advances in prenatal care was the discovery that folic acid can prevent neural tube defects, a devastating type of congenital malformation. It has only been in the past few years that we have come to realize that folate supplementation before and during pregnancy will prevent ASD. Ongoing research examines many, some over-the-counter, medications commonly taken during pregnancy that seem to be linked to neurodevelopmental disorders. The research remains preliminary. One very compelling finding is the discovery of antibodies to fetal brain tissue that are found in the mothers of children with ASD. It is hypothesized that the maternal immune system is activated to produce antibodies that interfere with fetal brain development, a finding that has been confirmed in animal models.

One area of research that is exploding is research into gastrointestinal ecology. The development of ASD has been directly associated with disruption in the gut microbiome, and other research has suggested that disruptions in the macrobiome, such as helminths and fungi, are related to the rise in ASD and other chronic childhood diseases. Very compelling is the link between the maternal microbiome and the development of childhood disease, a finding that highly suggests that maternal health and diet are very important in the development of the child.

ASD is associated with many physiological abnormalities, some of which are not well understood. Many children with ASD have problems with function of the powerhouse of the cell known as the mitochondria, but the exact nature of this mitochondrial dysfunction is not clear. Although 5 percent of children with ASD have a mitochondrial disease, 30 percent or more appear to have mitochondrial dysfunction in which the mitochondria does not produce the needed energy to support cellular function. We are only beginning to understand the nuances of mitochondrial dysfunction, and studying ASD will surely help us expand our understanding of the physiology of the body and the cells. This theme is echoed in other physiological abnormalities associated with ASD such as disruption in redox metabolism and immune function.

In this book, Dr. Lyons-Weiler takes on these complicated topics and presents them in an organized and understandable fashion so the reader can understand how the pieces fall into place. The book highlights not only the complicated nature of ASD, but also the many different lenses through which ASD can be viewed. For example, ASD is a behaviorally defined disorder, but the behavioral definition itself is not that straightforward, leading to complications in the way in which the diagnosis is made. ASD is associated with many genetic, environmental, physiological, and brain-based alterations, all of which are complicated within themselves. Thus, the challenge at integrating these many pieces of information is multiplied. Dr. Lyons-Weiler integrates many of these ideas into the Toxin Liability Sampling Concept, which he explains may be responsible for the rise in many disease conditions associated with genetic environmental interactions. Briefly, a diversity of genetic variants found to be important in ASD can be expected to reflect and reveal distinct susceptibilities to an increasing variety of toxins found in the environment. The Toxin Liability Sampling Concept helps explain the apparent precipitous rise in ASD and the apparent difficulties associated with nailing down singular causes.

Dr. Lyons-Weiler suggests that large, biologically informed, prospective studies are needed to better understand the potential causes of ASD, and better endophenotyping is needed to understand the subtypes of ASD. Thus, ultimately, the most effective way of curing ASD is to prevent it from developing in the first place, so it will be important to understand that multiple complicated interacting risk factors can lead to ASD. The inspiring news is that there is a path to preventing this devastating disease if we decide as a society to do the work that is required to understand it better.

Clearly, until research starts to uncover the nature of the physiological abnormalities associated with ASD and their underlying cause(s), almost every hypothesis will continue to be entertained. This book provides insight into the complicated nature of the search for the cause(s) of ASD but mostly highlights the incredible complex nature of this research. One clear fact is that looking at ASD through only one lens will severely limit our ability to come up with answers. Currently, and in the past, genetics has dominated the field of ASD research, but this has been less fruitful than expected, most likely because the important piece of the full influence of environment has not been added into the equation. In the same vein, the complicated nature of ASD itself most likely arising from multiple causes needs to be embraced. If funding organizations continue to fund reductionist research, rather than integrative and transitional research, it will be a long time before the necessary answers are found. In the future we must advocate for better research into the causes of ASD so we can treat and prevent this disorder. ASD overlaps with many other chronic childhood diseases and other neurological and psychiatric diseases, so a better understanding of ASD will no doubt lead us toward insights into understanding and treating many disorders that have, to date, eluded us.

—Richard E. Frye, MD, PhD
Director of Autism Research
Arkansas Children's Research Institute

PREFACE

No one doubts that some toxins cause autism. The basic and clinical science supports unequivocally that toxins such as thalidomide and valproate cause autism, and that science is at least as strong as the science that shows how and why additives used in vaccines, including mercury and aluminum, can also cause autism. In fact, the mechanisms are nearly identical in every detail. After reviewing more than two thousand peer-reviewed autism research studies, I can no longer support the notion that vaccines—as currently formulated—do not cause autism. Other causal factors include acetaminophen, which is especially dangerous and for which the evidence of causality is extremely strong. This book represents many of the conclusions from those studies, which have involved tens of thousands of patients and hundreds of thousands of person-hours spent by autism researchers. I have been told that I will endure withering attacks as a result of publishing this book. Frankly, I don't care. I invite detractors from the truth of immunoexcitoxicity due to vaccines and mitochondrial dysfunction due to acetaminophen to take it up with the army of thousands of researchers who have contributed forty years of research in molecular biology and medicine. That knowledge base is their legacy, their contribution to society—and it cannot be ignored.

But I didn't write this book just to defend the science showing immunotoxicity and other mechanisms by which environmental factors and genes cause autism. I wrote it to defend science. The interesting thing about the truth in nature is that it never goes away, no matter how inconvenient. The fact that some of us are doomed by the vaccine industry to acquire autism, and by reluctance of regulatory agencies to label clearly dangerous drugs, must no longer be ignored by the CDC, or by anyone else, including pediatricians, lawmakers, and parents. Our government has decided to protect that industry from lawsuits due to vaccine injury. Shame, I say, shame on them for performing pathetically weak science and for choosing to ignore the rest of the community's mountain of evidence in the formulation of public health policy. Now let's move on. Let science be done to protect the unborn, our babies, and our children. Let's make safe vaccines that really work. But let's use them wisely. Let's find and optimize biomarkers that can be used in the clinic to pinpoint individuals who are at highest risk of not just autism, but those who are at highest risk of any type of serious adverse events. If we as a society enjoy collective benefit from protection from infectious diseases due to vaccines, then we as a society share the collective responsibility to protect those who are at the greatest risk of harm from vaccines. Enough with the propaganda that says there is no risk, enough. Genetics and careful attention to reliable risk factors will play a fundamental role in protecting those among us who are most susceptible to neurotoxicity from vaccines via freedom of choice and, when possible, medical exemption. Policy shifts and reform in vaccine safety will protect the rest of us.

The Environmental and Genetic Causes of Autism

INTRODUCTION

Throughout this book, I refer to patients with autism as *autistics.* To some, this may appear cold or clinical for not addressing the person first (i.e., *persons with autism,* or *children with autism*). The origins of the use of the term *autistic,* however, comes from autistics themselves—especially some highly vocal individuals in the "neurodiversity" movement who have expressed their preference for the use of this term. It is not natural for me to refer to patients of any disease by the name of the disease (see the person, not the disease). For example, we do not refer to cancer patients as *cancers* or *cancer people;* we refer to them as *patients with cancer.* Autism, like cancer, is medical. At stake is the ability of society to recognize on the one hand the expressed preference for a vocal group of autistics and to be able to see autism as a primarily medical condition, without offending those who strongly identify with their condition. Autism has a genetic component, but it is not necessary for those born with a risk of either developing autism or remaining autistic. At least half of the liability for the occurrence of autism at the population level is environmental.

Autism is a spectrum of clinical disorders called autism spectrum disorder (ASD). A review of four studies that sought to detect G × E interactions in ASD (Bowers and Erickson, 2014) found that each study that focused on a different environmental factor led to different genes. Organophosphates seemed to interact with the PON1 gene, pregnancy-related stress interacted with variation in the ADRB2 gene, and traffic-related particulate matter (pollution) interacted with variation in the MET gene. Periconceptional maternal prenatal vitamin usage interacted with variation in three genes, two with variants in the mother (MTHFR, CBS) and one in the child (COMT).

ENVIRONMENTAL TOXIN LIABILITY SAMPLING

A major theme in the literature on the genetics of autism is formed by multiple lines of evidence that support the hypothesis that autism is the direct result of the failure of the body's natural inborn metabolic defenses against damage from the environment to the central nervous system (CNS) and to other metabolic systems that share afflicted pathways. Thus, the environment to which we subject our developing young, from conception to adulthood, can profoundly affect their neurological phenotypes. Failures of these neuroprotective proteins and pathways are also very likely at the heart of age-related cognitive decline. Thus, treatments designed to bolster these innate protective mechanisms will also likely prove to be useful in reducing age-related cognitive and metabolic decline.

Autism used to be found in one in three thousand people. The rate before age six is now one in sixty-eight. It seems likely that the best explanation for the dramatic rise in autism is an increase in environmental toxins. In her book *Outsmarting Autism,* Patricia Lemer refers to a total "load" that some of us cannot endure. Genetics adds another dimension to this: as we put greater amounts of toxins into our environment, we will find more individuals who have an otherwise neutral variation in their genomes in a gene that together—the mutation and the toxin—induces autism in that individual. And the more toxic our environment becomes, the more likely we will all experience new (de novo) mutations. With this book, I propose this idea as the *Environmental Toxin Liability Sampling* (ETLS) concept for the rise in ASD, schizophrenia, Alzheimer's disease, and other diseases and conditions that modern corporate chemistry has rendered unto our population. ETLS is more than a compilation of hundreds of findings at many scales of inquiry; it is a coherent framework in which a process model explains the "whys" and "hows" of causality in autism. It explains why not everyone becomes autistic after exposure to specific types of toxins. It explains how both chronic microglial activation and environmentally induced mitochondrial dysfunction and other distinct types of damage can cause the same disease phenotype (autism). In simple terms, individuals and families with different mutations "sample" an increasing diversity of toxins in their environment at different rates, depending on local concentrations, and due to their varying mutations, the outcome is benign for some and dramatically different for other families or individuals.

The scientific evidence is clear: autism is primarily an environmental disease with numerous and diverse genetic predispositions and susceptibilities. A study in 2014 found that individuals with specific MTHFR mutations are more susceptible to the toxic effects of mercury (Austin, 2014)—but no single gene in the entire genome accounts for more than 1 percent of ASD, and many common variants exist that confer weak risk. ETLS reconciles that apparent paradox of high heritability and low genetic liability found in all of the genetic studies. It extends the two-hit hypothesis into a multihit hypothesis, rules out environmental factors as "triggers," and instead places focus on both environmental and genetic causal factors and their interaction. It explains the numerous apparent paradoxes of many independent genes, each conferring distinct susceptibilities in different families. Under this process model, there is no missing heritability, and the "either-or" question is replaced by the interaction of G and E. There is spatially and temporally aggregated E and G × E risk, recognizing that G risk alone is at the population level very, very low. It also makes specific, testable predictions: that rates of autism should decrease when toxins are removed; that autism is a reversible condition, at least in some people; that different individual toxins can be expected to be root causes of autism in different families; and that, ultimately, such susceptibilities will be known and predictable based on an individual's genetic profile.

It is certain that genes do not always define our fate. We humans are remarkably good at modifying our environment, and we should attempt to reverse those changes we have made to our environment, which place even the smallest minority of us at risk of disease or disorder that reduces that minority's quality of life—especially if the rest of us have benefited from the risks others have endured. I have come to see autism as a profound test of our right to genetic freedoms. We have the right to express the genes with which we were born without fear of injury, harm, or damage due to medical, agricultural, or industrial practices that place any percentage—minority or majority—at risk of injury even if that risk benefits the many. Some will disagree, of course, and to them I would point out that we can, if we change medical, agricultural, and industrial practices in a manner that allows us to enjoy the greater benefit and not impose massive undue health and economic burdens upon a genetic minority. I am not counting any "burden" autistics might be perceived to bear on society. Any such burden should be borne by those of us with shoulders broad enough to recognize the debt we owe those injured by our poisonous environments for the benefits we enjoy as a result of their sacrifice. Those who have benefited the most should bear the greatest load for those already injured, and we must do all we can to reduce the risk of harm to the susceptible in the future.

Heritability of susceptibility to toxins in our environment is not evidence of genetic liability for autism per se. It is merely reflective evidence of neurotoxins in our environment. We can currently reasonably distinguish among which mutations in which functional gene classes are most likely to reflect independent, direct genetic risk of autism susceptibility, as well as which are likely contributors to inherited environmental susceptibility. Only outright, frank, sublethal, rare, compound heterozygotes with mutations in certain genes not related to susceptibility to artificially created or artificially concentrated neurotoxins can be considered candidates for true genetic liability.

This explains why the true genetic liability is so low: the environment determines which gene mutations are unsuitable for life. Autistics are well suited to living in a clean environment. Rather than change our pool of genetic diversity passively through selective abortions, high morbidity, high mortality, and low fecundity, we can, with less cost, change the environment we live in, we eat, we breathe, we drink—and the environment we inject into our pregnant women, babies, toddlers, and youth.

I call upon our governments and the corporations that run them to do it now.

Reference: see envgencauses.com

Chapter 1.

BACKGROUND AND CONCEPTS

What causes autism?

Genetic factors or environmental factors? Nature versus nurture?

Three things are certain. First, these questions pose a false and grossly misleading dichotomy given the breadth of published knowledge available. Second, false dichotomies can misdirect research funding priorities away from understanding the true causes of autism and can even warp public health policy and reduce priorities for the care of autistics. Third, the existence of mutations that confer risk does not automatically exonerate environmental factors in autism any more than mutations that confer cancer risk exonerate carcinogens. In developmental toxicology, risk due to exposure is cumulative.

If only autism were so simple as to give those questions significant meaning. Given the weight of the available evidence in objective scientific studies, no fruitful discussion about the causes of autism can rule out genetics as an important factor in autism. The same is true for environmental factors. Focus on one to the exclusion of the other reveals bias toward a particular agenda, ignorance of the massive published literature available on the genetics of autism, or both. In short, there is ample room for the discussion of both genetic and environmental factors.

In 2008, a survey of physicians found that many thought genetics played a weak and limited role as a causal factor in autism (Hoop et al., 2008). In a way, they were correct: no single gene can be found that, by itself, contributes to more than 1 to 2 percent of autism cases. Thus far, specific mutations can account for only perhaps 10 percent of individual autism cases. Throwing percentages around without a firm reference point can be confusing, however, because at the same time, genes and environment each share approximately one-half of the liability for autism in twins (Hallmayer et al., 2011; Sandin, 2014).

At the beginning of this century, all known identified Mendelian genetic factors—the sense of genes with mutations that were found to be associated with autism—were rare. This was in part due to a lack of research. Now that a great amount of research has been conducted, we know that in the sense of frequencies in the population and in the sense of frequencies in the ASD population, genes with mutations that are found to be associated with autism are rare. This was initially puzzling, because autism was also observed to have a very high heritability—at least a high concordance, which suggested high overall heritability. An awakening of sorts has occurred that involves three important observations:

1. Identical, monozygotic (MZ) twins show a significantly higher concordance of autism diagnosis than fraternal, dizygotic twins for autism, even though siblings grew up together, sharing many environmental influences.
2. No single gene has been found to have a large effect, and studies have resulted in the discovery of numerous genes, clustered in specific pathways, each explaining a minor percentage of cases of autism ASD.
3. First-degree relatives of affected individuals are often found with subthreshold autism or ASD symptoms, indicating that autism and ASD is a heterogeneous, variegated set of conditions, as opposed to a discrete (all/none) genetic disease.

In the terminology of genetics, these observations led to the conclusion that a simple autosomal or X-linked dominant model, or even a recessive mode of monogenic inheritance, was insufficient to describe the patterns of inheritance of risk of autism. They pointed to autism risk as a complex trait, involving many loci and many genes, with likely interactions among genes (epistasis). However, although the number was not known, an early estimate by modeling suggested approximately 15 loci (Newschaffer et al., 2002).

As complex as ASD appears, it is also common for pedigrees to appear "bottom heavy" for ASD diagnosis (see Figure 1). This is inconsistent with poor diagnostic accuracy in past generations. However, it is consistent with the appearance of new factors in the latest generation. Brandler et al. (2016) found that ASD diagnosis was associated with increased rates of copy number variations (CNVs), but not increases in large chromosomal rearrangements. In contrast, Chen et al. (2016) found idiosyncratic structural mutations to be important in autism. The finding of increased number of de novo CNVs in ASD would seem to indicate that something, or things, are in fact different in the environment.

Compared with what was known in 2002, the number of suspected genetic factors is now much larger, and there is even more evidence for heritability of

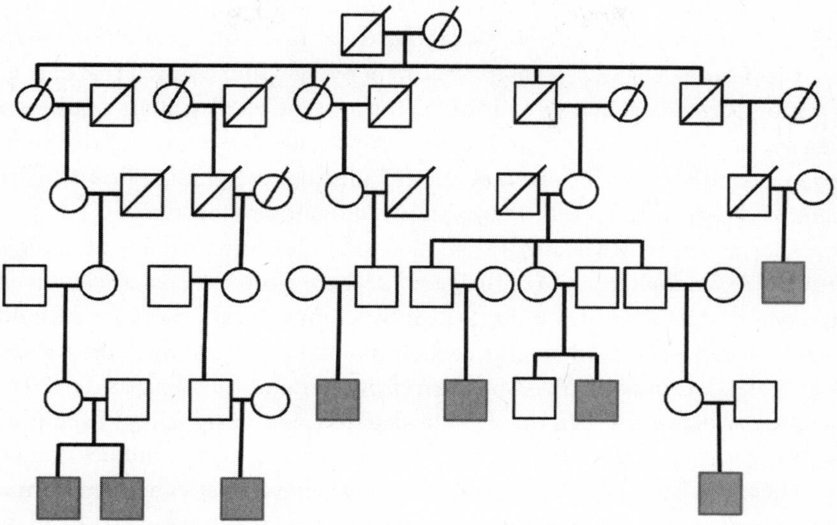

Figure 1. Typical pedigree tracking autism in a mapping study (after Allen-Brady, 2009). Males are squares, females are circles. Autistics with diagnosis are in gray; deceased subjects are indicated with a slash. Neurotypical phenotype (unaffected) are white shapes. Note that lack of ASD in the past generations and that the prevalence of ASD is highest in the last generation. It is reasonable to assert that even if risk alleles are inherited, the high prevalence in the final generation is due to the fact that something in their environment has changed. (Squares are males, circles are females.) The investigators noted a great deal of variation in the specific manifestation of ASD across the pedigree. Within affected, intelligence quotient (IQ) scores ranged from 41 to 124 for verbal IQ (VIQ) and 45 to 140 for performance IQ (PIQ); three had language delay; one had nonfebrile seizures, but the other six did not. (*Allen-Brady, K., et al., 2009. A high-density SNP genome-wide linkage scan in a large autism extended pedigree. Molecular Psychiatry 14:590–600; doi:10.1038/mp.2008.14)*

numerous genetic factors, each weakly contributing to risk at the population level. The Simons Foundation's SFARI Autism Database Human Gene Module contains, as of July 2016, over 790 genes potentially related to autism in some way, based on data from 1,266 curated references and 1,268 noncurated references. While many of the reported findings are individual reports of single individuals with mutations that may be clinically related to ASD, the resource is incredibly valuable for quickly determining the level of and type of support indicated by the literature variations involving any specific gene. In spite of systematic analyses of the literature to find "common variants" (e.g., Warrier et al., 2015), no gene contributes more than 1 percent to overall ASD prevalence.

A variety of common (inherited) variants account for 17 percent of the liability in ASD and up to 29 percent among other psychiatric conditions (Cross-Disorder Group, 2013). The large amount of overlap in the causal role of genetic variation across psychiatric conditions means that many genetic markers and even specific variations are not disease specific. The high frequency of common variants compared to the low frequency of autism indicates significant environmental liability: parents with these variants did not develop autism.

A large study by Matsunami et al. (2013) identified twenty-four regions with CNVs, and while some of the genes in the regions affected are involved in interesting parts of neurobiology, the most common variations were found in areas with genes involved in basic cellular functions. For example, the ANKRD9 (RAGE) variation is involved in ionic transport and signaling and OTUD7A variation, which is in turn involved in deubiquination signaling. Even housekeeping genes have to work properly for the CNS to function and develop well.

There is a big lesson here for understanding how genetics and environmental factors can induce autism as well as for picking targets for general and individualized treatments. This informs projects targeting development as well as those for evaluating the role of non-CNS specific genes in autism.

The risk of a newborn being autistic is higher in families that already have an autistic child, and the intensity of autistic symptoms is more pronounced in families with more than one autistic child. These facts would seem to further indicate a genetic risk. Not all of this risk can be considered genetic, however. Families share environmental factors. Numerous additional familial risk factors have been identified, such as parental age and birth order. Mutations new to a population, which occur during gamete formation (de novo mutations), are extremely rare but are more likely in gametes from older parents; and the incidence of autism is higher for babies born to older mothers and fathers, with the age of both genders contributing independent increased risk (Shelton et al., 2010). Note that Shelton et al. removed 324 parents because the variable "education level" was missing.

Some shifts associated with age of parents may reflect shifts in the methylation programming during sperm and oocyte formation. If this is increasing due to the environment, it spells increasing trouble. It could, however, also be due to overall cohort effect reflecting vaccination trends: autism has been steadily increasing since the 1980s; the CDC began expanding the pediatric schedule in 1983. We are now up to seventy-two injections before age 16—sixty of these before the age of twenty-four months. Knowing that methylation differences are involved in parental age does not tell us why methylation changes in parents, nor does it tell us if those changes are due to factors increasing in our environment.

The contributed risk from each additional familial factor is small. For example, advanced maternal age contributed to only 4.6 of the 600 percent rise in reported cases of autism in the 1990s. Demographic and socioeconomic factors are assumed to be additive but are notoriously correlated with one or more other, more ultimate causes. Birth order, for example, is a risk factor. Later-born children have a higher risk, but then they also tend to have older parents. The birth order factor seems to suggest biological causes such as aberrant methylation patterns during the formation of gametes in aging parents, and this hypothesis has been tested and is at least partly supported by data.

But increased risk due to birth order during the past fifteen to twenty years could also be a cohort effect—younger children in families receive an ever-increasing number of vaccines, or ever-increasing exposure in an increasingly toxic environment, or both. Despite the official CDC "party line" of no association between vaccines and autism, the studies conducted outside of the CDC point squarely at metal adjuvants in vaccines, which activate the immune system, as likely causal factors and not only for autism.

Data from the Vaccine Safety Datalink of the CDC found association between vaccine exposure (thimerosal + aluminum) and any neurodevelopmental disorder (National Academy of Science, Institute of Medicine [NAS/IOM], 2001). The many other neurological disorders and other health conditions are now increasing in frequency. Of course, familial factors can also include other shared environmental factors. And a more recent study (Frazier et al., 2014) demonstrated that the levels of social and repetitive behavioral symptoms were strongly influenced by common genetic factors, whereas the heritability of categorically defined ASD diagnosis criteria was comparatively low. Similarly, most emotional issues within ASD are explained by genetics (Tick et al., 2016).

As with genetic factors, numerous shared environmental factors are likely. A common statement made in popular writings is that "no one knows the cause of autism." Year after year, study after study, the body of scientific evidence mounts, and yet this myth is perpetuated by an increasingly willful ignorance on the part of the CDC. Each year, US taxpayers foot the bill for $30 billion worth of medical research. Nearly all of the peer-reviewed research is captured in scientific journals and by a branch of the government called the National Center for Biotechnology Information. One resource in particular, PubMed, is available for all researchers and the public to search the abstracts and full research articles published by thousands of scientists. PubMed is a product of the US National Library of Medicine and the National Institutes of Health, and it contains abstracts of more than 25 million scientific studies, many available as full-text versions of the published study.

Much of this research is not new. But it is richly varied in focus and form.

For example, a parent survey study conducted in 2008 (Schultz et al., 2008) reported that

> *Acetaminophen use after measles-mumps-rubella vaccination was significantly associated with autistic disorder when considering children 5 years of age or less.*

There is no warning on the CDC website to not give your child acetaminophen after vaccination. Instead, the CDC reports "Vaccines do not cause autism" and "Ingredients in vaccines do not cause autism" (CDC, 2016).

Granted, the Schultz study is just one study. However, given some research conducted since 2008, there is little to no doubt that vaccines can contribute to autism. Given the rest of that same body of research, there can also now be no doubt how.

Rossignol and Frye (2012) conducted an extensive analysis of the biomedical research and found the following:

- 416/437 (95 percent) of studies on immune dysregulation or inflammation in ASD found a positive result;
- 115/115 (100 percent) of studies on the role of oxidative stress in ASD found a positive result;
- 145/153 studies that examined mitochondrial dysfunction in ASD found a positive result;
- 170/190 studies on environmental toxicant exposures in ASD found a positive result.

They also found 95 publications that discussed possible association between vaccination and ASD in the immune dysregulation and inflammation group of studies; most of these were editorials and added no new data (Rossignol and Frye, 2012).

The CDC has failed consistently to utilize *any* of this valuable resource in the formulation of their policy. Instead, they rely on their own deeply flawed internal and contracted external studies. They cite "dozens" of studies that exonerate vaccines. Rather than allow the full body of scientific evidence to inform public health policy, they "cherry-pick" the studies that support their chosen policy.

The primary focus of this book is not those studies, nor what is wrong with them. Most of them (17/22) were determined to be flawed in 2012 by the Institute of Medicine (National Academy of Sciences, 2012), and they are currently the subject of inquiry for malfeasance and scientific fraud (see "Vaccine Whistleblower: Exposing Autism Research Fraud in the CDC," Barr, 2015).

Instead, the focus of this book is the rest of the science: what the CDC has so egregiously ignored. We cannot expect to understand and therefore prevent or treat autism unless we ask old questions with new data, and refuse the fast-and-loose practices used in the vaccine safety research studies in the 2000s. We need to pay attention to the rest of science, not just the corrupted bits of science the CDC wants us to accept as valid and as the whole story. As a result, it has prevented the public from knowing the truth about neurotoxicity of vaccine additives.

This book is about the *rest* of the science. It includes more than 900 key references on both the genetic and environmental causes of autism. It includes perspective peppered throughout the discussions of genes, regulatory pathways, and neurobiology. It is a call for attention to *all* of the science that US taxpayers have paid for and a call for reform.

VACCINE SAFETY RESEARCH REFORM

For starters, I believe that the CDC should no longer be in the business of conducting vaccine research science. I believe five independent trials are needed for each vaccine, three chosen for funding by lottery and two by competitive grants. All five should conduct their own studies and analyze their data independently, and the results should be communicated to the US Food and Drug Administration (FDA).

Similarly, no one with financial conflicts of interest—or even a hint of a possibility of a conflict of interest—should be allowed to weigh on the vaccine schedule.

The Vaccine Board should be disbanded and replaced by a Congress of Patient Representatives from each state that votes on each change to the schedule. The first Congress should be composed of people who either have themselves been injured by vaccines, or have loved ones who have been injured. The Congress could elect a panel of pediatricians to provide guidance and advice on the medical matters, but they should also have panel of research scientists who work independently from the pharmaceutical industry in vaccine safety research, to provide guidance and advice as well.

I also believe the CDC should change its tune. The sooner, the better. Let the people know that *vaccines can cause autism in some people.* Rather than propagating the myth that "no one knows what causes autism," by far, a much more accurate statement would be that some environmental causes of autism are known, that many more are suspected, and that additives in vaccines, especially mercury and aluminum, are likely to cause autism in some people. The CDC is woefully negligent in their activities and concerns over other environmental factors as well. For instance, autism is known to be induced by gestational exposure to certain environmental factors such as valproic acid (Christensen et al., 2013; Williams et al., 2001), a histone deacetylase inhibitor used to treat seizures and bipolar disorder (Christianson et al., 1994; Rodier et al., 1997; Williams and Hersh, 1997; Ingram et al., 2000). Intraperitoneal injection of valproic acid induces morphological changes in microglial cells in the hippocampus and amygdala within 24 hours (Wang et al., 2015). They seem to not be aware or to care about the science showing other compounds and exposures that might lead to autism via microglial activation, such as the science showing that glyphosate may be a causal factor and acetaminophen/ASD links.

They are asleep at the wheel on these other important factors, but they are actively misleading the public on vaccine safety. Other necessary changes to the conduct of vaccine safety research are noted throughout the book.

Aluminum has long been a suspected cause of neurodegeneration (e.g., Meiri et al., 1991) and is undisputedly a neurotoxin. According to Bhattacharjee et al. (2013):

> *Once biologically available aluminum bypasses gastrointestinal and blood-brain barriers, this environmentally-abundant neurotoxin has an exceedingly high affinity for the large pyramidal neurons of the human brain hippocampus . . . endothelial cells that line the cerebral vasculature may have biochemical attributes conducive to binding and targeting aluminum to selective anatomical regions of the brain, such as the hippocampus, with potential downstream pro-inflammatory and pathogenic consequences.*

The toxic effects of aluminum are best described as widespread and pernicious. Inside the cell, aluminum shuts down the transcription of protein-coding genes and miRNA genes in two ways, via direct and specific interaction with H1 linker histones and by suppressing global gene expression by down-regulating RNA polymerase II (see review in Bhattacharjee, 2013). Aluminum causes a buildup of glial fibrillary acid protein (GFAP) filaments near the cell nucleus and destruction of the actin cytoskeleton (Theiss et al., 2002). Structural effects of aluminum in rodents include the appearance of neurofibrillary tangles that resemble those from Alzheimer's patients (Uemura et al., 1984; Somova et al., 1997).

The same neurofibrillary tangles without amyloid or neuritic plaques are seen in autism patients at postmortem autopsy (e.g., Hof et al., 1991).

While the degree of toxicity to astroglial cells varies with which species of aluminum is present (Lévesque et al., 2000), this damage to astroglial cells impairs their ability to function in their role of keeping microglial cells under control. Astroglial cell communication with astrocytes is disrupted by aluminum and the cytokine interleukin-6 (where IL is commonly used as a shorthand for interleukin) is increased. Astroglial cells uptake glutamate; damage to their function will cause a buildup of glutamate and induce excitotoxicity of microglial cells. The same changes in brain chemistry (increased glutamate) and increased microglia caused by valproic acid have been seen in many animal studies of aluminum. Animal studies have also demonstrated higher susceptibility of young rats to aluminum toxicity (Veiga et al., 2013).

Aluminum, an adjuvant in some vaccines, ended up deposited in distant organs, including the spleen and brain, where it was still detected one *year* after injection (Khan et al., 2013). Experiments with mice show neurological and behavioral deficits due to adjuvant aluminum (Shaw and Tomljenovic, 2013). Aluminum has been demonstrated to remain in the body for decades, and aluminum accumulates in the brain as humans age (Roider et al., 1999). It seems likely that one route is the increased extra-axial cerebral spinal fluid (CSF) found by Bradstreet et al. (2010). Uptake of aluminum is biased toward macrophages, and thus the carrier and conduit into the brain are both suspected and demonstrated.

Appreciation of the dynamic roles of microglia in the healthy and injured/infected brain is now widespread (see, for example, Bilimoria et al., 2015). As we will see, glutamate-driven chronic microglial activation (immunoneuroexcitotoxicity) is an out-of-control body response to toxins that is critical to our understanding of numerous other environmental factors and causes of autism. In fact, a clinical trial with memantine, targeting glutamate neurotransmission in autism, is under way (Häge et al., 2016). There are now dozens of review articles on the role of the innate immune system in autism and in psychiatric disorders. Such studies may be well-informed by biomarkers that predict response.

Exposures in early pregnancy to thalidomide, at twenty to twenty-four days' gestation (Miller et al., 2004; Strömland et al., 1994; Trottier et al., 1999), and misoprostol (Miller et al., 2004) are both known causal factors (Miller and Strömland, 2011). Topotecan, a chemotherapy agent, reduces topoisomerase, critical for the expression of long genes (King et al., 2013), and may cause autism. Prenatal exposure to serotonin reuptake inhibitors (taken by pregnant mothers for depression) has been found to be associated with autism, even after correcting for head size at birth (El Marroun et al., 2014). Hill et al. found that the CHD7 gene, which is essential for neural crest cell migration and patterning, was found to be hypomethylated in animals exposed to common environmental pollutants or valproic acid. This finding may be a rare instance in which a very specific genetic risk—mutations leading to loss of function (LoF) in two genes, CHD7 and CHD8—could have the same effect as environmental exposures. In fact, many environmental exposures can have precisely the same negative effect as deleterious mutations (phenomimicry).

Teratogens aside, environmentally induced phenotypes can be expected to be more reversible than phenotypes that are primarily genetic in origin. The theme of phenomimicry recurs throughout research in autism. Understanding phenomimicry leads to the conclusion that if one rejects the basic evidence demonstrating how environmental factors cause autism (association), one must then also reject the basic science that demonstrates how mutations cause autism (also association). Thus, those who will reject autism as environmentally induced (e.g., adjuvants and additives in vaccine cause autism) because autism "is a genetic disease" arbitrarily prefer one type of association study over another. In so doing, they unknowingly undermine the support for the "genetic cause" position as well as the environmental inducement theories. For all but the ultimate cause, the mechanisms of the genetic and environmental processes that render autistic phenotypes are *identical.* Whether one lights a match, sparks a fuse, or implants an explosive device, a powderkeg still explodes.

So let me introduce three types of autism: *endogenous autism,* caused purely by genetics; *environmentally induced autism,* caused purely by environmental toxins, including the environmental effects on genes and methylation; and *mixed-cause autism,* caused by a combination of genetic and environmental factors. These delineations help not only in the study of individual cases, but also in thinking about causal factors at the population level and defining meaningful study designs.

Natal autism is thought to result from diversions in the brain development program within the first trimester of gestation, approximately the time of the folding of the neural tube. This body of background knowledge alone gives all kinds of environmental factors a seat at the table of candidate factors for primary (natal) autism: there are many ways to disrupt neural tube folding. In natal autism, once environmental triggers are set forth, the pathogenesis of autism continues to be greatly influenced by the genetics.

Exposure to a group of flame retardants, chemically polybrominated diphenyl ethers (PDBEs), has been linked conceptually to Rett syndrome in a mouse model. Mice with a truncated methyl CpG binding protein 2 gene (MeCP-308 model) exhibit a number of characteristics that resemble those of Rett syndrome in humans, especially in the social domain (e.g., abnormal home-cage diurnal activity without motor skill deficits and reduced nesting behaviors and less time near other mice; Moretti et al., 2005). An initial study of the mice showed that they

> *appeared normal and exhibited normal motor function for about 6 weeks, but then developed a progressive neurological disease that includes many features of RTT:*

tremors, motor impairments, hypoactivity, increased anxiety-related behavior, seizures, kyphosis and stereotypic forelimb motions.

MeCP-308 mice exposed to PDBEs developed disorders similar to Rett syndrome, but mostly in the females. MeCP female pups spent approximately one-half the amount of time with their mothers as MeCP pups and pups not exposed. MeCP pups exposed to PDBEs have impaired memory and learning abilities. Perinatal exposure to BDE-47 in offspring of MeCP-truncated mice bred with wild-type mice caused hypomethylation in the brain. Both BDE-47-treated MeCP-308 mice and BDE-47-treated wild-type controls showed more pronounced Rett-like symptoms (Wood et al., 2012). The concentrations of BDE-47 in postmortem mice at the low dose of BDE-47 were similar to that found in human postmortem brains.

This provides an excellent example of a genetic predisposition matched with an environmental primary cause. However, it also provides a good example of how genes and environment can interact, how a gene can act alone, and how environmental factors can act alone.

We now also know that BDE-47 causes an increase in extracellular glutamate (Costa et al., 2016). Antagonists of glutamate ionotropic receptors diminished toxicity of BDE-47, but antagonists of glutamate metabotropic receptors did not. Remarkably, stimulation of the serotonin receptor 7 in mice heterozygous for the MeCP truncation also showed improvement (De Filippis et al., 2015). As we will see, increased glutamate is a key indicator of environmentally induced autism through chronic microglial cell activation. Polybrominated diphenyl ethers are among the numerous chemicals suspected of adding to autism risk by environmental scientists (Nevison, 2014). Other lines of evidence offer strong support (Hertz-Picciotto et al., 2011).

Polycyclic aromatic hydrocarbons induce change in mitochondrial gene copy number with teratogenic effects (Kim et al., 2014). They are also a large component of air pollution and, along with dose exposure to fine particulate matter, are associated with ASD and other neurodevelopmental conditions (Suades-González et al., 2015).

Ultrasound has been suggested as a source of growth factor stimulation leading to a simplified, singular columnar brain structure phenotype common in autism (Williams et al., 2011). The use of inhaler-delivered beta agonist drugs during pregnancy appears to increase the risk of autism by 30 percent; however, this may be confounded genetic risk (susceptibility/sensitivity to environmental factor, or immunological factors). In the study, no nonasthmatic users of these drugs were available to see if the detected association confounds the known genetic/environmental risk of asthma (i.e., probability of being placed in the "case" group) and drug exposure. The fact that use in each trimester was independently significant and consistent with "asthma + drug exposure" is at least partly confounded with genetic risk, as natal autism is thought to be the result of exposure in the first trimester only. This is a good example of the limits of knowledge from retrospective case-control studies on causality assessment or the lack thereof.

Exposures to mercury, aluminum, and other neurotoxins, in utero and after birth, are cumulative. Holmes et al. (2003) found that mothers of autistic children had higher exposures to mercury from vaccines and from dental mercury amalgam. Exposure of the fetus to mercury derived from amalgams is particularly dangerous. Consider the work by Mutter et al. (2007), who were responding to an article suggesting safety of mercury in amalgams. Mutter et al. pointed to a bias in the article, noting that the authors

> *do not present all the relevant studies in their review. The additional data provided here show that: (a) Dental amalgam is the main source of human total mercury body burden, because individuals with amalgam have 2–12 times more mercury in their body tissues compared to individuals without amalgam; (b) there is not necessarily a correlation between mercury levels in blood, urine, or hair and in body tissues and none of the parameters correlate with severity of symptoms; (c) the half-life of mercury deposits in brain and bone tissues could last from several years to decades and thus mercury accumulates over time of exposure; (d) mercury, in particular mercury vapor, is known to be the most toxic nonradioactive element and is toxic even in very low doses and (e) some studies which conclude that amalgam fillings are safe for human beings have important methodological flaws. Therefore, they have no value for assessing the safety of amalgam.*

In two separate analyses in the United States and from seven Western countries, strong correlations were found between the cumulative aluminum exposure and the number of ASD cases (Shaw and Tomljenovic, 2013). In addition to there being strong correlations, the studies fulfilled 8 out of 9 of Hill's causal criteria (Hill, 1965). Thimerosal was phased out of use in vaccines in the pediatric schedule when it was realized that the dosage in the schedule exceeded the limit of mercury exposure allowed by the FDA. Unlike drugs and other medical procedures, vaccine safety assessment then, and now, depends on unreliable postmarket surveillance. In this regard, the pediatric vaccination schedule resembles an uncontrolled experiment. For years, repeated calls (e.g., AAPA and PHS, 1999; Ball et al., 2001) to remove thimerosal were all but ignored by the CDC.

Pesticides and organic pollutants are recognized as likely cause of autism, as they interfere with acetylcholine (Ach), γ-aminobutyric acid (GABA), and dopaminergic neurotransmission. Studies that show that these transmissions are altered in subsets of autistics were reviewed, along with immunological factors, by Pessah et al. (2008). A study of McCP2 mice exposure to common flame retardant polybrominated biphenyl ether led to deficits in sociability, early postnatal growth, and brain DNA methylation in the female mice, which also influenced spatial learning (Woods et al., 2012).

Exposure to the organophosphate insecticide chlorpyrifos is strongly suspected due to association of prenatal residential proximity to high agricultural use (Shelton et al., 2015). The fact that autism-like features are found in BTBR T+tf/J mice exposed to chlorpyrifos (De Felice et al., 2015), but not in mice in general (Williams and DeSesso, 2014), strengthens the case for chlorpyrifos as an environmental trigger set by underlying genetic risk factors. Maternal infection during gestation is also accepted as an environmental cause of autism (Ciaranello et al., 1984; Hwang and Chen, 2010), perhaps involving maternal immune system irregularities (Brown, 2012).

Mazina et al. (2015) found evidence of an interaction between maternal infection and genetic CNV for autism symptoms (increased rates of social communicative impairments and repetitive/restricted behaviors). In so doing, they provided an exemplary case study by which future studies of putative causal factors in autism and other neurodegenerative diseases should be conducted. The consideration of interaction terms during models has been rare in studies seeking association between autism and environmental factors. Synergy among causal factor counts and multiplicative effects can be more important than the effects of individual factors. It is important to note that although increased rates of social communicative impairments and repetitive/restricted behaviors could be attributed to CNV and maternal infection, Mazina et al. (2015) did not find any interactions between CNVs and prenatal maternal infection, and cognitive and adaptive functioning of individuals with ASD. They did conclude, however, that ASD-related CNVs are not likely to be related to general neurodevelopment, but rather to increased risk of ASD due to maternal infection and febrile episodes in pregnancy. Under this interpretation, the genes set the risk, and the environment fulfills the sufficient and necessary conditions.

Genetic variation related to nonpathogenic phenotypic variation in neurotypicals can be ruled as autism genetic risk.

BREASTFEEDING AND ASD RISK

One ecological study points to undernourishment due to exclusive breastfeeding (Shamberger, 2011) and recommends continuation of prenatal vitamins during breastfeeding. Women with all but one MTHFR mutation should avoid folic acid during pregnancy and during breastfeeding.

Many other indications support the idea that longer breastfeeding times could reduce the rate of autism. One Japanese study by Tanoue and Oda (1989) found that 24.8 percent of ASD babies, compared to 7.5 percent of the neurotypicals, had weaned by the end of the first week. "Mother's condition" was responsible for a majority of early weaning in 17.9 percent of ASD and 5.8 percent of neurotypicals, suggesting that early weaning was a causal factor in the outcome of ASD. However, genetic contributions to difficulties in breastfeeding on the part of both mother and child could be contributing, and the weaning outcome could be correlative (as with all retrospective studies).

Mahurin-Smith et al. (2013) found that breastfeeding duration may be protective against persistent stuttering; the neurological basis of stuttering is similar to one of those for ASD: a high excitatory/inhibitory synapse ratio. The authors attributed the protective effect to the fatty acid profile of human milk; however, aluminum exposure (however small) from formula may be additive to the risk of neurological damage overall.

Schultz et al. (2006) found that lack of breastfeeding significantly increased the odds of both ASD (all cases) and regressive autism (RA). They also found that use of formula without omega-3 fatty acids (docosahexaenoic acid or arachidonic acid) increased the odds of ASD overall and for RA. Thus, parents who must use formula should ensure that the formula includes omega-3 fatty acids.

There could be some women who secrete a high load of toxin in their breast milk, however. In January 2015, Germany's Green Party reported that breast milk in German mothers is unsafe after finding high amounts of glyphosate in the range of 0.210 to 0.432 nanograms per milliliter (the safe limit in drinking water is no more than 0.100 nanograms).

A study in 2015 found liver and kidney damage in rats with chronic exposure to ultra-low-dose Roundup™ exposure (Mesnage et al., 2015) and reported:

> *Observed alterations in gene expression were consistent with fibrosis, necrosis, phospholipidosis, mitochondrial membrane dysfunction and ischemia, which correlate with and thus confirm observations of pathology made at an anatomical, histological and biochemical level.*

They noted mechanistic target of rapamycin (mTOR) signaling disruption, which, for the nervous system, means loss of macroautophagy, that is, a dearth of microglial pruning of dendritic processes, essential for early brain development.

Concerned mothers can have their milk tested for toxins.

Ornoy et al. (2015) provides a full review of known and suspected teratogenic causes of autism. If all of these are plausible possibilities, then surely metals such as mercury, aluminum, and nickel might cause autism in a percentage of people, given their toxicological profiles.

In all of these examples, the research on "how" is extensive and yet is not considered in the formulation of vaccine policies in the United States. Given this massive knowledge base, it is unconscionable that the CDC remains silent on how to minimize risk of ASD. The organization has abdicated its responsibilities in autism.

Parents who report "regression" as part of their children's symptoms tend to hold vaccines responsible (Goin-Kochel et al., 2015). In no other area of medicine are conditions and factors reported by parents more dismissed. The common charge is "correlation does not imply causation." If this applies to the thousands of pediatricians' experience of hundreds of recent cases of regression after vaccines, then surely the same applies to the retrospective correlative epidemiological studies of the CDC that (ostensibly) failed to find a correlation? If the presence of a correlation cannot be used to support evidence of a link between vaccines and autism, then the retrospective correlational studies themselves do not constitute a critical test of the hypothesis: a positive result can always easily be rejected as a mere "correlation."

Failure to find a correlation does *not* imply noncausality in epidemiologic correlation studies, especially when the data have been analyzed to death, as described by Dr. William Thompson and as confirmed by internal communications on recalcitrant association findings that were eventually made to disappear by statistical shamwizardry (Barr, 2015; and below).

Far from exonerating vaccines from their fair share of liability, these other known causes help shine intense, bright light on key molecular pathways and molecular circuitry disruptions that lead to autism due to environmental exposures. This knowledge actually makes understanding how mercury and aluminum can cause autism easier. It also aids in the interpretation of the genetic data and points to ways that vaccines could cause autism. This knowledge enhances biological plausibility, shining light on mechanisms of injury.

The FDA's published product information package for the Tripedia vaccine product Diphtheria and Tetanus Toxoids and Acellular Pertussis Vaccine Adsorbed (DTaP) lists autism among the adverse events, as well as other conditions:

> *Adverse events reported during post-approval use of Tripedia vaccine include idiopathic thrombocytopenic purpura, SIDS [sudden infant death syndrome],*

anaphylactic reaction, cellulitis, autism, convulsion/grand mal convulsion, encephalopathy, hypotonia, neuropathy, somnolence and apnea.

The vaccine contained thimerosal, an ethylmercury-based preservative, at the time the insert was written.

Prior to the removal of thimerosal from most pediatric vaccines, numerous studies indicated that vaccines can cause autism and related neurodevelopmental conditions in certain individuals (Holland et al., 2011). A threefold increase in the risk of diagnosis of autism was found in male neonates receiving hepatitis B vaccine during the first month of life, which included 250 μg of aluminum in addition to thimerosal (cohort time frame 1997–2002; Gallagher et al., 2010). According to the FDA, the adult safe dose of methylmercury is 0.1 μg/kg body weight per day.

The toxicity of thimerosal is unquestioned in serious scholarly treatments in the scientific community. It has been shown to be toxic and to affect phagocytosis at very low levels (Rampersad et al., 2005). In public discourse, however, the solid knowledge foundation is sometimes misrepresented as equivocal.

The best description of the state of knowledge of the toxicity of thimerosal is by Duszczyk-Budhathoki et al. (2012), who showed, among other findings, that the ethyl form of mercury, like the methyl form, leads to excess glutamate in the mammalian brain, signaling microglia activation. They showed that administration of dehydroepiandrosterone sulfate (DHEAS) ameliorated the neurotoxic effects of thimerosal.

Thimerosal is still present in some influenza vaccines, and it is present in pediatric vaccines shipped overseas in developing countries. The CDC has recommended thimerosal-containing vaccines preferentially for pregnant women—with no scientific basis for that recommendation.

HOW TO THINK ABOUT GENETIC FACTORS

Clearly, not everyone vaccinated with thimerosal- and aluminum-containing vaccines develops autism. What determines who will react to environmental triggers and who will not? This question is useful for prevention, but does not imply that genes hold special liability over environmental factors. The environmental factors may strongly interact with genetic variation.

Thimerosal toxicity is an excellent example. The toxicity of thimerosal is now known to involve disruption of the endoplasmic detoxification and immune response pathway. Thimerosal is now known to be a selective inhibitor of the protein endoplasmic reticulum aminopeptidase 1 (ERAP1), a proteolytic enzyme that targets and shortens a wide variety of proteins, including some involved in the adaptive immune response (Stamogiannos et al., 2016). The effects of altering ERAP1 can be devastating to health, in ways that can depend on an individual's genotype, including causing varied types of severe autoimmune responses (Cifaldi et al., 2012). At least one of the conditions that result from specific function-altering variation in the ERAP1 gene has also been observed after vaccination (i.e., Behçet disease; Bilgili et al., 2011), leading to concern that other long-term disabling autoimmune conditions that can also derive from genetic variation in ERAP1 may similarly be causally associated with thimerosal (e.g., ankylosing spondylosis; Kenna et al., 2016).

Another expected effect of low ERAP1 function would be improper processing of immunoglobulins. A study by Grether et al. (2016) reported low immunoglobulin levels in mothers of autistics compared to neurotypicals. They attributed these low levels either to "suboptimal function of the maternal immune system" or "reduced maternal exposure to common infectious agents." Further, researchers are noting "protein intrinsic disorder" in a range of psychiatric conditions, including attention deficit hyperactivity disorder (ADHD) and ASD (Tovo-Rodrigues et al., 2016).

The effects of ERAP1 dysfunction may explain the utility of C-reactive protein (CRP) as a putative biomarker for predicting autism in pregnancy, as found by Zerbo et al. (2016), who attributed the change in CRP as likely due to "alterations in the immune response to infectious agents."

Given the impact that thimerosal is known to have on ERAP1 function, it would seem that thimerosal should be removed from vaccines altogether, and ERAP1 dysfunction caused by environmental toxins such as thimerosal should be included in the list of likely causes of maternal immune system dysfunction in the mothers of autistics. While specific genetic mutations may induce this specific thimerosal susceptibility, the discovery of the highly specific mechanism of disruption of such critical normal cellular processes should be grounds for the removal of thimerosal from vaccines altogether, since current medical practice does not include a screen for ERAP1, or any other type of genetic susceptibility, prior to vaccination. Other pathways in protein transport and modification such as the endosome (Partak et al., 2016) may similarly be affected by toxins.

Nearly all of the genetic risk factors for ASD can be found in the general population (Robinson et al., 2016). This means that most of the inherited genetic contribution to autism exists solely as risk and does not become manifest as a factor in action until there is an environmental trigger. However, the high heritability of ASD diagnosis should not be misinterpreted as placing all sources and types of genetic variation as *the* causal factor with primary liability before environmental factors. For example, some of the apparent heritability is from shared environmental factors, some mediated via epigenetics (changes in the methylation of specific regions of chromosomes).

Also, not all genetic variation found to be involved in ASD should be considered evidence of genetic liability in the sense that most people tend to think. Measured genetic variation is split into de novo variation (new to the individual) and inherited. Within these two classes, the nature of specific individual risk may be further discerned as reflecting primarily genetic risk, environmental risk, or an interaction between the two (G × E). I have studied the categories of genes for which variants are known in ASD and offer the following:

1. **Environmentally induced de novo alleles (mutations).** Some percentage of the de novo mutations are induced by mutagens in our artificial environment. They do not represent heritable variation in the generation in which they first appear. Genes impacted by methylation repatterning also fall into this category. Copy number variations, for example, increase in response to exposure to toxins (e.g., Kim et al., 2014). Somatic CNVs, which affect pathways that are involved in autism, represent a type of environmentally induced genetic risk. Kinney et al. (2010) explored the literature on this issue and identified five mutagens of nine likely environmental risk factors for autism. The five mutagens were mercury, cadmium, nickel, trichloroethylene, and vinyl chloride.
2. **"Bad luck" de novo mutations.** Another percentage of de novo genes are evidence of bad luck. These likely involve structural genes such as synaptic genes and cell adhesion genes only, however, and are unlikely to involve genes involved in detoxification or microglial activation signaling. Important exceptions are genes that under LoF cause glutamate buildup or shut down microglial cell deactivation (cytokine signals) without environmental intrusion, such as glutamate transport and receptor genes.
3. **Inherited susceptibility to neurotoxins alleles.** A large proportion of inherited environmental susceptibility alleles confer risk to neurotoxicity from recently developed or concentrated neurotoxins in our environment. These are not autism susceptibility alleles per se; their contribution is realized only when there is an environmental challenge and, if so, they fall into category E, in a G × E interaction. These include detoxification pathway genes.
4. **Inherited ASD risk alleles.** Like "bad luck" de novo mutations, inherited ASD risk alleles confer risk without any requirement of environmental insult. These are the "genetic fate" genes. They contribute to risk in the classical Mendelian sense. They may be dominant or recessive

(typically the latter, as homozygotes will tend to be lethal). They are independent of environment and would show no G × E effect. Their occurrence, however, may be the result of environmental exposures in prior generations.

5. **G × E interaction alleles.** Because genes and environmental factors interact and share targets, common and preventable environmental factors can reasonably be considered primary causes. A root-cause consideration leads to that conclusion because many genetic contributors actually depend on environmental exposures to have an impact. In cancer, mutations do not exonerate carcinogens. Mutations do not exonerate neurotoxins as a causal factor: they provide the setting into which neurotoxins fulfill the necessary and sufficient conditions for autism (and other disease).

Gene × gene interactions and protein × protein interactions are made very complex by protein isoforms (Corominas et al., 2014). This gives insight to the complexity of establishing a fully comprehensive knowledge base even within molecular biology, independent of environment factors. Third-order interactions are almost certainly at play, and thus, while it is important to study statistical interaction terms, direct knowledge of the functional roles of genes and variations can yield further specific insight into which risk categories specific genes most likely fall.

Given these genetic risk categories and a solid foundation upon which the functional significance of any specific allele may fall, any case of ASD may involve none, some, or multiples of these types of alleles. For an individual case of ASD, the degree of nonenvironmental genetic liability can, in principle, be estimated, leaving the rest as an estimated environmental liability.

The effect of the environment is apparent at the neuroanatomic level in the brain as well. Mitchell et al. measured via functional magnetic resonance imaging (fMRI) volumes of regions of the brain in identical twins concordant for and discordant for autism and found no differences in the neuroanatomical characteristics, but large differences between autistic and nonautistic monozygotic twins.

It is important to remember that our genes don't define us. To do that, they would have to exist separate and apart from us and us from them. We *are* our genes and our genes are *part* of us. An injury to our genes is an injury to ourselves.

Similarly, a toxic environment does not (always) determine risk of exposure-induced disease. We are what we eat, but we are also what we are enabled by our genes with our food.

CAUSE OR PROCESS?

Intermediate processes, such as inflammation, are phenomenological, proximate factors. Detailed descriptions of molecular processes involved in the processes of neurological damage are a great source of understanding of disease, but should not be confused with ultimate causes. Aberrant development processes are an intermediate outcome, clinically manifested as disease. Root causes are the factors that, if removed from the equation, would not set those processes in motion. Modifier genes affect degree of severity, and causal genetic variation causes autism.

POPULATION-WIDE ESTIMATES OF LIABILITY

The estimates of 50 percent genetic and 50 percent environmental have been questioned as overestimating environment due to statistical artifact of overinclusion of concordant dizygotic twins (Tick et al., 2015). The revised estimates by Tick et al. reported monozygotic twin concordance of 98 percent and dizygotic correlation of 53 percent when ASD prevalence rate was set at 5 percent (roughly the Broad Phenotype of ASD), but increased to 67 percent using a prevalence rate of 1 percent. They provided an estimated range of heritability from 64 percent to 91 percent and concluded that liability due to shared environmental effects ranged from 7 percent to 35 percent.

To understand how geneticists think about assessing the degree to which autism is genetic, one move toward that direction is the comparison of the sibling recurrent rate (or risk) to the prevalence in the population (Jorde et al., 1999). The sibling recurrence risk is the probability of autism occurring in a child from the same parents of one previous autistic child. This estimate is driven by data (frequencies) in the population and is the same as the rate of families that have two autistic children.

In nearly all studies, the sibling recurrent risk is much higher than the prevalence, indicating that autism is clustered, or aggregated, into families. This does not mean it is genetic; it just means it tends to be clustered in families.

Hallmayer's estimates of heritability and liability are in line with a realistic assessment of the state of knowledge on overall genetic and environmental contributions, from a molecular biology point of view considering the pathways involved. They concluded that a large proportion of the variance in liability can be explained by shared environmental factors (55 percent for autism, 58 percent for ASD), whereas genetic heritability (and therefore Mendelian liability) was lower (37 percent for autistic disorder [AD], 38 percent for ASD). Other studies report high heritability with very little room for shared environmental liability; however, these conclusions ignore the statistical confounding of heritability of all quantitative traits.

Even their estimates of concordance do not parse out the degree of apparent heritability shared by concordant and discordant twins due to shared genetic variation and that which is due to environment on a gene-by-gene basis. Liability estimates do not parse the lines with degree of functional granularity in the genetic risk categories that I have laid out from a deep reading of the literature. Much of the genetic variation that is found to be associated with autism to date is CNV. These are defined as the gain or loss of genomic material greater than 1 kilobase (kb) in size (Iafrate et al., 2004). Some CNVs are common variants in the population, with low penetrance in ASD risk (low or no effect in carriers), and most have existed for a long time. Gaugler et al. (2014) estimated that common, inherited variants make up 49 percent of the so-called genetic risk (Figure 2). Many of these cannot usually be pathogenic, however. They are certainly not dominant; otherwise, many, many more people would have autism. They estimated that de novo variants make up 3 percent and are rare.

Inherited ASD variants accounted for only 3 percent of the genetic risk. De novo CNVs in genes functionally related to autism are more common in sporadic compared with inherited forms of ASD (Sener, 2014).

Another 41 percent of the "genetic" risk is as yet unaccounted. This is sometimes considered "missing heritability," but that is an assumption. These may be immunomodulated mitochondrial dysfunction, as yet undiscovered additional CNVs, LoF mutations, miRNA mutations and miRNA recognition site mutations, and mutations in long noncoding RNAs (lncRNAs), as well as mutations in noncoding regulatory regions (e.g., Turner et al., 2016). That risk also likely includes separate and overlapping environment and epigenetic components and one other category, which is very important: alleles for environmental susceptibility to neurotoxins. These alleles do not determine ASD per se, as they require environmental causes.

Another category includes environmentally induced de novo variants. Any additional rare bona fide inherited (i.e., dominant) genetic autism risk alleles likely occur in similar proportions to those already discovered. Hallmayer and colleagues' (2011) and Sandin and colleagues' (2014) attribution of ~50 percent liability to shared and unique environmental factors in twins did not include the environmental root cause consideration of some of the de novo mutations, nor did they distinguish between common variants as necessarily including nonautism genes. Some unknown percentage of common variants surely reflect "autism genes" as well, but only in combination with other rare ASD variants. Taking inherited dominant ASD variants as our guide, they are also likely to be at most 4 percent of common variants.

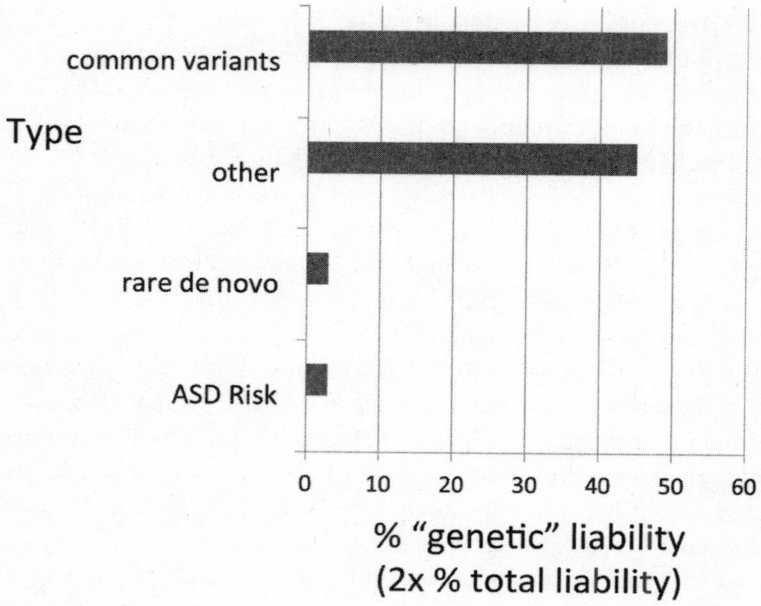

Figure 2. Percent "genetic" liability contributed by mutation class type (estimates from Gaugler et al., 2014). Pure "genetic" ASD and de novo variation represent the least amount of liability. Common variants set the stage and are thus not "autism" genes; "other" represents undiscovered variants in the other three classes and ASD modifier variation (protein function altering nonsynonymous substitutions, miRNA and miRNA elements, mutations in lnRNAs), semi-heritable epigenetic changes (reflecting environmental) with liability manifested via G × E interactions. These liabilities add up to 100 percent for the "genetic" liability, some of which are environmental by consideration of root cause. That 100 percent is then roughly only 50 percent of total liability, as both Hallmayer et al. (2011) and Sandin et al. (2014) attributed 50 percent liability to environmental factors and 50 percent to heritable genetic variation without discernment for these types by environmentally induced genetic risk. Studies of contribution of de novo variation range from 4 percent to 24 percent (Tick, 2015); however, many of the CNV are not functionally related to ASD or ASD phenotypes. Observation of occurrence is not proof of causality. This leaves some private allelic causes of autism at risk of never acquiring causal status until criteria for levels of evidence are developed, as has been seen in breast cancer, in which some alleles never reach "clinical status." Going forward, I recommend combining predicted LoF mutations and significant microdeletions in the same gene into one category and not make families wait until other families are found with the exact same predisposing mutation to confer "clinical" status. This will inflate the apparent dominant genetic component of autism; therefore, the functional categories provided should give suggestions on how to proceed in accounting risk versus cause.

In fact, the Sandin et al. (2014) analysis concluded that for classic autistic disorder (AD), only nonshared environmental factors and dominant genetic factors combined were relevant for understanding concordance patterns in families. This would mean that different environmental factors served as causes of autism in families with more than one autistic child, with an underlying dominant genetic risk. However, a close look at their model selection process shows that another model is very nearly as good a fit: the model in which the dominant genetic factor is left out, leaving only shared and nonshared environmental factors. Given the large confidence intervals in the range estimates of variance components, either model could easily be accepted. Either way, the dominant genetic contribution is small compared to environmental factors, and a variety of environmental factors appear to be at play within families.

The de novo variations—arising during gamete formation in the mother or father (with only ~2.6 percent liability)—are recent. The common variants are relatively ancient; they certainly predate modern medicine and the expanded and accelerated pediatric schedule of the CDC. Because they likely represent variation that predated the emergence of modern medicine, they represent that part of human variation that contributes a necessary (contributing) but not sufficient factor in causal analysis. They are, therefore, risk alleles, true "autism alleles," *whether their nonlethal contribution to phenotype shows a dominant pattern or not, with or without leading to autism diagnosis in some individuals.*

Girirajan et al. (2013) found increases in both rare and common CNVs in ASD and concluded that CNVs may predispose individuals to ASD. It is not safe, however, to presume that any particular CNV or that increased rates of CNVs are "genetic." Similar to the effect of certain environmental toxins on methylation patterns, mutagens and teratogens can induce changes in CNVs (e.g., Kim et al., 2014). It is very important, therefore, to consider gene function when assessing liability. In the absence of gene function, individual contribution by mutations of unknown origin could be estimated from the percentages of variations of the same class (point mutation, microdeletions/insertions, inherited CNVs [with caution; many are nonfunctional]) and de novo contributions.

Consider the view of Parisi et al. (2009):

> *[A] teratogenic exposure can mimic a known Mendelian genetic syndrome and caution is urged in presuming a genetic etiology for infants with potential teratogenic exposure to relatively new drugs with limited published animal data.*

The number of genes found with CNVs in ASD is growing with every study, making functional assignment and causal inference difficult. For example, Glessner et al. (2009) found hundreds of CNVs in total in a study of ASD versus controls and highlighted some that are likely to be of functional significance (NRXN1 CNTN4, NLGN1, ASTN2, and various ubiquitin genes). The finding of individual CNVs that are likely—even highly likely—to contribute to the autism phenotype is not sufficient evidence that a variant is playing a causal role. Genotype and haplotype both matter, too, and it is well known that much variation may be functionally neutral. In clinical genetics, the observation of a single mutation alone is insufficient evidence to ascribe causal status. However, the evidence of the influence of CNV in non-ASD traits in the general population means that many CNVs are modifiers of the ASD phenotype, not risk alleles or environmentally susceptibility alleles.

Van Daalen et al. (2011) considered the issue for CNVs as follows: for cases in which ASD-contributing CNVs arose de novo in families wherein both parents scored within the normal range (on the social responsiveness), those CNVs were then assumed to be one of the primary causes of ASD. (Notice they did not suggest that the CNVs were *the* primary cause of ASD for that case.) However, for all other cases, they suggested that ASD-contributing CNVs be considered a secondary contributor, within a "background of other putative susceptibility alleles." I think that is partly right, depending on the specific nature of the CNV, the rest of the genome and exposure. While CNVs are more prevalent in autistics, people homozygotic for CNVs may in fact live their entire lives without autism if they are never exposed to neurotoxins or other inflammatory substances: this is why they are not "autism risk genes," but rather, "environmental susceptibility genes." The same is likely true for many nonsynonymous nucleotide substitutions (which change amino acids but do not truncate a protein). I suspect, therefore, that the majority of the "other" in terms of the missing genetic concordance will prove to be shared environmental insults, reflected by low penetrance.

Since autism is so highly controversial and our thinking has been influenced by governmental information paradigms that do not by any measure reflect the full body of valid scientific knowledge, it is helpful to consider the same problem apparent in another condition that has similar findings, at least in terms of de novo variation. Consider the work of Boshes et al. (2015) on the matter in schizophrenia:

> *The overwhelming majority of SNPs and CNVs are post-fertilization mutations, occurring in somatic tissue, not germinal tissue. These mutations are a normal aspect of somatic cell division but occur more frequently in patients with schizophrenia.*

The cause of the increase in postfertilization mutations in schizophrenia is unknown. One can postulate about molecular mechanism that are heritable that make CNV more likely (unstable genome hypothesis). However, absent any data demonstrating slippage of DNA replication, that is mere speculation. The incidence of schizophrenia has been found independently to be on the rise in Denmark and in Australia. A survey in 2007 showed a lifetime prevalence of schizophrenia of 0.6 percent in the United States (CDC data). The National Institute of Mental Health 2015 estimate was 1.1 percent, an 83 percent increase.

Whatever proportion of increases in schizophrenia are due to environmentally induced CNVs, the ultimate cause of that percent liability is not likely "genetic" (i.e., there is not likely a common genetic risk for de novo CNV production independent of environmental insults). Still, the most relevant genes that show up in ASD (and SZ) with either copy number variants or point mutations in multiple studies are found that are functionally related to phenotype. There is some circularity here that should be avoided; every "discovery" study highlights those genes that make the most "sense" (involved in neurological developed synaptic genes, glutamate receptors, etc.). As important as general function genes are, that strategy is very much a major factor in determining which genes are highlighted in this book. Thus, it is a biased look at the biology inherent in the risk of ASD.

That said, it provides a way forward through the quagmire of too many genes. They can be parsed into various categories. From a look at the published data, there is no doubt that some LoF de novo variants may in specific cases play a primary role in the etiology of ASDs. Loss of function mutations, which may include any of a myriad of nonsense, frameshift, or splice site mutation, have been found to be significantly associated with ASD (Samocha et al., 2014).

Some (but not many) of these are rare and dire "double knockouts" in humans, contributing a 2 percent risk increase of autism in females and 5 percent increase in risk males (Lim et al., 2013). Most of these included complete loss of genes on the X chromosome. MeCP2 (methyl CpG binding protein 2), used as a marker for Rett syndrome, was among these genes.

MeCP2's role in non-Rett ASD is becoming increasingly apparent (Loke et al., 2015). A thorough examination of Rett syndrome from molecular viewpoint is Banerjee et al. (2012). The clinical course of ASD patients with LoF MeCP2 could be greatly informed by their work. Research on the effects of MeCP LoF and duplication mutations is just beginning (Tropea et al., 2016). Some ASD mutations (MeCP2 duplications) are found in some patients with Rett syndrome. Keeping Rett syndrome on the spectrum would help avoid syndromizing ASD given the immense etiologic overlap that has been observed among subtypes. The unique clinical features of specific molecular subtypes (e.g., AUTS2 "syndrome"; Beunders, 2016) can be studied by valuable molecular stratification studies. A literature review of autistic cases with CHD8 mutations resulted in a finding of high clinical variability within that group (Merner et al., 2016).

MICRODELETIONS, MICRODUPLICATIONS

Classically, molecular syndromes involved portions of chromosomes missing, duplicated, or rearranged. Technologies now can exist that can identify small regions or segments involving single genes. This could "blur the lines" between chromosomal and monogenic diseases (Kashevarova et al., 2014), making clinical "syndromes" restricted to large-scale chromosomal rearrangements.

Genetic overlap among neurodevelopment disorders has led to the concepts of "contiguous gene syndromes" (CSG's; Weise et al., 2012) and "genomic sister disorders" (Crespi et al., 2009). CSGs were originally conceived of as conditions involving gains/losses or mutations in critical regions involving two or more genes, located in close proximity to each other. Because not all genes in a microregion may be involved in the phenotype of a disorder, the idea has generalized to the concept of "microdeletions and microduplications syndromes."

It has also been generalized to the concept of "genomic sister disorders" for when two or more clinically distinct disorders result from the same microdeletion/microduplication either due to pleiotropic effects of a single gene or due to the independent effects of variation in different genes simultaneously lost, mutated, or duplicated.

These concepts are useful because they maintain the conceptual demarcations among clinically distinct disorders, while allowing that they can both result from the same genetic event. They can also share a portion of specific genes contributing risk and phenotypes.

However, while I support the importance of individualized medicine, I caution against and question the utility of deconstructing or fractionating conditions like ASD into millions of individual "syndromes." In any individual patient, the observation of a specific mutation, such as a microdeletion/microduplication, may be consistent with specific disorder, but it does not always demonstrate primary or exclusive causality. Zygosity, epistasis, and environmental exposures can determine whether the effects of a specific mutation are seen clinically. This is common in dietary disorders such as phenylketonuria (PKU), which, of course, is a good example of a condition that can be alleviated by minimizing exposure to a causal factor in the environment (dietary phenylalanine).

In terms of environmental syndromes, similar concepts are at play. Two or more separate environmental injuries could result in changes in the same phenotypes, or in distinct phenotypes that co-occur in a patient. Damage to the kidneys, for example, by exposure to one toxin could be accompanied by separate, environmentally induced gastrointestinal issues. It is more difficult to identify specific environmental contributors, and this is why the development of highly specific biomarkers of toxic exposure is important. The environmental factors, of course, can then add to or even interact with any genetic variation predisposing to risk, susceptibility, or modification of extent of the manifestation of a specific disorder.

LOSS OF FUNCTION MUTATIONS

Recent whole-exome sequencing (WES) studies of ASD families have revealed LoF mutations in numerous, individually rare risk genes. Observations of independent de novo LoF mutations occurring in the same gene in different individuals are compelling.

Sanders et al. (2012) found 279 LoF de novo mutations in autistic families, only one of which showed LoF mutation in the same gene in two individuals: SCN2A (sodium channel, voltage-gated, type II, α subunit). The individuals with the mutation had no history of seizures.

Neale et al. (2012) found that only 46.3 percent of ASD cases has an LoF de novo variant and concluded that missense mutations in genes CHD8 and KATNAL2 (katanin p60 subunit A-like 2) were likely autism risk factors.

O'Roak et al. (2012) also observed LoF mutations in KATNAL2 in families. They found that most de novo mutations were of parental origin (4:1), with incidence correlating with paternal age. They reported that 39 percent (49 of 126) of the serious disruptive novel mutations were in genes involved in the β-catenin/chromatin remodeling protein network. This implies possible defaults in the epigenetic regulatory role that impact several fundamental biological processes. They found more frequent protein-altering mutations in genes CHD8 and NTNG1, and they also observed de novo, protein-altering mutations in GRIN2B, LAMC3, and SCN1A.

Iossifov (2012) observed a great deal of overlap of de novo mutations in ASD shared with fragile X syndrome, pointing to synaptic plasticity, and estimated between 350 and 400 low-penetrance autism risk genes. Among many other mutations, they found the genes NRXN1 and MTHFS harboring LoF variants. They also found a variant in CACNA1G, which was found to be associated in a cohort study (Strom et al., 2010). The found a mutation in the gene GRM5, which encodes mGluR5, a glutamate receptor. Noroozi et al. (2016) found variation in marker GRM6 to be associated with ASD. As signal for microglial activation, glutamate is extremely central to many cases of autism.

Iossifov et al. (2012) also noted a bias in the contribution of fathers to de novo mutations: they estimated that 75 percent of de novo mutations come from fathers. They attributed 16 percent of the ASD differences between autistics and their sibling controls to de novo mutations as an underestimate (by approximately half); their study did not survey the entire genome, for example, a point the authors take pains to point out.

There are many other similar studies; these are but a sample. Each of these studies also found hundreds of additional idiosyncratic LoF mutations, unique to each patient, in different genes. Attributing causal status to these mutations is difficult, but we know that large tracts of homozygosity in CNV and increasing numbers of CNV are associated with increased risk of ASD diagnosis in a largely vaccinated population.

GENETICS × ENVIRONMENT

These studies are each truly a cause for celebration. However, as informative as these genetic studies may be, if they are conducted in isolation from environmental exposures, they are doomed to identify only genetic culprits. Without consideration of possible exposures, G × E (genetic × environment) interactions cannot begin to be considered.

The genetic (heritable) components of parental personality may also inflate apparent genetic heritability of some classical ASD traits, as can a shared placenta for monozygotic twins (Correles et al., 2011). It is well known that in humans and other social animals, not all measured heritability is genetic; some is cultural and some is due to shared environment (e.g., shared womb). We now also know that new genomic variations, which do not necessarily originate via inheritance of genetic variation in the classic Mendelian sense, contribute as much to the risk of autism as inherited genetic variation. These variations, which include de novo mutations, personal CNVs, and chromosomal rearrangements, are not always "genetic" for a given person. Environmental factors have a strong effect on genomic methylation patterning in both somatic and germline cells, which can influence gene expression in highly idiosyncratic but apparently heritable ways. Some of the "heritable" variation in autism risk is epigenetic, which can in turn result from environmental exposures as a root cause. We know also know that both heritable and de novo mutations themselves can effect changes in the methylation, including genomic and mitochondrial mutations.

This view is contrary to that of those who would like to portray genetic variation as a cause of an adverse event after vaccination such as that espoused in the article "Vaccination Triggers, Rather Than Causes, Seizures" published in *Epilepsy Currents* (late 2015). This is an unusual—and unjustified—position. Vaccines are not part of our species' natural environment. The human species (*Homo sapiens sapiens*) is approximately two hundred thousand years old. Vaccines with aluminum and mercury are a scant eighty-five years old. The increase in the pediatric schedule of the CDC is a mere thirty-five years old. How is the ancient genetic variation in the human population the primary cause of ASD, when the clear root factor has been vaccination-induced neurotoxicity in so many instances?

The heritability in trait categories that, in the extreme, represent autism is the same in the unaffected neurotypicals as in those clinical extremes (Robinson et al., 2011). This means that in autistics, naturally existing variation in the population contributes to the expression of phenotypes in autism via the same non-pathological pathways that are involved in the unaffected population. Much of what we see in autism is therefore environmental alterations of naturally occurring phenotypic variation. I think the philosophical, ethical, and legal implications for this knowledge are profound. It means that many genetic variants involved in variations or subgroups within autism reflect subgroups that exist in the general population. Parents of autistics know this—they recognize familial personality traits in their kids—they see the person, not the disorder.

This means that the genes involved in subtypes in autism will be modifier genes, not causal (in the liability sense). It means that in spite of the few specific risk variant genes some autistics have in their genomes, autistics have as much going for them biologically as do unaffected people. And, most important for some families, it means that most of the variations found among autistics that contribute to the autism phenotype do not contribute liability in the causal or legal sense.

Understanding cause and precursor conditions is simple. A terrorist setting off a bomb causes building damage, not the failure of the building to sustain the damage. It is not the engineer's fault the terrorist defeated their design. A man comes home drunk and beats his wife. She dies. To say that the woman's body's failure to withstand the onslaught caused her death, even if she were already ill, would be to blame the victim. Cyanide acts on proteins that are not adapted to the presence of cyanide and causes death; cyanide, not the failed ability of the proteins to withstand its effects, is the cause of death at toxic doses. The foreign, artificial, industrial factors that abrogate normalcy in biological systems are the causes of disease, not the range of functions observed in the population upon which they act.

Overly simplistic representations of genetic contributions that lead to that portrayal of genetics as the sole cause of autism, that suggest that it is therefore deterministic and that we can forget about environmental factors, are similar exercises in blaming the victim. The *Diagnostic and Statistical Manual of Mental Disorder, Fifth Edition* (DSM-5) correctly refers to any discovered genetic basis of ASD as a risk factor or as a specifier, not a differential diagnostic marker that automatically denotes a private syndrome.

In positions aimed at administrative dismissal of RA altogether, as a tactic to remove from sight the consideration of RA after vaccination, genetics are also sometimes referred to as an "underlying cause," which in itself reveals a misunderstanding of the logic of causality and injects an air of mystery to the autism (or seizures) puzzle. In considering unusual and rare events such as onset of autism, seizures, fainting, hearing loss, and other adverse events that can occur after vaccination, the baseline in a specific case is the genotype of the individual for any susceptibility loci. On the morning before the vaccine, an individual has a particular genotype, but not ASD phenotypes. After the vaccine, the individual develops ASD. It takes abilities beyond science to conclude that autism or ASD would have resulted in such individuals without exposure to neurotoxins in vaccines.

People have the right to carry their genetic diversity safely without being blamed for their autism when it is caused by environmental insult.

It is logical to conclude, in the context of the massive body of current knowledge of the effect of aluminum on pathways involved in autism, that many individuals suffering any of a myriad of adverse events would not had have that event, or disease onset, without vaccinations. Consider that most individuals with high genetic susceptibility and developed AD had parents without AD (because AD is associated with low fecundity) and that many of the risk loci are common variants. The genes alone provide the context (setting), and the vaccine or other environmental exposure becomes the cause.

By the end of this book, the reader will understand that were it not for the advent and introduction of neurotoxins included in vaccines and thus their addition to the environment of our species, many individuals would not have developed autism. That is, at the population level, vaccines share liability with other neurotoxins and with genes, for the increased rate of autism. The reader will also understand precisely why and how these toxins can cause lifelong, self-sustaining damage. This has nothing to do with vaccine efficacy, other than that the use of aluminum, a serious neurotoxin, is an immune-activating adjuvant included to increase efficacy at low cost.

THEORIES EXPLAINING AUTISM

The field is ripe to move beyond denial, beyond blame—to move into high gear toward understanding the causes of ASD, thereby preventing it and enabling the development of effective treatments.

There are numerous theories on how to best synthesize and interpret the data from genetics and molecular studies into a coherent framework.

One of the best theories, supported by the bulk of the published data from genetic studies is that variation contributing to autism involves genes that encode proteins that normally provide antioxidant protection, or remove toxins from cells, the bloodstream, and the body (excretion). Glutathione levels are reduced in the serum of autistics (Al-Yafee et al., 2011; Frustaci et al., 2012), providing evidence of weakened defenses against neurotoxins, including mercury (Mutter et al., 2005).

Neurotoxins' defeat of these protective mechanisms leads to a poor intracellular environment, in which the rest of an individual's genetic variation is also expressed and interpreted. In some people, the outcome is autism. The published data support this general idea in a diversity of forms.

Another well-supported theory is one of dysfunctional synaptic biology. Synaptic biology is extremely complex, involving a huge number of proteins. Genes for synaptic proteins have been studied (Zoghbi et al., 2012), revealing a large number of genes with function-altering mutations, associated with local neurological dysfunctions. Among the first of these was the GABA-β3 receptor subunit gene, which is perturbed also by cellular responses to pesticides. Evidence exists for a large number of functionally disruptive mutations in genes involved at the synapse. Mechanisms of dysfunction include loss of nerve cell extensions and connections, loss of inhibitory synapses, overgrowth of excitatory synapses, and overall alteration of the control of synaptic formation, growth, and function.

Numerous studies have found mutations in genes involved in the birth/death processes of synapses as well. The connections between neurites have been found to be lower in some areas of ASD brains, at certain ages, leading to reduced connectivity (hypoconnectivity). This is detectable in early childhood by electroencephalogram (EEG). Connections among nerve cells involve growth and recession of nerve cell extensions (i.e., neurites, which are axons and dendrites). From this perspective, autism may be seen as a "synaptic neuropathology" (Canitano and Bozzi, 2015).

Even looking at the synapses, however, a reasonable mechanism for hypoconnectivity is the overactivation of the innate immune system (microglial) cells, which act to prune new neurite extensions. Microglial activation, via any of a number of environmental factors (peripheral nerve injury, trauma and stroke, inflammatory disease, and neurotoxicant-induced neuronal injury), can lead to numerous downstream effects, including a helper T cell (Th1/Th2) immune imbalance and excessive interleukin (IL)-6 cytokine release, reflecting a shifting toward Th2-type immune activity. Increased glutamate in the brain and chronic IL-6 expression is a marker reflecting microglia "stuck" in their activated form, in which they chew away at nascent and existing brain tissue. This condition (excitotoxicity) is a form of innate autoimmune disorder.

Signals that keep microglia activated cause them to act in the deconstruction of these neuritic extensions and neural precursor cells. These include the excitatory amino acids (EAAs) such as glutamate. One of the functions of astrocytes is to remove EAAs via the glutamate-glutamine pathway. This prevents the extracellular accumulation of the excitatory EAA and neurotransmitter glutamate. Gestational and early infection can lead to glial priming, a type of sensitivity in which the microglia become too easily activated.

Anything that causes harm to astrocytes or reduces their capacity to uptake glutamate also leads to glutamate buildup, which leads to sustained and chronic microglial activation (CMA), a form of immunotoxicity. Mercury is preferentially stored in astrocytes and has been shown to reverse astrocytes' abilities, causing them to swell and to release glutamate into the extracellular environment, instead of removing it (Aschner, 2000). This signals microglia to stay activated. Overactivation or underactivation of microglial cells leads to overgrowth and hyperconnectivity (initially in ASD), or overpruning (as the condition progresses), leading to hypoconnectivity. Both of these aberrations are evident at different developmental stages and are reliably detectable by EEG. Aluminum is toxic to astrocytes in a manner that specifically disrupts the glutamate-glutamine pathway (Struys-Ponsar et al., 2000). There is extensive evidence that both aluminum and mercury can lead to chronic microglial activation that lasts the lifetime of autistic individuals, ultimately destroying dendritic extensions and neural precursor cells. Mutations in the astrocytic glutamate receptor gene can similarly prevent proper uptake of glutamate by astrocytes, and the outcome is not always ASD. Van Amen-Hellebrekers et al. (2016) found increases in copy numbers of the solute carrier family 1 (SLC1A3, aka glial high-affinity glutamate transporter) in patients with ADHD and/or autism behavioral problems, noting the gene's role in glutamate transport. Gliosis is a root cause of intellectual disability in Fragile X syndrome (Higashimori et al., 2016).

A third well-supported theory is one of developmental hyperconnectivity—too many connections among brain cells, too soon. This may occur with and could explain macrocephaly (large head), which occurs in 15 to 35 percent of natal autism cases. Head circumference at first appears small at birth among autistics followed by a sudden increase in head size sometime between one to two months and six to fourteen months (Webb et al., 2007). Hyperconnectivity seems to follow, reflecting aborted learning processes, in which connections are made but too many are retained in spite of a standard learning environment. Mutations leading to dysfunction of mTOR signaling appear to lead to extra synaptic processes compared to controls via loss of macroautophagy, indicating a *lack* of self-pruning of dendritic processes (Tang et al., 2014). The result is a change in the architecture of the number of connections successfully made during reinforcement (learning). Some of this is seen in the imbalance in the inhibition-excitation (I/E) synapse ratio. The excess spines are free to interact independently with individual axons as singular one-to-one synaptic connections, and the local structures show a dearth of the many-to-many synapses that reflect proper microglial-guided reinforcement learning. The numerous and simple one-to-one synapses perform an excitatory function but lack the opportunity for feedback inhibition made possible via the more complex local many-to-many synaptic networks. Because microglia are "distracted" in the defense mode, they are not available to facilitate proper, healthy pruning of weak one-to-one connections during which spines, too, are pruned. Macrocephaly is also found in a subset of ASD patients with function-disruptive mutations in the ASD-linked chromodomain helicase DNA binding protein 8 (CHD8) gene or deletions in 17q12 (Bernier et al., 2014; Moreno De-Luca et al., 2010).

Both environmental and genetic factors can play roles in the manifestation of autism involving pruning processes. As we will see consistently throughout the features of autism, given a backdrop of genetic risk, environmental triggers are all liabilities (Hallmayer et al., 2011). Thimerosal has also been shown to deplete glutathione in a manner directly pointing to thimerosal neurotoxicity (James et al., 2005) and the mechanisms for both chronic microglial activation and protein disorder via disruption of the protein ERAP1.

A fourth theory is the lack of communication among specialized areas of the brain, suggestive of failure of long-range connections and pathfinding (axon guidance) during development (Bakos et al., 2015 et al., 2015; Sbacchi et al., 2010). This is due to the reduction in the quantity of reinforced synapses between adjacent cells, so that proper long-range connectivity cannot be established during development. This is not merely gestational—the human brain undergoes its development program during the course of a quarter of a century. At any time, if aberrant reinforcement of connections takes place, the outcome can be dramatic. Local regional homogeneity and long-distance connectivity appear to be separate manifestations (Dajani and Uddin, 2015); still, it is difficult to conceive of how long-range connectivity could be effective when local synapses are few and tenuous.

The drastic simplicity that results (many one-to-one connections between cells, few many-to-many connection) belies a lack of dynamic synaptic plasticity. This type of altered, simplified connectivity is seen in fMRI brain imaging studies, and the findings include a biologically plausible neurological explanation of some autistic phenotypes (e.g., Jiang et al., 2015). This shines a light on the recurrent question of autistic phenotypes: are the individuals merely sensory-disabled, or are there also underlying brain process disruptions? This question is examined for each major phenotype. The number and weakness of synaptic processes play an important role here and, developmentally, successful axon guidance is required for interregional connectivity and the development of canonical brain functions that involve multiple regions. The simplified morphology of nerve connections in AD may also present difficulties in inhibition of impulses. Mirror neuron deficits are not always present in ASD, even in "classic" autism (Fan et al., 2010; Gallese et al., 2011). Altered communication among and through brain regions with different functions appears to be key to some behaviors in autism in which input (perception) signals are mistaken for motor activity signals.

A fifth theory is one of alterations of generalized regional functional homogeneity and incorrect specialization among different regions of the brain. This is supported by evidence from both gene expression (Voineagu et al., 2010) and fMRI (Paakki et al., 2010) studies and from studies of brain scans of word sound processing. Voineagu et al. (2010) found a lack of regional patterns of gene expression that typically distinguish frontal and temporal cortex, suggesting "abnormalities in cortical patterning." Paakki et al. (2010) found significantly increased regional homogeneity of resting-state brain activity in some brain areas compared to neurotypical controls and significantly decreased regional homogeneity in others areas.

Genes encoding perception inputs appear to play an important role in ASD severity. Genes coding for input processing signals appear to be important, as well. For example, some studies have indicated that phonemic perceptual narrowing, which is the normal reduction of an initially rich ability to detect all phonemes, is absent or inconsistent in autism. In a more recent study, this ability was similar across autism/ASD and low-risk groups—however, lateralization (hemispheric specialization) of event-related potentials (responses to word sounds) was aberrant in the autistic group (Seery et al., 2013). A number of studies have demonstrated that autistics may have superior, not inferior, skills of perception under controlled conditions (Gliga et al., 2015; Kemner et al., 2008; Mottron et al., 2006; Plaisted et al., 1998). One gene, Syntaxin 1A, shows higher expression in high-functioning autistics (Nakamura et al., 2008).

Local connectivity, like aberrant long-distance connectivity, is important to consider, as it may add to understanding the phenomenon involved in the cascade of developmental trajectories and trade-offs among skill sets. For example, as infants develop, the network of regions dedicated to processing language becomes more efficient, narrowing from four to five regions into primarily the temporal cortex, potentially freeing the frontal areas for higher-level processing (Blasi et al., 2015). This level of understanding is helpful for guiding intervention, and given that deficits in sensory perception and learning are cumulative for later social development, the earlier pathway disruptions play an important role in terms of understanding later development.

The effects of local functional heterogeneity appear to be split geographically in the brain by autism domain. Communication and the stereotyped behaviors and restricted interests are positively correlated with lower functional connectivity within the right superior temporal sulcus, whereas general autism diagnostic characteristics positively correlated with lower functional connectivity in the right middle frontal gyrus (Jiang et al., 2015). This no doubt reflects the simultaneous contribution of autism risk genes (e.g., SHOX microduplications; Tropeano et al., 2016) and modifier genes. Variations in modifier genes may exist and modify phenotypes within the general population and may be working in same way in ASD, but on different fundamental substrates. Modifier genes, their markers, and variations within them should not necessarily be considered to be "disease" genes, markers, and alleles unless they exacerbate core diagnostic domains. In this way, a person's genetic individuality can be considered first as "variation" and not necessarily "pathological."

It is also important to keep in mind that some traits, such as homogeneity of activity and lack of functional specialization, may be more accurately thought of as important intermediate outcomes (endophenotypes) rather than as causes. They do not compete with possible root causes, such as individual gene mutations and environmental triggers. Thus, while primary causal genetic variations exist (rare autism without environmental influence), genes that would have merely contributed to variation in these characteristics without neurotoxin-induced CMA are considered modifiers, not causal. An excellent example of this is found in the polymorphisms in the gene Dectin-1, a gene that mediates innate immunity against fungal infection. Specific nucleotide base positions in Dectin-1 appear to be related to the degree of severity of ASD, but not to ASD itself (Bennabi et al., 2015). It is possible that fungal infections may pile on the innate immune response hyperactivation, which turns out to be key for understanding the role of neurotoxins in autism.

An example of support for the theories involving synaptic genes is a study by Lu et al. (2012). On the basis of biological plausibility, their team targeted calcium channel genes and found variants associated with autism. The function of calcium channel proteins is essential for nervous impulse transmission and for proper synaptic transmission; the calcium channel proteins are highly sensitive to metal toxicity. There are many other findings that support disruption of synaptic function via LoF mutation in synaptic genes (Giovedí et al., 2014).

A sixth theory is an adaptive autoimmune theory, in which individuals' adaptive immune systems attack parts of the nervous system in a chronic assault that prevents normal development, normal maintenance and functioning, or both. There is good evidence that immune activation during gestation may activate mothers' immune systems. Maternal antibrain antibodies are more often present in mothers of autistic children than in mothers of typically developing children (Rossi et al., 2013; see Braunschweig et al., 2012, for a review). These antibodies react to proteins that are highly expressed in fetal brain tissue, and the immune response has negative impact on neural development. Neural development disorders involve pathogenesis initiated during childhood and adolescence. This may provide a reasonable potential explanation for the birth-order effect (similar to Rh factor exposure—older children experience fewer infections). Mothers' cytokine profiles may also provide insight into autism risk. Immunoglobulins that recognize self-antigens can also cross the placenta and reach the CNS before blood-brain barrier formation. Goines et al. (2011) correlated the presence of anticerebellar autoantibodies with diagnosis of autism, lower adaptive and cognitive function, and aberrant behaviors.

It is clear that the immune system is critical to understanding autism, with roles for both adaptive and innate immunity. Indeed, direct evidence of both types of autoimmunity has been known since the late 1990s. Singh et al. (1997) found circulating autoantibodies to both neuronal and glial filament proteins. What causes this is the focus of intense research. Antibodies against glial filament proteins are known to reflect traumatic brain injury (Zhang et al., 2014); however, neurotoxin-induced autoimmune disorder can render the same signature by keeping microglia active. Indeed, a glial signature was found in a transcriptomic analysis of ASD brains.

Some cases of autism may be similar to Rh-factor incompatibility. Infection in pregnant mouse dams leads to ASD features and hippocampal synaptic deficits without evidence of microglial activation (Giovanoli et al., 2015). That said, maternal immune activation (MIA) can introduce reactive oxygen species, inducing microglial responses (Le Belle, 2014). The innate and the adaptive immune system interact via T-cells (Filiano et al., 2015) and myeloid dendritic cells, which are found to be increased in autistics and correlated to amygdala volume and repetitive behaviors (Breece et al., 2013). Once activated against paternal brain proteins, the mother's immune system may be more likely to reactivate in later-born children.

The occurrence of MIA, however, does not automatically rule out subsequent, independent, environmentally induced CMA as a second environmental hit, independent of MIA even years later, with cumulative effects on the developmental program. CMA, which involves primarily innate immunity, can be induced from vaccines given at birth and via secondary activation, even in late early childhood and early adolescence, via environmental factors that disrupt normal microglial cell activation. The act of repeatedly reactivating innate immunity is not exonerated due to later adaptive immunity. It depends on the exact history of the individual. Clearly, the risk of CMA is additive—if not multiplicative—with increasing doses of microglial activators.

The two types of immunological theories (adaptive and innate) can be considered noncompeting causal theories, as the actions are events that occur early in development, or via repeated exposure and activation, both consistent with profound lifelong effects. Importantly, the evidence that improper neural pruning may occur after birth and can also act to *maintain* autism throughout life is supported by numerous lines of evidence from a multitude of independently motivated and executed studies. Once triggers are identified, exposure to microglial activators such as glutamate should be minimized to prevent increasing severity. Monosodium glutamate is one activator; nitrates are another. A good list of excitotoxic foods is available online (American Nutritional Association, 2016).

In fact, due to cumulative risk, and especially the accumulated effects of repeated exposure to risk of chronic microglial activation, none of these theories are mutually incompatible; for example, unusual patterns of connectivity trajectories and/or the lack of development of specialized function could be an emergent result of aberrant local-scale aberrations in neurite functioning, caused by damage to nerve cell growth and function processes, which could be due to microglial aberrations. Further, the literature is filled with references that point to both genes and environment as clear central causal roles in all of these theories. However, it is important to keep in mind that common variants were part of the genetic landscape long before the advent of environmental toxins.

Allowing the field of autism research to progress requires a firm grasp of potential causal factors in autism and autism genetics. This means letting go of a lot of "either/ors." It means putting the pieces of the puzzle together. It is not useful either to throw one's hands in the air and give up because "everything" causes autism: this is not a position from which we can progress toward prevention. No serious scholarly research study can be conducted on causes of autism without considering interactions among genes and interactions between genes and environmental factors. A specific environmental trigger may indeed have caused a specific phenotype, but only given the specific genetic predisposition of an individual. A critical example in the study of autism is the finding that individuals with mutations in the MET receptor tyrosine kinase gene *and* high exposure to air pollution have a higher risk of developing autism (Volk et al., 2011). A variant that disrupts MET transcription was found to be associated with autism (Campbell et al., 2006).

This does not relieve other environmental exposures of their liability in individual cases. Also, it is well accepted that lifetime risk of many diseases from environmental exposure is cumulative and also that autism is developed by plenty of other people without exposure to high levels of air pollution. Di Renzo et al. (1993) found a potential role of HGF/MET in microglial reactions to central nervous system (CNS) injuries; therefore, it seems likely that air pollution is one of many repeated insults that lead to microglial activation, leading to CMA.

Most models of interaction of genetic and environmental risk factors have multiple possible outcomes. For some lucky people, it's mutation plus no environmental trigger → no autism. For other individuals, it's no mutation + trigger → no autism. Combining the G and E factors, of course, leads to increased specific (individual) risk of autism. This is where the models are tricky, because with a large enough environmental load, we would all develop autism. The "naughts" (those with 0 risk-conferring mutations) are the lucky ones (or are they?) and those with autism characteristics show a wide range of variation in the combination and intensity of the expression autism traits—even within monozygotic twins. The distribution of autism traits in the diagnosed population certainly also invokes a good deal of chance. This has led to an interesting and important epistemological parallel between cancer and autism.

Long ago in cancer research (Knudson et al., 1971; Nordling, 1953), researchers posited a two-hit hypothesis. These "hits" are mutations that are either inherited or occur in normal somatic tissue. Individually, neither hit is sufficient to cause cancer. Combined, however, the two genetic changes may push a normal cell further toward the cancer phenotype. The idea, known at the "Knudsen hypothesis," has matured into a *multiple-hit hypothesis* based on the knowledge that most people carry a significant genetic load—a number of silent genetic variants inherited from one of their parents.

The variants can be inherited from either parent, and the cancer-related effect is usually masked by a normal variant from the other parent during early life. However, a number of people may then develop two or more cancer-related variants via somatic mutation (mutation in the tissue). Even these individuals are not necessarily destined to acquire cancer. However, they also accumulate additional somatic mutations, making them more susceptible as they age. Of course, during their lifetime, people experience cumulative environmental triggers that generically add to the risk. Age-related accumulated mutations play a central role in the Knudsen hypothesis, as it is thought that people become more susceptible to environmental insults as they accumulate mutations as people age. Environmental and other nongenetic factors still play absolutely essential and central roles in our understanding of cancer.

The same seems to be robustly supported by the data from autism. Multiple mutations, inherited or de novo in gametes, may make individuals more susceptible at a very young age to damage from environmental insults. The specific nature of the interactions between environmental triggers and the genetic load may vary from person to person. It has been long established that many so-called "cancer genes" can be interrupted or changed in a myriad of ways. The average human gene is approximately 3,000 nucleotide bases long, and any of those base positions can be different from the most frequent variants. The moniker "cancer gene," of course, is a misnomer—these genes may encode for DNA repair proteins, such as the BRCA1 gene, which is associated with breast cancer, and therefore they are now considered "proto-oncogenes." There are now hundreds of genes suspected of contributing to the risk of cancer occurrence and progression, many of which are confirmed by many studies, and genetic testing in cancer is now a billion-dollar industry. There are hundreds of genes suspected of contributing to the risk of autism, many in the same pathway, and vaccinations are ubiquitous. I cannot imagine an area more ripe for genetic testing. The American College of Medical Genetics now recommends that all children with an ASD receive a genome-wide microarray and undergo an evaluation by a clinical geneticist.

Understanding the genetic results can be challenging, and numerous conceptual frameworks have emerged. A two-hit hypothesis in autism as posited by Picci and Scherf (2014) involves a first genetic "hit" followed by one or more environmental hits. Their model is focused on the genetic and environmental causes of failure of autistic individuals to develop adult cognitive capabilities, although they specifically contrast their model with those that encompass the regressive autism (RA) phenotype (approximately 30 percent of cases of autism are RA; Miles et al., 2003).

Multiple vaccinations can precipitate developmental regression in susceptible individuals (e.g., Poling et al., 2006), and routine vaccination has been associated with a variety of autoimmune conditions (Agmon-Levin et al., 2009; Girard et al., 2005). Evidence exists that multiple vaccines in one visit increase the risk of morbidity and mortality due to vaccines (Miller, 2016).

ASD DIAGNOSIS: HIGH GENETIC OVERLAP CLARIFIES DSM-5

Regressive autism has historically also been called secondary or late-onset autism (between two and three years). After reviewing three thousand studies on autism and after careful analysis of the changes from DSM-IV to DSM-5, I can find no basis for the exclusion of RA from a comprehensive framework of autism. While the criterion of earlier signs of autism exist in DSM for a diagnosis of ASD, not all criteria of autism are required for diagnosis. RA was formerly a recognized form of ASD, along with childhood disintegrative disorder (CDD), in DSM-IV.

DSM-5 is most generally understood as combining AD, Asperger's, CDD, and pervasive developmental disorder not otherwise specified (PDD-NOS) under the ASD umbrella (Fig. 3). It clearly includes late-onset regression in autism, if you read between the lines and pay attention to some very important qualifiers. For example, excerpts from DSM-5 are full of qualifiers:

> "The age and pattern of onset should be noted for autism spectrum disorder."
>
> "Symptoms are **typically** recognized during the second year of life (12–24 months of age) but may be seen earlier than 12 months if developmental delays are severe, not noted later than 24 months if symptoms are more subtle." This reflects the ideas that the majority of cases that regress do so before 24 months. Late-onset regression (after 24 months) is allowed.
>
> "The pattern of onset description **might** include information about early developmental delays or any losses of social or language skills." The caveat *might* indicates that it is expected that sometimes parents will report not only no developmental delay, but that their child was ahead of their peers in terms of language and cognitive development.
>
> "In cases where skills have been lost, parents or caregivers **may** give a history of a gradual or relatively rapid deterioration in social behaviors or language skills." This is not prescriptive—parents will report what they see. It does inform pediatricians, however, to expect that some cases will seem to occur suddenly.
>
> "**Typically**, this would occur between 12 and 24 months of age and is distinguished from the rare instances of developmental regression occurring after at least 2 years of normal development (previously described as childhood disintegrative disorder)." The link to CDD leaves the incorrect impression that RA is rare in ASD. ASD is not synonymous with CDD; regression can occur in and lead to AD (most notably), CDD, Asperger's, and PDD-NOS as well. Note that there is no mention of any particular environmental factor here.
>
> "The behavioral features of autism spectrum disorder first become evident in early childhood, with **some** cases presenting a lack of interest in social interaction in the first year of life. **Some** children with autism spectrum disorder experience development plateaus or regressions, with a gradual or relatively rapid deterioration in social behaviors or use of language, **often** during the first two years of life." The DSM would be improved with percentages, or ranges of percentages.

The sentence in DSM-5 on the first evidence of appearance of behavioral features in autism, with only some cases showing social deficits is a critical point in which the DSM-5 contradicts itself; the criterion of prodromal (early) signs for ASD is clearly not meant to be an absolute requirement. Pediatricians cannot rely on all parents to recall or accurately represent earlier signs when asked

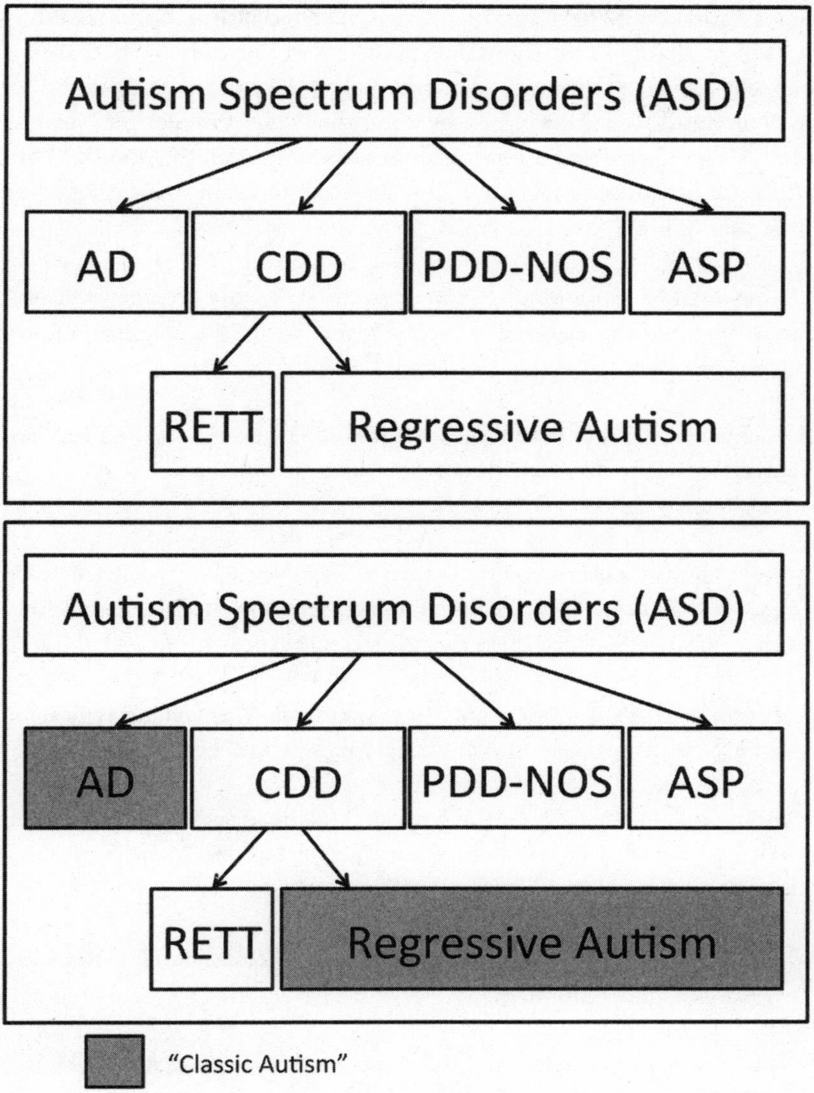

Figure 3. A molecular view on regressive autism within ASD. DSM-5 does not specifically distinguish between AD and RA and hints that for a diagnosis of AD, earlier (prodromal) signs should be present. That leaves RA out of AD. Given the etiologic similarities and genetic overlap between RA and RETT, RA could be a subtype of CDD; however, pediatricians are taught that CDD is very rare. Most pediatricians would diagnose RA as simply as "AD," keeping in mind the caveats and exceptions sprinkled throughout DSM-5. For research on effects of genetic and environmental factors, however, classic AD and RA should be kept separate.

during a short screening diagnosis. Retrospective confirmation bias can cause parents to recall, out of the thousands of instances, one or two where their child will appear to have withdrawn, or "spaced out." This likely "happens to" every child! The recall bias is amplified by an undue weight on earlier "instances." Most AS screens take five minutes, and thus it is important that the DSM be read carefully. Only some cases will present a lack of interest in social interactions in the first year of life.

> "**Some** children with autism spectrum disorder experience developmental plateaus or regression, **often** during the first 2 years of life." Here, again, the caveats are important.
>
> **"Such losses are rare in other disorders and may be a useful 'red flag' for autism spectrum disorder."** This means that regression is so rare outside of ASD, it nearly always indicates ASD.
>
> "Much more unusual and warranting more extensive medical investigation are losses of skills beyond social communication (e.g., loss of self-care, toileting, motor skills) or those occurring after the second birthday."
>
> "Autism spectrum disorder is not a degenerative disorder and it is **typical** for learning and compensation to continue throughout life."
>
> "Symptoms are **often** most marked in early childhood and early school years, with developmental gains **typical** in later childhood in at least some areas (e.g., increased interest in social interaction)."
>
> "A small proportion of individuals deteriorate behaviorally during adolescence, whereas most others improve."

It calls for caution in differential diagnosis between Rett syndrome and ASD because Rett syndrome most often includes delayed social skills, is usually restricted to girls, and usually resolves with age. DSM therefore cautions that (for this particular comparative diagnostic task) only when "all diagnostic criteria are met." However, this does not apply to direct diagnosis of autism without consideration of Rett syndrome, and Rett syndrome is nearly exclusively found in females.

Persons with Rett syndrome can still be also diagnosed with ASD, noted with a specifier of "with known genetic or medical condition." A major review of research on regression in autism (Ozonoff et al., 2008) concluded, "The research literature reviewed in this paper suggests that signs of autism emerge over the first year and a half of life and are not present in most cases from shortly after birth."

The history of RA diagnosis (Spratt and Asper, 2015) begins with Heller, who in 1908 described autism occurring in the third and fourth years of life in six children. Late regression is sometimes called Heller's syndrome. He labeled the disorder *dementia infantalis.* Kanner, in 1943, considered autism a distinct condition requiring a separate diagnosis.

The use of the term *disintegrative* began with International Classification of Diseases (ICD)-9, while DSM-III listed RA as childhood-onset pervasive developmental disorder (COPDD). This was carried over into the DSM-III-R, in which childhood disintegrative disorder patients were included as "autistic disorder—onset in childhood."

Childhood distinctive disorder was first used in the ICD-10 and DSM-IV, in which childhood disintegrative disorder fell under the general category of pervasive developmental disorder.

In DSM-5, RA is not specifically called CDD, but with the intent of moving all pervasive developmental disorders under the umbrella of autism spectrum disorders, severe RA will most frequently be diagnosed as ASD, specified as AD with late onset. Some cases could fall under CDD, but pediatricians are taught CDD is rare. Given the room for RA afforded by the caveats, RA should fall squarely into ASD.

For diagnostics, ASD is defined by specific sets of behaviors, not etiologies. That will almost certainly change in the future. Etiology-based diagnostics may become routine as they enhance understanding of the condition in a given individual. For some, it would appear that "no mutation + environment" may be the only explanation for their ASD. For these individuals, no first "hit" seems needed. No genetic mutation is needed for autism from valproic acid or thalidomide, for example—the congenital effects lead to the autistic state in a rather uncomplicated manner, and thus many animal studies have been used to tease apart the developmental anomalies that derive directly from those environmental injuries. Early hyperconnectivity measured by EEG may prove useful in predicting which patients may develop autism (Orekhova et al., 2014).

Other animal studies of environmental effects may miss the "big picture" of autism altogether. Low-powered studies with wild-type animals and small sample sizes will not likely reveal a main effect of some neurotoxins, such as mercury and aluminum. Moreover, since genetic subgroups are strongly suspected of being susceptible to such toxins, then studies that use animal models that mirror genotypes associated with autism risk, such as those described by Schroeder et al. (2015) would seem to be much more well designed to the problem of understanding autism in humans.

AUTISM RATE INCREASES

Autism rates are increasing at an alarming rate. This increase is not administrative or due to changes in diagnosis. In fact, use of DSM-5 criteria is expected to result in a *decrease* in the diagnosis of autism by one-third, particularly AD and PDD-NOS (Kulage et al., 2014). Initial studies attempted to show that autism diagnosis itself was "contagious" because individuals tended to learn about autism from people they knew; however, it is well established that private information travels in social networks, not randomly, and that process is a characteristic of private information flow regardless of increases or decreases in incidence of disease. The fact that doctors are being trained that autism is primarily genetic may cause borderline symptoms to be reevaluated once a full case of ASD is diagnosed in a family. Autism (ASD) rates are now one in fifty-eight by the age of six years in the United States, and the increase shows no sign of slowing.

The bulk of the literature on differential diagnosis warrants separation of various subtypes but with substantial overlap (Tsai & Ghaziuddin et al., 2014). The boundaries are not distinct and, given the role of environmental factors, it seems likely that continuous rediagnosis would see patients move from category to category as the condition progresses. Most clinicians perform diagnosis of ASD as subtypes with specifications. DSM-5 is highly specific, but may leave out some patients from ASD without intellectual impairment (McPartland et al., 2012; Huerta et al., 2012).

During the build-up to the changes in DSM-5, certain changes were proposed that would lead to an administrative disappearance of RA. A careful read of the final DSM-5, however, shows that past cases of regressive autism still fall in ASD, just without (or with weak) earlier signs of autism. For the study of causality, of course, there are many reasons to study natal autism and regressive autism as separate conditions. Among these reasons is the increasing prevalence of regressive autism and similar conditions with no evident genetic prior risk. Brain development is most rapid by the time of birth and undergoes successive bouts of devolution and reconstruction at approximately ages two years, five years, and during adolescence. Brain development continues until approximately age twenty-five. During this time, development of many brain functions accelerates at a remarkable rate—in speech, the acquisition of language and the expansion of vocabulary; in cognitive thinking, acquiring one's own identity of self, development of symbol-based abstract thought, and so on. The sudden loss of speech and language processing, accompanied by apparent losses of cognition at any age greater than two years old, is, clinically, a very different manifestation of symptoms than a baby born who showed delayed speech and should be treated as such. The data from molecular studies, including cell lines; animal studies, including mice, rats, and monkeys; and the type of genetic variations predominantly associated with autism strongly support the idea that a small percentage of people may be at high risk of RA due to absence of any number of neuroprotective phenotypes. Pulled together in one place, in this book, the evidence is simply overwhelming. The cumulative effect of vaccination and other sources of neurotoxins may produce autism in susceptible children at a much younger age than would have occurred without widespread infant vaccination. Importantly, early regression in autism (less than thirty-six months) has been observed to occur in 23.9 percent of patients (Parr, 2011), and the evidence shows that when ASD exists at birth, the toxins/autoimmune exposure would have occurred in gestation; if ASD onset is late, exposure was cumulative.

The existence of autism-like traits prior to the onset of RA is sometimes used to try to exonerate environmental toxins. Given the widespread knowledge in environmental epidemiology that cumulative lifetime risk is due to cumulative lifetime exposure, this perspective represents tortured logic. Early (gestational) exposure and genetic risk do not make vaccines (or other exposures) less dangerous; in fact, they likely make the effects of continued, additional insults more likely to be pathogenic. Going forward, research on autism and other neurodegenerative conditions should focus on cumulative exposure and cumulative risk.

Those who pitch the idea that autism is nearly "entirely genetic" are ignoring the available data. It is also a gross misrepresentation of the data from published studies, and such reports are misleading the public and causing grave harm. A genotype, and even familial risk, is often not predetermined fate. The public should not be misled by individuals who would like to turn a continuous risk variable into a duality (all or nothing). The literature is filled with evidence of room for environmental factors, with perhaps as much as 50 percent liability going to environmental factors (Hallmayer et al., 2011; Sandin et al., 2014).

But contrary to a growing trend in representation, autism and ASD have not historically been widespread. I have read numerous recent treatments describing autism as "common." In genetics, "mutations" that appear in the population at 3 percent or higher qualify as "polymorphisms." Any values less than 1 percent are classified as "idiomorphisms." If anything, autistic disorder (AD) itself is, under normal conditions, a rare, genetically and phenotypically heterogeneous idiomorphic condition. In a toxic environment, it becomes more prevalent, expanding in the population as ASD. In an environment with an increased diversity of toxins, individuals who otherwise would not be at risk are suddenly and increasingly at risk, in varied ways that reveal a diversity of genetic tolerances for toxin. It is certainly increasing in prevalence. Conditions on the autism spectrum, or the broad autism phenotype (e.g., autism traits in undiagnosed siblings), however, are not rare at this time. ADHD, for example, is as high as 20 percent in African American males in the state of Georgia in the United States. I have a chapter in another book, *Cures vs. Profits: Successes in Translational Research* (World Scientific, 2016), in which the story of how the first reports of ADHD overdiagnosis led to the destruction of a clinical psychologist's career. The CDC now concedes, after many years, that ADHD is overdiagnosed. However, the CDC also found results showing strong association of overall ADHD risk and vaccines and also of ASD risk and vaccines (see Barry, 2015). The report was made public after enforcement of the Freedom of Information Act (FOIA). Another internal CDC report (Verstraeten et al., 2000) included a finding of positive association between the CDC vaccination schedule and ADHD. A Senate committee that looked into allegations of whether this positive association was "covered up" concluded no cover-up, but reported that in a meeting, "Simpsonwood participants generally agreed that the VSD data set was weak, it was difficult to assess causality and further study and investigation were warranted." Dr. Thomas Verstraeten had presented data showing that infants exposed to vaccine Hg during the first six months of life had 7.62 higher risk of developing autism. This result never made it into the final publication, which, like many CDC-sponsored studies, included results after repeated rounds of analysis after initial association was found.

The "weakness" here results from the fact that all ASD conditions had to be lumped into a single group before a significant association was found. However, this is not unexpected given the low prevalence and heterogeneity of the conditions; there are some instances in which important and real significant result appear weak due to poor study design. Studies for rare conditions caused by heterogeneous factors (such as autism/ASD and ADHD) should take positive associations seriously because they are difficult to generate by chance under such conditions. These issues are addressed in a chapter on study design.

AUTISM ANALYSIS

Single-factor explanations are easier to understand, but they may not reflect the truth in any specific case. Particularly sensitive people may not be able to endure as large or as frequent doses, and a small dose of exposure may be sufficient. Two or three mutations plus gestational exposure may appear "congenital" but is more accurately "natal." Similarly, one large dose of neurotoxins may be sufficient.

ASD may show itself later in people who have intermediate sensitivity, perhaps with one risk mutation and multiple risk factors. The entire remainder of the population could be at low risk of ASD at any time of life, with increasing lifetime accumulated risk. This may explain part of the incidence of Alzheimer's and other age-related neurodegenerative conditions.

There is strong support by studies that show that of the genetic contribution to risk, a proportion is due to inherited variation and the remainder is due to de novo variation. De novo variation occurs during the formation of gametes (sperm and egg), and the mutations are therefore highly unique, except in the case of identical twins. The idea in a multiple-hit model for autism occurrence involves any type of variation—inherited or de novo, or both. Sometimes the genetic hits are both inherited and sometimes a combination of inherited and de novo. It does not rule out the possibility of two or more de novo mutations that confer risk, although most geneticists would expect that that probability of such an occurrence would be very low.

Much of the genetic variation contributing to autism risk includes ancient "common variants." It is unlikely that all or even many of these variants are by nature deleterious, or even slightly deleterious—although balancing selection (Sewall Wright) can lead to the maintenance of somewhat deleterious alleles at moderate to high frequencies. It seems much more likely that the common genetic variants may in fact be beneficial in the absence of mutations that break neuroprotective mechanisms, and their presence modulates the intensity of a given phenotype. An example of this has been found in alleles that, in persons without autism, appear to confer a slight cognitive edge. In one study (Clarke et al., 2015), researchers found that individuals with the largest number of autism-associated genetic variations showed an edge in tests of cognitive ability, including verbal fluency, logical memory, and vocabulary, as well as in general assessments of cognitive ability. The study was based on the reanalysis of data from three prior studies. However, more than 99.5 percent of the variation in cognitive ability in their study was located in genes that do not contribute to autism risk.

The environmental hits that may be relevant are also myriad. These are enumerated throughout this book, which is arranged by phenotype, as is appropriate for a work on genetic traits. Importantly, however, simply because there may be numerous environmental causes of autism does not remove any from the list of suspects. The degree of severity of autism (in terms of both number of characteristics and their degree) appears to be also controlled by both genetics and the environment, although the latter may be subtle and nefarious. Imagine, for example, a child born to parents who each have partial autism phenotypes. They may be less able or likely to engage their child socially; thus, genetics determine, in part, the developmental environment. Also, the human mind is self-programming; our individual decisions about what to watch on television, what to read, where to go, whom to associate with are all factors in our social environment. This makes attribution of severity to environment causes difficult but not impossible. Grave concerns exist regarding the shift in the pediatric vaccination schedule and the addition of so many vaccines, each one an occurrence of immune system activation. Are we expecting too much from our infants?

Just as no serious work on the genetics of autism could leave out consideration of environmental factors, neither could one avoid exploration of the myriad of phenotypes involved in autism. The neurobiological basis of autism appears to involve a number of manifestations, some rendered during early and late (postnatal) brain development. These range from aberrant local cell-to-cell synaptic communication to failed long-distance neuronal connections via failed axon guidance among regions of the brain. These phenotypes can be examined at the molecular, cellular, morphological, and behavioral levels. Studies indicate an absence of sufficient functional specialization of different areas of the brain, while in other instances the autistic phenotype expressed may involve dysfunction of synaptic genes, leading to overactive and/or lack of inhibition function at synapses, forming the hyperconnectivity phenotype. That type involves a failure of the pruning of synapses by the innate immune system cells called microglial cells, which are types of macrophages, key actors in the CNS immune system that engulf and digest aberrant proteins and foreign invaders during infection. These cells are the resident "macrophages" of the immune system in the brain and also serve to prune extensions of neurites. Neurobiology is fascinating, and autism is at least as complex.

Some phenomenological theories of autism have also been proposed. These include *theory of mind* (i.e., the ability to attribute mental states to oneself and others; Baron-Cohen, 1988; Tager-Flusberg, 1996, 1999), weak central coherence (inability to process information in context for interpretation of global meaning; Frith and Happe, 1994), and an absence of social reward for learning language and other skills (Dawson, 2001). These are descriptive and useful in the sense of satisfying the clinicians' and parents' minds to knowing what is going on in the minds of autistics, but they are not causal theories. They are also useful as starting points for proposing new hypotheses of likely effective methods for education, behavioral therapies, and some treatments; however, they also (mostly) describe a system already in motion, that is, the consequences of causal factors. We must avoid confusing descriptions of autism with discovery of its causes.

In Chapter 16, I extend and formalize all of these ideas to a more generalized, discrete, multifactorial risk class category model, which is incomplete to the extent that it does not encompass every aspect of the expression of modular autism: different pieces of the puzzle fitting together differently in different people. That model does not fit neatly into a box; instead, a multidimensional tesseract model seems more appropriate. This level of complexity of autism demands rigor in thinking, time for deep study, attention to details in defining phenotypes and study populations, and, above all, objectivity. No specific agenda should be introduced during the formulation and testing of hypotheses and explanatory models. Given that autism is at least 50 percent genetic, models that describe internal cellular processes only and ignore environmental causal factors are incomplete.

The evidence accumulated to date requires the consideration of the environmental liability sampling process. The field of autism research is moving from an exercise in diagnostic discord toward a consensus of multiple, as yet not well defined subtypes of autism. Whereas medical experts may prefer "domains" because they give the doctors something to target with treatment, geneticists prefer "phenotypes" because they give us something to try to understand via genetics that may sometimes be independent of a fixed diagnosis category. It is evident, however, that some domains cosegregrate in families (Oerlemans et al., 2013), meaning they are likely linked, inherited together via the same segments of chromosomes.

Because strong evidence points to an ongoing assault by the immune system on synaptic architecture in nerve cells, as well as attacks on other cells in the nervous system, we have clinically actionable knowledge. A misbalance in the formation and pruning of structures at the synapses by microglial cells—important during both development and normal brain maintenance metabolism—can lead to excesses of some structures as well as deficits in others, as a birth/death process is in constant play, with pruning mediated by microglial activities. Immunological responses by the mother to brain proteins, which may result from infection during pregnancy, is evident in mothers of autistic children (Patterson et al., 2011). This indicates that some cases of natal autism are likely due to autoimmunity acquired in the womb or even via breastfeeding. A screening program for brain protein antibodies in blood and breast milk should be explored as a way to reduce the incidence of autoimmune-mediated autism. However, such cases are early-first-trimester prenatal cases. Studies are needed of high-risk pregnancies to study the immunological dynamics during pregnancies of the risk of natal autism, both for characterizing the timeline of brain protein antibody appearance and for identifying useful tracking biomarkers and environmental triggers involved. The presence of maternal antibrain antibodies should be a red alert for vaccination. Due to cumulative risk, other risk factors of autism should easily accepted as medical exemptions as well.

As fascinating as the immunological factors may be, there is equally strong evidence for a role of other factors, such as disrupted proteins and CNVs. These endogeneous molecular characteristics should not be seen as predetermined fate, however, because many if not most represent weakened neuroprotective mechanism. Although there are many low-penetrance genes involved, many individuals are at high risk of being susceptible to autism environmental exposure. I explore the multitude of specific manifestations damage caused by environmental factors in the presence of weakened neurodefenses.

VACCINE SAFETY

Given the breadth and depth of research studies explored, I also have concluded that we need vaccine safety research reform, including an endgame strategy in the pediatric vaccine safety schedule. There are hundreds of vaccines under development.

Dr. Paul Offit shamelessly defends his outrageous conflict of interest for voting at three out of four opportunities to add the rotavirus to the pediatric schedule. Rotavirus is a disease for which Offit partly owned a patented vaccine while serving on the federal Advisory Committee on Immunization Practices. We are told by a government report that Offit participated in the discussion, but abstained from the final vote for "general use." He also infamously claimed that babies could tolerate 100,000 vaccines at one time. He later revised this estimate downward to 10,000. It would appear that he neglected to include in his consideration the various additives to vaccines, especially aluminum. State Senator Pan of California similarly made an outlandish comment in 2015, stating that the most dangerous ingredient in vaccines is water. Pan, a medical doctor, was similarly apparently unaware of the nearly 400 studies on aluminum neurotoxicity, readily available via a web search of the National Center for Biotechnology Information resource PubMed.

Subsequent to his votes, Offit sold the patent for his rotavirus vaccine for millions. The hyperbolic claims by Offit and Pan and others are not based on science, are the epitome of irresponsible rhetoric, have no place in scientific discourse, and are damaging to meaningful, progressive consideration of the facts.

The same type of irrational thinking goes into consideration of adding new vaccines by the members of the Advisory Committee on Immunization Practices. Wholescale changes to the vaccine schedule—including the move to vaccinate from birth to two years—have not been subjected to prospective randomized trials and are therefore experimental. The safety profile of the vaccine schedule is unknown, yet epidemiological risk due to exposure is cumulative.

Every time a new vaccine is added to the schedule, we are conducting an uncontrolled experiment on our children.

STUDY DESIGNS

In the 1980s, autism was rare. Studies of vaccine safety were typically powered to detect a main effect that was prevalent in the population. However, autism was and is rare (although many authors refer to it as "common"). Individuals on the ASD may be "common," in some areas as high as 20 percent. Each study that reported "no association" really was reporting "no universal main effect." This practice continues in more recent animal studies that recapitulate the vaccine schedule of 2003, when most childhood vaccines included thimerosal. Designed with small samples and not powered for the given prevalence, such studies are of limited or no value in asking the question: can vaccines cause autism in some people?

This practice of studying for a main effect continues in studies that focus on overall rates of autism in populations (e.g., Jain et al., 2015; Uno et al., 2015). Knowing there is a low prevalence and heterogeneous genetic risk, enrichment studies should focus on individuals with mutations that predispose individuals to autism and focus on the combined risk using the distribution of molecular risk of environmental susceptibility. The effect of ignoring these factors during the design of studies is predictable: negative finding after negative finding, due to design artifact, not due to lack of effect.

The outlay of information from genetic studies demonstrates that many of the studies that sought, or seek, to understand environmental causes such as vaccines were doomed to find no effect when they seek to find a population-wide response from individual alleles. When no major loci exist, but instead many low-frequency alleles contribute to risk, the hypothesis stated, study design and the design of analysis of a simple population-wide association study are not well placed. This information is not new: Hardy et al. (2008) described this issue in great detail in the early days of genome sequencing.

APPLICATION OF UNIVARIATE THINKING IN THE FACE OF ETIOLOGICAL HETEROGENEITY

In case control discovery studies, significant factors that influence only a subset of patients can be missed under conditions of etiologic heterogeneity. Methods have been developed to address this issue, allowing significance of difference or association for multiple factors that produce the same phenotype (e.g., Lyons-Weiler et al., 2004; Zheng and Pepe, 2008; Ernst et al., 2008; Tong and Coombes, 2012; Wang et al., 2012). Similarly, use of additive linear models (e.g., logistic regression) assume that all markers are informative in all patients. This assumption is violated for the molecular basis of autism and perhaps for environmental factors as well. Major algorithmic advances have also been made in this area.

GENETICISTS ARE DOOMED TO FIND GENES . . .

The fact that the assumption of monogenic mode of inheritance might apply has led a few researchers astray on assessing the significance of certain genes with structural variation and with low-frequency variations found in ASD. Before I give the examples, I want to remind the reader: finding association with ASD does not confer disease-locus status to a gene. In cancer, hundreds of mutations are found, but only those that reach a certain percentage of the population are considered "clinical." In ASD, I advocate that LoF genetic mutations be considered at the whole gene and perhaps pathway level when they are counted by frequency, as, for example, the data on colon cancer genes like MSH2 and BRCA1 have resulted in hundreds of mutations not considered to be "clinical" because they do not appear in a large enough proportion of the population. This is wasteful and based on a legacy of limited knowledge.

SEEING ENVIRONMENT THROUGH PATTERNS OF INHERITANCE

In 2003, Bill et al. found association of variants in the RBFOX1 locus and wrote:

> *However, a significant proportion of the observed structural variation is inherited from phenotypically normal individuals, raising questions regarding overall pathogenicity of variation at the RBFOX1 locus.*

What would make an allele appear, in one generation, to be associated with an ostensibly heritable condition? A change in the environment from one generation to the next could do that. We see this type of shift in phenotype all the time in animal studies. An animal, say a mouse, that inherits a mutation from its parents is given a changed diet, and we see a major shift in the metabolism. Perhaps the change is an iron challenge or a folic acid challenge. It happens so often in biomedical research, it's common knowledge.

This may be an example of an important miss, because environmental factors were not studied. RBFOX1 is a neuron-specific splicing factor gene that regulates a number of important processes during brain development. Variation in RBFOX1 may not contribute to ASD risk specifically. Mikhail et al. (2011) found it to be among those tied to developmental delay, mental retardation, and/or autism spectrum disorder.

Sometimes when two genes or more are involved, the effect is spread out. But when a single mutation confers risk and the environmental challenge is presented, we can see large effects. The same issues exist for studies of environmental factors uninformed by genetics. Autism itself is rare (between 1 and 2 percent in the United States), and therefore association studies should have been powered to detect a relatively rare condition with heterogeneous genetic influences. This flaw, as well as sampling biases, make having confidence in the negative results from retrospective population-wide association studies extremely difficult. Those who continue to conduct such overly simplified study designs and interpret such studies but ignore the rarity of autism fall into illogical extensions and can pose a threat to sound public health policies. Ethnic or racial subgroup analyses, a form of stratification, only address genetic variation distributed uniquely within the subgroup. Positive results for a specific subgroup might point to shared heritable risk, or shared environmental factors, or both, making attribution of a positive result difficult. Nevertheless, such discoveries, while unexpected, represent very promising discoveries of important factors that influence variation that can help render etiological understanding of diseases. Standard practice in such studies would dictate additional studies for validation with larger studies.

AUTISM PREVENTION AND TREATMENTS

There are social impediments to understanding via research. Some in the autism community have expressed the desire to eschew "cures" for autism—they would prefer to remain who they are. This so-called "neurodiversity" movement wants us to celebrate autism as a normal expression of human genetic variation. However, while their variation itself may be celebrated, like anyone else's, their condition often exists due to the intrusion of environmental factors on the human genetic landscape, which is (at least) two hundred thousand years old, sprinkled with idiosyncratic de novo mutations.

Our fates are not determined by our genes. We have the uniquely human capacity to change our environment. As a by-product of our ingenuity and industry, we have made neurotoxins, including those present in vaccines, an unnecessary part of our environment. We can make better choices.

There are some precious inroads to translationally actionable discoveries, which have, in some cases, clinically actionable knowledge. For example, a reasonable recommendation would be that pregnant women with one autistic child should certainly not receive a thimerosal-containing influenza vaccine. They would do well to avoid activating the immune system via any vaccinations during pregnancy in light of the massive amount of data supporting a causal role for MIA in autism.

Prevention means in part avoiding neurotoxins. It also means real vaccine safety reform. In no other area of biomedical science can so many animal studies point squarely to a medical procedure with such abject failure in terms of its safety profile. Yet translation to clinical use proceeds with only a hope that the aggregate effect on humans is safe, merely because humans are not mice. If that is a rationale, then why bother noting safety profile data in animal studies for any drug? In ethics, we are taught to generalize our maxims—no special pleading allowed. Human studies also show lifelong chronic microglial activation in autistics. The concern here is not any individual vaccine; it is the entire schedule. Laws passed to compel vaccination via the threat of loss of access to public education are unquestionably unethical; they violate the letter and the law of volunteerism in matters of informed consent. Threats by doctors to patients that would deny health care services, regardless of the nature or severity of their disease, unless they are vaccinated, is coercion. Forced medical treatment and coercion are both illegal under US federal law and under the Nuremberg Code.

The fact that the entire schedule has not been subject to the proper types of science necessary to study efficacy and safety means that the use of the schedule is experimentation on subjects in an uncontrolled clinical trial. Subjecting individuals to participate in medical experimentation without informed consent is likewise illegal.

Treatments are needed for those who want them, so family members and society can enjoy more of a good thing. Some parents wish their children could suffer less (not having a lifetime of seizures) and be more engaged. The entire discipline and principles of bioethics and our own morality guide us in these areas, with limits. Genetic testing has already led to prenatal screening. But do we know enough to warrant those options? The moral questions on that issue are immense. However, there is at this time little chance of an accurate gene-informed prediction of infantile autism within the first three months of life in the uterus. For some couples, it may be appropriate to consider genetic testing to understand the odds of one-, two-, or three-plus-hit pregnancies. For others, fate, destiny, or God's will serve as their guide. As to the morality of the questions these issues raise, I offer this: all children have merit and all have potential. Hopefully, treatment options will emerge based on this new knowledge that will allow all autistics to express themselves to their full potential.

Concerns regarding eugenics could be replaced with a drive for prevention and informed consent. Genetic studies of individual patients is also paving the way to understanding both genetic and environmental etiologies of autism for individual patients and, of equal importance, shining light on pathways for tailored therapy, diet changes, and other ways to improve the quality of life for individual patients. The knowledge of the pathways points a way to modular treatment, which, of course, is most granular in the form of completely individualized treatment given genomic variation and knowledge of the environmental exposures.

Focus can also be placed on improving the quality of life of those born with autism, or who may regress into autism (risk minimization), all the while respecting the individual patients' personalities and the consenting parents' wishes. It seems likely that developing and offering optional treatments for specific phenotypes, rather than seeking "cures" for autism, will be found to be most tractable and more acceptable to all concerned.

There is also mounting evidence that we can learn a great deal about autism from many other diseases, in part because they often share a genetic component. I examine ways of thinking about comorbidity and relate the issue of disease classification to the issue of study designs. It is important to define study populations and control populations and handle variables appropriately as either cofactors or control variables. In the past, important studies on the causes of autism have not always handled these issues correctly, yielding misleading results and incorrect inferences. Instances exist in which unintentional selection bias has made interpretation impossible. Ascertainment bias can result from the inclusion or exclusion of types of individuals with certain subconditions, and yet interpretations are (inappropriately) generalized to all autistics (overdrawn inferences). This has been common in numerous studies and is a serious flaw, widely recognized as a sign of poorly conducted science with an agenda.

Also moving forward in considering environmental factors, we must also look at published data that impeaches "established notions" of what we "know" about environmental factors and autism. Discussions of the safety of mercury in vaccines often cite studies that show that ethylmercury—the form found in thimerosal, an additive in vaccines—is cleared from the blood of animals faster than methylmercury. At face value, this observation is taken to mean that the exposure time is lower for ethylmercury than for methylmercury, forming a critical foundational observation by which policy on the use of thimerosal in vaccines has been based. Take, for example, the American College of Medical Toxicology (ACMT) statement of 2009:

> *Much of this concern was based on methylmercury-related neurotoxicity, the timing of vaccination during the first year of life when the blood-brain barrier is more permeable to heavy metals and a model that equated intermittent exposure to ethylmercury to cumulative dosing of methylmercury. Recent research has confirmed that the ethylmercury component found in Thimerosal is less hazardous than methylmercury. These are different compounds and should not be considered as equivalent neurotoxins.*

The only statement that is incorrect here is the claim that recent research has confirmed that the ethylmercury component, found in thimerosal, is less hazardous than methylmercury. With respect to neurotoxicity, the reverse seems likely. An important study had already shown that the alleged clearing is more likely due to prolonged sequestration of mercury in organs, including the brain

(Burbacher et al., 2005). Unfortunately, these policies ignored the Burbacher study findings. Sequestration of mercury in brain cells seems likely if any of number of key pathways to removal of mercury by brain cells is broken. The glutathione pathway is certainly one; in other patients, detoxification via endoplasmic reticulum seems to be unable to function properly, preventing proper trafficking of toxins and protein truncation. Alaei et al. (2016) traced regressive autism to a mutation in the BSCL2 gene, which encodes a protein involved in endoplasmic reticulum. Keeping mercury (and other toxins) in brain cells longer will cause deficits in the growth of apical cells because the mercury robs the cell of the energy it needs to continue to grow. The retention time of mercury in the brain is vastly underestimated. Mutter (2011) observed: "The half-life of mercury in the brain can last from several years to decades, thus mercury accumulates over time of amalgam exposure in body tissues to toxic levels."

Mercury also causes microglial cells to become overactivated (Charleston, 1994; Eskes, 2002) and in that state they overprune dendrites, leading to a cytokine storm, which keeps microglia activated—a positive feedback loop. Depending on their state, microglia secrete both proinflammatory molecules, such as tumor necrosis factor (TNF)-α, IL-1β, nitric oxide (NO), and glutamate, as well as anti-inflammatory effectors, such as IL-4 and IL-13. They also express glutathione reductase (Gutterer et al., 1999). Variation in many enzymes related to glutathione, a source of cellular defense against reactive oxygen species (ROS), is observed in the autistic brain (Gu et al., 2013).

When the mechanism of excitotoxicity and its role in autism becomes more widely appreciated, everyone will know how vaccines can induce autism in some people.

This realization undermines completely the justification for the use of thimerosal in vaccines. Moreover, such policies have moved forward, all but ignoring any literature other than the "research" developed to prove original concerns regarding vaccine safety wrong. These studies were agenda-driven from the beginning. In 2012, an IOM report found that seventeen out of twenty-two studies used by the CDC and others to justify the continued use of thimerosal were fatally flawed. Among those studies were some conducted by the CDC itself, including the now infamous DeStefano et al. (2004) study that was thrust into the limelight when Dr. William Thompson stepped forward and confirmed that significant results were omitted for idiopathic autism cases as well as for male African American cases (see Barry, 2015).

The potential harm in hiding this result is astonishing: it has led to a stagnation of comprehension of causes, risk prediction, prevention, and treatment, and not just in autism. There are two populations that appear to be at increased risk of schizophrenia: immigrants and people of African descent (Bresnahan et al.,

2007). It is reasonable to propose that the battery of vaccination updates received by immigrants may induce symptoms of schizophrenia and that schizophrenia is an additional burden of morbidity on African Americans for an unknown reason. Vitamin D deficiency may play a role. Low vitamin D levels (especially low serum 25(OH)D; Mazahery et al., 2016) appear to be associated with autism. In a preliminary study, variants in the vitamin D receptor gene have been shown to be associated with ASD (Coşkun et al., 2016).

The ACMT statement also cited Madsen et al. (2002), which was identified by Dr. William Thompson as another example of CDC abuse of statistical methodology via par-for-the-course data cooking (analysis to desired result); I looked into it very closely. Indeed, Madsen et al. (2002) inappropriately used many highly redundant covariates in their modeling as control variables instead of cofactors. Worse, studies have used multiple highly collinear variables as control variables, many of which are redundant. The removal of variance in functional-related factors, such as both gestational age and birth weight, will certainly lead to problems with the residuals for the main effect, as will their use of both age of mother and income of mother. These variables are causally linked to each other. The effect of modeling out redundant variables is to chip away at overall variance in an arbitrary manner, leaving less variation to be explained by a potentially real main effect. In data analysis rounds for another study (Verstraeten et al., 2003) with initial reports of a strong association of autism with vaccine, the eventual lead author (Thomas Verstraeten) pleaded with his colleagues to keep in the name of "objective science" in a smoking gun email titled "*It Just Won't Go Away.*" These studies have all of the signs of wanton statistical shamwizardry designed to lead the study to a predetermined conclusion by overanalysis and what people in the field of bioinformatics and biostatistics call "overfitting the model."(The "*It*" in the Verstraeten 1999 email title is the significant association of autism and vaccines after repeated rounds of analysis.)

At the time of this writing, the CDC is "investigating" the issues raised by Thompson's and Congressman William Posey's repeated calls for congressional hearings have fallen on deaf ears in the US House of Representatives.

The current push in the United States for universal vaccination is not based on scientific need when the levels of immunization required for herd immunity is not 100 percent. Instead, it is nothing more than a power play for profit—and for passing the buck of liability for safety, away from the CDC and pharmaceutical companies and onto the government. However, liability begins with the definition of the schedule, which is supposed to be based on consideration of both safety and efficacy. Adding vaccines to the schedule will ensure continued increases in adverse events, which are incompletely captured and highly unreported as it is. There is no real need for universal vaccination for every vaccine.

Avoiding combined vaccines such as measles, mumps, and rubella (MMR)—and makeup or catchup days in which five to nine vaccines are given at once—is essential to reducing vaccine neurological injuries. Miller (2016) found that mortality was increased 650 percent among individuals with serious adverse events when multiple vaccines were given at once.

Once mercury and aluminum are removed, and accurate testings exist to determine who may be at high risk of adverse events from vaccines, "ring" vaccination around clusters of infection designed to ensure sufficient immunity could be considered, as it would minimize exposure of neurotoxins to infants and children. (It is interesting to note that the obituary of the inventor of ring vaccination stated that vaccination of the entire population was considered "superfluous.") Given that genetic studies strongly point to a subset of humans who may be susceptible to the increased, not decreased, immunoneurotoxicity of adjuvants in vaccines and that autism and the ASD are a likely canary-in-the-cage syndrome, we cannot consider research in autism without taking the warning signs seriously. Any cost/benefit of analysis of utility of vaccines has to include the severity of the morbidity of the diseases versus the total costs of adverse events. The cost of autism to society is staggering, at an estimate of $2.4 million per individual when autism involves intellectual disability and $1.4 million when it does not (Autism Speaks, 2009). As individuals with autism age, their access to services becomes limited. I have been chided in discussions for being out-of-bounds for bringing up the cost of autism because I myself do not have any autistic children. That boundary is bogus—any rational discourse on priorities in public health issues must include full utility functions, all factors on the table. The maxim fails to generalize, so it's a pretentious and false moral high ground. For example, having lost my mother to breast cancer, I would never eschew anyone who has not lost loved ones to cancer from discussing the toll of cancer on society. I would thank them for their efforts to spread the word.

Shame plays a large role in the marketing of vaccines. The argument is that people who do not vaccinate are putting others at grave risk. This is based on the assumption that vaccines are perfectly safe. They are not. The "Special Masters" Vaccine Court has paid damages for vaccine injuries to families of patients who decided they would give the CDC vaccine schedule a try. Many families may have believed they were mandatory.

Vaccines are not off the hook as potential causal factors in autism. Indeed, the FDA lists "autism" as one of the potential adverse events on hepatitis B virus vaccines; the special masters in "vaccine court" have found autism and autism-like symptoms to have resulted from vaccines in at least two, and likely many more cases all but in name. Hannah Poling's family was awarded $1.5 million for vaccine-induced autism (indirect), and Bailey Banks's family was awarded more than $800,000 for vaccine-induced acute disseminated encephalomyelitis (ADEM) leading to PDD-NOS, which falls in DSM-5 on the ASD spectrum. Other awards for vaccine-induce neurological damage include Richelle Oxley (encephalopathy), Eric Lassiter (diagnosed with autism), Elias Tembenis (PDD), and Ryan Mojabi (diagnosed with autism, asthma, and encephalopathy).

There is a thorough PACE Law Review very much worth reading on this issue (Holland et al., 2011). Their examination of court records in 1,300 cases of childhood vaccine-induced brain injuries for which the Special Masters made awards revealed twenty-one cases that specifically mentioned "autism" or "autism-like symptoms." After 150 additional compensated families were contacted, sixty-two more cases led to a total of eighty-three cases of autism, thirty-nine of which involved medical confirmation of autism other than parental report.

The Poling case has been fraught with pushback on whether she actually has autism. Her neurologist, Dr. Zimmerman, gave her a diagnosis of autism. The backlash has been ferocious. Clearly, the vaccine court has ruled that vaccines cause autism—at least indirectly. In fact, the Poling case was originally supposed to be one of the five omnibus cases. After the finding, her case was removed from the omnibus set, and replaced with another case, with court records sealed.

A growing number of physicians are also willing to break with the pack and state concern regarding vaccine and neurological injury. According to the *New York Times* (February 4, 2015):

> *Dr. Jane Orient, the executive director of AAPS, which is based in Tucson, said that she believed the science behind vaccination risks was far from settled and that hundreds of parents had reported that their children had had severe deficits after an inoculation.*
>
> *"We have a lot of observations that are not otherwise explainable," said Dr. Orient, an internist. "I don't think we can dismiss it out of hand."*

The vaccine court tends to offer findings of encephalopathy as an alternative diagnosis to autism. Medically and biologically, it is not. Encephalopathy after vaccinations a recognized route to vaccine-induced autism, for example: "Documented causes of autism include genetic mutations and/or deletions, viral infections and encephalitis following vaccination" (Ratajczak, 2011). Such cases could appropriately be called "Vaccine-Induced Encephalopathy-Mediated Autism" (VIEMA).

Ratjczak's statement drew fire for ostensibly conflating cause and correlation. However, as the rest of the vast body of science shows, it is difficult to get to autism without systemic brain inflammation: any diagnosis of autism would likely also involve a mention of encephalopathy. Encephalopathy is a broad, nonspecific diagnostic category of diseases; autism is a specific endpoint diagnosis. Settlements from the court that mention encephalopathy also often mention autism or "autism-like features" as somehow "secondary"; however, making word salad out of medicine in court does not help families who hold a diagnosis of autism in their hand, nor does it help society or science.

In conducting research for this book, I interviewed a pediatrician, who requested not to be identified. He is considered "vaccine-flexible" and advocates privately to parents of autistics that they should at least space out the vaccination schedule. For this position alone, the doctor reported being "isolated, ostracized, threatened, and reprimanded" because his position cuts into profits from his practice's vaccination program.

There is excellent biological plausibility for vaccines as candidate environmental factors. For years it was thought that the ethylmercury in thimerosal was safe relative to methylmercury. That is now understood to be reversed. Many of the vaccine safety studies upon which current policies are based were flawed. Therefore, our understanding of neurotoxins in vaccine adjuvants may well be completely upside-down. Quite simply, we must forget most of what we think we know about the metabolism of ethylmercury and other adjuvants, such as aluminum. As a major work on the topic has suggested, "Let the Science Speak" (Kennedy et al., 2015). Claims of a lack of biological implausibility ignore the vast amount of basic research indicative of a direct causal initiation of neuroexitoxicity of microglial cells by both mercury and aluminum. Such claims are agenda driven and are often made by those who are alleged to have fudged key vaccine safety research studies; their claims are not at all based on the balance of available knowledge from science.

Edward R. Murrow Award–winning journalist Sharyl Atkisson reported that between October 1, 1988, and March 4, 2008, a total of 1,322 children were compensated for encephalitis/encephalopathy and seizure disorders. All of the science on autism is consistent with co-occurrence or single phenotype of encephalitis, encephalopathy, or seizures as phenotypes caused by environmental injury in individuals with specific genetic predispositions to being sensitive to the toxins.

Increases in regressive autism have been driving the increase in autism during the past two decades. This problem still demands a viable, tractable solution. Given the model the vast literature supports of a loss of neuroprotection followed by environmental trigger as a main driver of regressive autism, it is clear that vaccine adjuvants should be considered as one of many fundamental factors behind potentially millions of cases of autism.

The disclosures of Drs. William Thompson to Brian Hooker, presented in the book *Vaccine Whistleblower: Exposing Autism Research Fraud at the CDC*

(Skyhorse Publishing, 2015), are particularly damning of the scientists who conducted those studies, which includes the leadership of vaccine safety research at the CDC. Moving on with no charges filed—no resignations, no firings, and not even any censureship of the CDC by Congress—is difficult. However, science is resilient. Individuals in the rest of the scientific community have continued to move the field forward at an ever-increasing pace. Going forward with improved appreciation for the critical roles of environmental factors in autism, their interactions with proteins modified by genetics, let us not forget the original description of the experience of children with autism, who live in "extreme aloneness from the very beginning of life, not responding to anything that comes to them from the outside world" (Kanner, 1947). Vaccine safety research reform, including moving vaccine safety research out of the reach of those with a financial stake and new research toward a biomarker-informed risk screening program for vaccine safety, should be among our highest priorities.

I believe that if we move vaccine safety research into the twenty-first century and consider all of the relevant facts, not just the facts that fit one particular political or financial objective, we will find molecular biomarkers of sensitivity to thimerosal, aluminum, and other additives in vaccines. We already have hints in the involvement of gut peptides activating genes in the brain and evidence that the systems in brain cells designed to capture, neutralize, or excrete neurotoxins—when disabled by mutations, or by toxins—can make chemicals safe for most of us and yet extremely dangerous for some of us; those of us who are at most risk deserve to be protected by policies that consider the full body of scientific knowledge. Physicians, the press, scientists, and politicians have a moral obligation to get vaccines right, not just to promote universal acceptance of vaccine as a way to protect the masses from infectious diseases, but also to protect the minority of people who, through no fault of their own, happen to be unable to tolerate neurotoxins in their bloodstream as well as others. Failure to protect this minority, which may be as many as one in ten, may ultimately dictate the future for hundreds of millions of people worldwide to a future of autism, ADHD, and other conditions they otherwise may not have developed without exposure to neurotoxins in vaccines.

If mutations do confer sensitivity to certain vaccines or their components, let it be known and let the clinical workflow for vaccination adapt accordingly. Let us develop and adopt a conditional vaccination program that is concerned with safety outcomes for each and every vaccinated individual. Genetic screening for vaccine safety would be a logical imperative. This would help *define* our national vaccine safety program. Other aspects that can be improved include the use of virus-like particles, which do not require adjuvants and use single-dose vials. Any initial increased cost is worth protecting individuals at risk. Van

Herck et al. (2015) found that antibodies to hepatitis A were found long (at least 5.5 years) after vaccination with the aluminum-free virosomal hepatitis A vaccine. They estimated the protection to last approximately twenty-five years. Vaccines based on virus-like particles are also showing promise against ebolaviruses (Ohimain et al., 2016).

"JUST SAY NO" TO MORE CHERRY-PICKING RESULTS FOR PUBLIC POLICY!

The biased citation of literature is commonplace in the formulation of vaccine policy in the United States. Most of the science cited in this book is ignored by public health policy makers, and yet it represents most of the science on autism. Many of the studies cited in support of safety of the use of neurotoxins in medicine have serious methodological flaws. The practice of biased literature citation and reliance on flawed studies have also played a role in the delay of the removal of mercury amalgams from dental use in the United States, in Europe (Mutter et al., 2011) and worldwide, causing (literally) untold numbers of serious injuries and harm.

CONCLUSIONS AND CAVEATS

Given the immense number of genes found to date that may be important in autism, I have summarized themes by examples. The rest of the book provides details behind the major themes that emerged during my research. Where comprehensive reviews are available, I cite them and rely on a few clear examples. As a result of what I hope has been a comprehensive ingestion of autism research, I can offer some safe conclusions. First, there is a woefully harmful and wide disconnect between knowledge in the vast literature on potential, likely, and plausible causes of autism and public health policies. Second, other areas in medicine seems more primed for the development of individualized treatments, for those who desire them. Third, an industry of genetic screening for autism risk prior to environmental exposures may allow society to enjoy the protection of vaccines with fully informed consent. Specific genetic variants that weaken an individual's neuroprotective defenses may make some individuals much more susceptible to neurotoxic effects of adjuvants in vaccines, for example, while most of the population may tolerate such exposure better.

While it is understandable that society must avoid the development, use, and perpetuation of pejorative labels, continuity of terminology is also necessary for researchers to be able to relate current and past concepts in the study of neurological conditions. From the perspective of human development, measurements and terms reflecting delayed milestone aspects of autism are the purview of scholarly and medical research interests and are used without judgment or attributing special meaning to the value of any individual or groups of individuals. Any phrases or concepts found by anyone to be offensive are submitted without such intention. Words such as *disease* or *disorder* are reserved either for canonical use (i.e., as used in the primary and medical literatures), or for normative general discussions of genetics, without any assumption or implication that any autistic phenotypes are necessarily negative.

The literature on the biological basis of autism is immense. Genetic studies point to a heavy role for both genetics (mostly additive risk) *and* environmental factors. While I have tried to be comprehensive in terms of the scope of topics, I will certainly have overlooked important publications by colleagues. In that act, any oversight is not meant to diminish the importance nor is it a statement of the value of those contributions. Research on the impact of electromagnetic fields on voltage-gated calcium ion channels is underrepresented (see review by Pall et al., 2016).

While I have tried to be comprehensive, I cannot guarantee that I have been unbiased. I certainly set out to see if there was any evidence to support specific mechanism of ASD from vaccines. There have been some studies with negative and contradictory findings; for example, Dempsey et al. (2012) found no evidence of increases in internalizing and externalizing behaviors in typically developing siblings of autistics. Autism is complex, and the positive evidence for a genetic risk is compelling. I have tried to take the time to imbue the message that genes are not fate, that a molecular basis of disease is not grounds for recategorization, and that variations that we may call "autism risk variants" are present in individuals with no sign of ASD. These truths bear repeating and keeping in mind, but then variation in results from similar studies is nothing new to science.

The scientific literature is filled with references to "brain damage," "disabilities," and other terms at which many loud voices in the autism community take umbrage. Where I have failed to find the least offensive terminology, as in the normative use found in the context of these comprehensive citations, I humbly apologize. I hope it does not distract from the massive amount of research in autism that I have reviewed. My research included consideration of more than three thousand peer-reviewed studies and reviews. Since 2006, there have been at least seventy major studies on copy number variants in ASD alone. Where I have missed relevant and important citations, I also sincerely apologize.

Vaccines represent one of the most significant man-made alterations in a child's immunological and chemical environments. I ask my colleagues to consider, as they read this book, that chronic perinatal inflammation has serious negative effects on neurodevelopment in the brain (Chhor et al., 2012). The most common nonserious side effect of vaccines is fever. Knowing that fever is evidence of immune system activation and that both adaptive and innate routes exist to chronic microglial activation, I ask them to please consider: are we giving our children ASD to protect ourselves from contagious diseases? ASD? Asperger's? CDD? Rett syndrome? PDD-NOS? Schizophrenia? Alzheimer's? How many vaccines do we honestly believe our children can tolerate?

The corporations that hold high government influence have decided that the environment in which we try to raise our children should be filled with neurotoxins that are more toxic to some of us than to others. The more toxins they put in the environment, the more our population will respond by getting sick. The high genetic heterogeneity of autism is a mirror reflection of the heterogeneity of the toxins in our environment. Those with autism and ASD and other conditions are truly the canaries in the coal mine. We owe them and their families a debt of eternal gratitude that can never be repaid, for serving as the unwitting early warning system on the toxification of our air, food, water, and medicines.

The most important question is: since they have paid the cost so far, what are we going to do about it?

This will not be the first time we in the scientific community are called upon in history to risk asking impolitic questions to generate knowledge, to increase understanding, and to reduce human pain and suffering. I ask my colleagues in science, in medicine, and in industry to see the handwriting on the wall and to step forward against the campaign to shame and dishonor those who would seek that truth. You know who you are. You have met these ideas on your own. You simply dare not say them in public. You could lose your funding. Your job. Well, my friends, they cannot fire all of us. I say that we demand that the National Institutes of Health take control of vaccine safety research as an extramural program, I say we demand that they get aluminum out of vaccines, I say we tell industry to keep their glyphosate and other chemicals that make us sick. As Dr. Gary Null said, "I'd rather have a worm in my apple than to see another child suffer." I say we reform medical research with a high priority to detoxify ourselves and reduce the rates of Parkinson's, ADHD, ASD, Alzheimer's, schizophrenia, and cancer.

References : see envgencauses.com

Chapter 2.

SYMPTOMS AND DIAGNOSIS OF AUTISM

Our understanding of autism as a medical condition has been evolving since it was first described by Dr. Leo Kanner in the middle of the twentieth century. Early descriptions of autism often invoked a sense of a cohesive condition, characterized by late speech development; restricted, repetitive verbal and nonverbal communication; low social reciprocity (limited give-and-take interactions); stereotypical behaviors, including repetitive movement, unfocused gaze, lack of eye contact, hand flapping and tics, and echolalia (repetition of words); impaired language-processing abilities; pedantry; impacted cognitive ability (executive function limitations, 75 percent of AD patients); seizures (25 percent); and sensitivity to lights and sounds in the environment. Repetitive behaviors appear to break down further into *repetitive sensory motor* and *insistence on sameness* behaviors (Bishop et al., 2013). Other traits include concrete (literal) thinking, a lack of pretense, and an apparent lack of immediate humor. Other studies have confirmed the independence of insistence on sameness and repetitive sensory motor—e.g., Cannon et al., 2010, who also confirmed previous findings that repetitive sensory motor behaviors is more related to severity of autistic disorder (AD) than insistence on sameness behaviors. Loss of language and hand flapping in severe autism is identical to that from Minimata disease, which results from intense mercury poisoning.

For *natal autism*, less well-known symptoms include large body size at birth (macrosomy), transitional macrocephaly (large head size), permeability of the intestine and persistent inflammation of the intestinal tract (nonspecific enterocolitis), renal peptiduria and immune dysfunction (low adaptive immunity as measured by immunoglobulin levels), altered cytokine profiles (Li et al., 2009; Molloy et al., 2006), and altered T-cell activation (Ashwood et al., 2010). In addition to stereotypical behaviors, aggression has been observed and shown to be independent of intelligence quotient (IQ) and speech development. In a study of 1,380 children and adolescents with autism, aggression was found to be independent of severity of ASD symptoms but associated with repetitive behaviors (Kanne et al., 2011). Such behaviors may also be due to the whole-system response to the stresses of limited normative social interactions, self-image, and frustrations with executive limitations in problem solving. Medications such as beta blockers are known to help, but some medications cause aggression in autistics.

Parents may notice early in their children's development a few indicators that might suggest autism. These include:

- Marked reduction in eye contact.
- Delayed walking (on average, 1.6 months later than non-ASD peers; Shetreat-Klein et al., 2014).
- Not responding to their name.
- Not engaging in pretend play.
- Not pointing or waving.

Early childhood screening is important because ASD therapy is thought to be more effective at an early age.

The distribution of all of the above symptoms varies widely among patients and over time. When it occurs, macrocephaly (circumference > 97 percenttile) tends to be noticeable by mid-infancy, likely reflecting neurite overgrowth, excess glial cell formation, and inflammation. Head size typically returns to average in adolescence due to convergence of rates with non-ASD peers. Each of the individual symptoms seems to provide clues to the etiologies of autism, but the picture has been far from clear.

Specific genes and pathways have been identified that may contribute to these phenotypes. At least four studies found that individuals with macrocephaly tend to have a familial (inherited) PTEN mutation, which in one report was coincident with early age-of-onset cancer (McBridge et al., 2010). Loss-of-function mutations in PTEN suppress AKT signaling, the ability to regulate both cell body size and the length and density of dendritic spins in primary neurons (Spinelli et al., 2015). The mutations associated with macrocephaly appear to be distinct from those associated with cancer. Macrocephaly, however, is not evidence of PTEN mutation, and observance of PTEN mutation and macrocephaly does not rule out the involvement of other factors. Variations in the gene HEPACAM have also been associated with macrocephaly (Lopez-Hernandez et al., 2011).

Signs of inflammation and unusual immune system characteristics abound in autistics and, importantly, some also indicate Rett syndrome. For example, microglial activation without adaptive immunity-related neuroinflammation is seen in Rett syndrome—evidently activated by both genetic (mutational) and epigenetic (environmental) factors (Maezawa et al., 2011).

Neurological activity may be disrupted locally, at the connections (synapses) between brain cells within specific regions (intraregional connectivity), as can the formation of connections among brain areas (hyper- or hypoconnectivity). These two types of changes appear to be accompanied by a lack of specialization in regional brain function and aberrant synchronization of brain region activities. A variety of malfunctions have been observed.

Early ideas on causal factors, including those from Kanner and Bettelheim, attributed the lack of social reciprocity to emotionally distant, unattached "refrigerator" mothers. Removing blame from consideration, this unsavory characterization itself hints at a genetic correlation of social traits. For years, the public's understanding of autism was colored heavily by Dustin Hoffman's depiction of an autistic man in the movie *Rain Man.* It has long been recognized by clinicians that not every aspect of autism needed to be present for a diagnosis of autism. It also has been recognized that different characteristics may appear in individuals at varying degrees of severity and that autism can even exist in persons with some characteristics intensely *reversed* from pathologies (e.g., high IQ).

AUTISM: WHAT'S IN A NAME?

The diagnosis of autism and similar conditions has an unusual history in disease classification. Classical autism is usually noted by three years of age. Under the current *Diagnostic and Statistical Manual of Mental Disorders, Fifth Edition* (DSM-5), it is at the extreme range of a group of heterogeneous conditions known as autism spectrum disorder. Autism spectrum disorder also includes *Asperger syndrome* and *pervasive developmental disorder not otherwise specified* (PDD-NOS).

During the decade between 1991 and 2001, autism in US schools increased by an astonishing 1,700 percent (Yazbak et al., 2003). The prevalence of autism has increased dramatically in incidence from 1 in 2,500 in 1970 to 1 in 45 in 2015. Nevison (2014) studied the factors that might contribute to the increase, including chemicals—pesticides, flame retardants, and total adjuvants (immune-system stimulating compound vaccines—and concluded that changes in diagnosis was not sufficient to explain the exponential increase. She attributed 75 to 80 percent of the increase in autism since 1988 to an actual increase in the disorder, rather than to changing diagnostic criteria. Another study reached very similar conclusions, attributing approximately 25 percent of the increase in California to diagnostic artifacts (King and Bearman, 2009).

Certainly, genetics cannot change in less than one generation.

From a medical perspective, studying autism has become more complicated by including conditions that may reflect less extreme cases, or even completely different conditions than than those described originally by Kanner (1943). Asperger syndrome (AS), first described by Asperger in 1944, includes some, but not all characteristics of autism (mostly lack of intellectual disability). It is possible that AS left low intelligence out of his consideration to save children from the Nazi death hospitals. Autism and AS now fall under the ASD umbrella, with AS being considered by many to be a mild, or high-functioning form of autism. Others have referred to individuals with autism who show high cognitive abilities and adequate social perception as high-functioning autistics.

Certain classically recognized molecular syndromes have a high rate of autism. These syndromes include those with chromosomal alterations (e.g., Trisomy 21), microdeletion and microduplications (e.g. 22q11.2 deletion syndrome [22q11.2DS]), and monogenic (e.g., Fragile X syndrome and tuberous sclerosis). The high rate of ASD within the 22q11.2 deletion syndrome (14 to 25 percent) has resulted in a call for screening (Wenger et al., 2016), but calls for reduction of exposure to environmental toxins to this at-risk group via a reduction in vaccination are not yet acceptable. Sadly, inadequate response to vaccines is one of the characteristics of this syndrome; each revaccination to induce titers introduces an additional dose of vaccine adjuvants, including the neuro- and immunotoxic aluminum. Studies of the roles of environmental toxins, including the role of vaccines, in autism in molecular syndromes that show high rates are warranted. This includes Prader-Willi syndrome, wherein individuals with paternal interstitial duplications at 15q11.2-q13.3 have high rates of ASD (Isles et al., 2016). The question of indiscriminant use of vaccines must be readdressed overall, since past studies tended to focus on the general population.

Formal diagnosis of ASD under DSM-5 is made by observation of behaviors indicating clinically significant impairment in social, occupational, or other important areas of current functioning due to persistent deficits in, for example, social-emotional reciprocity or nonverbal communication, and absence of interest in peers, or inability to adjust in socially varying situations often accompanied by restricted or repetitive behaviors, interests, or activities. The patient may insist on sameness and adherence to routines and may show extreme distress at small changes or during transitions. The restricted interests may lead to obsessive-like fixation on objects, situations, or scenarios. The patient may also exhibit sensitivity to certain auditory input, sensitivity to light, or fascination with lights and movement. Important for this book, DSM-5 suggests these symptoms should appear in early childhood, but as many parents know, they do not always exist prior to environmental injury.

Classically, autism was divided into primary and secondary autism, with primary being evident at or near birth (natal/perinatal) and secondary occurring after some language development. In the DSM-5, autism is cast as a spectrum, including AD and childhood disintegrative disorder (CDD), which is subdivided into regressive autism and Rett syndrome. Given that the age of onset is an important consideration in the type of autism, both clinicians and researchers have continued to use the term *regressive autism* or *late-onset autism* to refer to cases in which losses of advanced cognitive functioning is obvious.

Other types of autism within ASD now include PPD-NOS and Asperger syndrome, which many consider a form of AD without intellectual disability. Diagnosis considers severity (need for services) and, unlike DSM-IV, perceptual processing (aka sensory aberrations), which is included as a key symptom (Table 1).

TABLE 1. CORE SYMPTOM CATEGORIES OF ASD

Core Symptoms	Key Symptoms	Frequently Observed Conditions
Language delay	Stereotyped behaviors, Hyperactivity	Inattention, obsessions
Lack of social/ emotional reciprocity	Insistence on sameness	Compulsions, picky eating
Lack of nonverbal communication	Insistence on sameness	Intellectual disabilities
Lack of developing/ maintaining	Sensory variance	Relationships

Given the epidemiological trends involved in increasing prevalence, a clear demarcation should be retained between autism that is evident at birth (infantile or natal autism) and autism that clearly appears later in childhood. The mean age of regression in RA is 19 months. Early screening is needed to distinguish cases of RA (no early sign) from AD.

Natal autism refers to autism that is evident in the first months of life. The DSM-5 criterion that language delay must be present at birth is hard to realize and is not empirically supported. The vast majority of cases of autism/ASD are diagnosed after the age of three years (e.g., Brett et al., 2016). The use of—and focus on—the term *congenital autism* should be eschewed because the concept lends itself (erroneously) to a determined fate. Any inquiry into causes of autism must not be limited by a particular diagnostic classification scheme, especially given that we will learn much more about interactions between environmental factors and genes as time progresses. We already better appreciate environmental exposures in the womb and their mechanisms. Numerous environmental factors during gestation, and during and shortly after birth, have been shown to contribute to autism, including valproate, thalidomide, maternal nutrition, infection and fever during pregnancy, use of antibiotics during pregnancy, and congenital rubella syndrome (secondary to rubella infection). The last three may be correlative to the onset of maternal immune activation against fetal brain proteins (maternal adaptive immunity), whereas the primary mechanism for toxins such as valproate, thalidomide, mercury, and aluminum is the onset of chronic microglial activation (CMA). Gestational and perinatal complications have also been noted (Glasson et al., 2004), but many of these may be intermediate outcomes of toxic exposures as opposed to risk indicators.

Perinatal conditions and risk factors associated with natal autism include obstetric conditions such as low birth weight and abnormal gestation length (preterm delivery; Kolevzon, 2007). Birth asphyxia (hypoxic-ischemic insult) is a likely cause. Concern regarding cesarean section mode of delivery as a causal factor in autism motivated a study in which the risk of autism was studied for various modes of birth. In an initial analysis comparing emergency cesarean section to vaginal birth and elective cesarean section (Curran et al., 2015), cesarean section is associated with increased risk of autism. However, when using sibling controls, the increased risk was not found. This suggests familial and/or genetic influences instead of emergency cesarean section. Although the study confirmed that children born via cesarean section are 20 percent more likely to be diagnosed with autism, the study ruled out mode of delivery as an environmental cause. Indeed, it makes sense: macrocephaly is found in approximately 20 percent of children with autism, and that condition is likely to lead to a need for emergency cesarean section. Ultrasound has been suspected, and animal studies have indicated that concerns regarding lack of regulation of its use may lead to neurological injuries associated with autism. A randomized trial did not find any difference between regular and intense use of ultrasound on rates of diagnosis of autism in humans (Stoch et al., 2012); however, rates of autism between cases in which no ultrasound was used versus those in which ultrasound was used were not reported. Parental occupational chemical exposures have also been associated with ASD (McCanlies et al., 2012), with suspicion of de novo mutagenic effects (Pino-López et al., 2013).

There has always been a fairly clear delineation between congenital autism at birth (natal autism) and secondary, or regressive, autism. The natal form may be environmentally induced, a product of genetics, or due to a combination of both factors. For parents who witness their children regress post-vaccination, the concept that the condition may be entirely genetic is a nonstarter. They have excellent reasons for their causal inference. Pediatricians have seen hundreds of cases themselves now where a parent points to vaccines as the cause. Much of the increase in autism is of the secondary, or late-onset regressive type.

Parents would do well, however, to also consider the hypothesis, that, for their child, a genetic risk of susceptibility to environmental toxins, including those in vaccines, may have also played a role in the occurrence of regressive autism in their child. However, if a genetic mutation or change in gene methylation status in genes confers risk, that finding does not exonerate environmental causal factors. Genetic factors are rarely primary causal factors, and the observation of mutation in an autism risk gene is not a sufficient level of evidence for that mutation to be considered a clinical mutation. Even if variants are found with sufficient levels of evidence (those in multiple families, for instance), their contribution cannot be assumed to be total, unless the variant is observed to cause autism in unvaccinated children as well.

The strictures of medical genetics set a high standard for a mutation to be considered clinical. But there is much more than that at stake here. On this issue, as well as that of natal autism, there is a basic human-rights issue at stake. All children should be free to be born with genetic variation (inherited or de novo) and be safe from harm from toxins that can cause autism. Moreover, when society imposes those toxins on that child, we are collectively responsible for the harm that would not have occurred, were it not for the exposure.

These risks are not engrained, however, because we can modulate the environment. The good news is that the search for possible genetic risk factors in a child is not likely to be as challenging as the unfortunately unrealistically high level of evidence required to conclude a vaccine injury. Confirmation of the risk should involve separate biochemical tests that confirm abrogation of the phenotype the mutation may impact. However, there is no a priori logic or scheme in the science of medical genetics, from its foundation, to reject environmental factors as an important cause of a disease phenotype simply because one identifies a mutation. "Either/or" argumentation simply does not apply, especially in any collection of phenotypes as complex and plastic as those in brain function. Certainly, there may be instances of strongly dominant locus patterns of inheritance that are largely independent of exposure; however, the heterogeneity model that the genetic data supports, and the absence of autism in the parents, dramatically lowers the acceptability of a hypothesis that inherited mutations, and only mutations, caused autism in a child. Combined with the two largest heritability studies, which attribute at the population level approximately 50 percent liability to environment and approximately 50 percent to genetics, the evidence is clear enough. De novo mutations can add to the likelihood of autism, but they, too, even in the presence of inherited variation in autism risk genes, do not completely exonerate environmental causes; in fact, environmental factors can increase the incidence of de novo copy number variation (CNV), which are submicroscopic chromosomal deletions and duplications of stretches of DNA in the human genome.

In specific cases, regressive autism may be caused by combinations of genetic and epigenetic risk factors and preventable causes (environmental toxins, including those in vaccines). With exposure to environmental causes beginning at least in the womb, some of the epigenetic changes can result from environmental exposure, whereas others are determined by mutations in genes that control methylation programming. With most mutations, one cannot know that a child would have regressed from the mere existence of one, two, or even three variations. There are exceptions: with some rare individual mutations, expressivity (how strong or severe a trait presents in a given individual) is very high (and would be matched by high penetrance). The same is true with some combinations of two or three mutations in genomic or mitochondrial genes. However, the frequency of multiple hits, by their nature, is expected to be an inverse function to their number, assuming they are independent events. As independent, rare events, the probability of their co-occurrence is a product of their low probabilities. This is precisely what has been found. Pinto et al. (2014) found an excess in every count category of number of genes hit by both copy number deletion and insertions in ASD in brain-expressed genes—and the larger the number of genes hit, the larger the risk of autism (measured by predicted odds ratio by Pinto et al., 2014; Figure 4). Combined genetic and environmental susceptibility explains variation in the age of onset of autism. The exact direct risk or susceptibility conferred by individual mutations is determined by how they impact the biology of the individual.

WHERE IS REGRESSIVE AUTISM WITHIN AUTISM SPECTRUM DISORDER?

Autism in childhood that occurs after otherwise normal development for at least two years has historically been called regressive autism (RA). DSM-5 combines

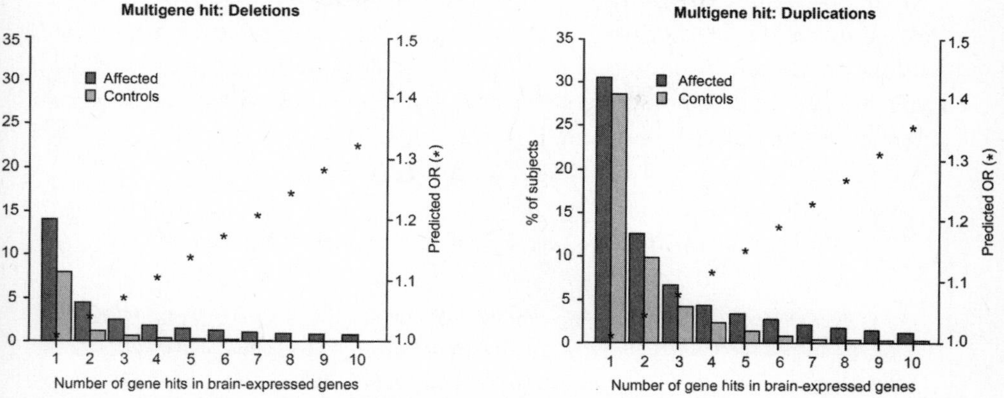

Figure 4. Overrepresentation of CNV hits in ASD affected vs. neurotypical controls is related to the risk of ASD diagnosis (predicted odds ratio, OR) for both CNV deletions and duplications. Data from Pinto et al. (2014). Copyright © Pinto et al., 2014, used with permission.

all types of autism, including natal autism, regressive autism, CDD, PPD-NOS, under ASD. In the past, some cases of regressive autism were considered to fall erroneously into CDD (Kurita et al., 2004) and some to Rett syndrome. Rett syndrome is characterized by normal early growth and development, followed by a period of slowed development, loss of intellectual ability, and loss of fine and gross motor skills (especially the hands). Differential diagnosis of RA and Rett syndrome includes the presence, in some cases of autism, of developmental abnormalities prior to regression (Kurita, 2011). The regression in autism is typically less severe than in Rett syndrome. Not all criteria need apply for a diagnosis of ASD and *previous developmental abnormalities* is not clinically measurable and thus not a diagnostic criterion. Development is complex, and although RA may be a form of autism reflecting genetics, or toxins, in other instances RA may appear suddenly, due to acute exposure. Because not all criteria for ASD are required for ASD diagnosis, DSM-5 thus allows the capture of late-onset regression.

Differential diagnosis between RA and Rett syndrome is also not clear-cut. Rett syndrome is supposed to be indicated by the presence of a specific chromosomal rearrangement and/or loss of methyl cytosine binding protein (MeCP2). However, false diagnosis of Rett syndrome without a genetic test could cause a missed case of regressive autism. Keeping in mind that the absence of MeCP2 in Rett syndrome causes a dearth of dendritic spines, and that aberrant pruning of dendritic spines by microglial activation is a core cause of autism, the molecular basis of Rett syndrome is very similar to that of ASD. Epigenetic aberrations involving MeCP2 are important in non-Rett ASD (Loke et al., 2015).

In the case of Rett syndrome versus ASD via MeCP2 mutation, the distinction of molecular mechanism—mutation versus epigenetics—confuses cause and manifestation. Amputation of a limb is still amputation regardless of the type of blade used; although the severity may differ and one form may require more extensive medical treatment, it is still "amputation."

Consider the view of Pelphry and Westphal (2012):

> *. . . we believe that childhood disintegrative disorder represents a process sufficient to cause autism, but that it is different from the mechanism that leads to autism in children without regression. As such, it is an important example of the heterogeneity of the autism spectrum. Doing away with a separate diagnosis of childhood disintegrative disorder would hinder research efforts into better understanding autism . . . we believe that the late-onset, well-defined regression found in childhood disintegrative disorder is an example of a well-differentiated phenomenon. Any muddiness about the diagnosis is related to the diagnostic tools rather than the disorder itself. . . .*

The writers point out that CDD is usually accompanied by regression in multiple domains of experience, whereas regressive autism is usually restricted to a step backwards primarily in language ability. However, the medical literature reports many cases of regressive autism in which multiple domains of experience are hit. Because one cannot presume to know which underlying connections and biological pathways are disrupted, and perhaps more important why they exist, the utility of the clinical differential diagnosis of regressive autism and CDD is unclear. It is therefore more useful to consider RA and Rett syndrome as subtypes of CDD.

The ability to focus on regressive autism is of great importance, not only to the medical community, but also to the research community studying cause and etiology. Legal ramifications exist as well, for access to services and for assessment of liability. A major concern for research into genetic and environmental causes of autism is the possible administrative removal of regressive autism to CDD, or outside of the spectrum. This is an important concern for many patients who look for environmental liability, although DSM-5 allows that the increase in severity of symptoms may occur at a later developmental age.

As with AD, both types of CDD also involve deficits in communication, including receptive language skills (language understanding) and expressive language skills (spoken language) and social or self-help skills and motor skills, such as repetitious activities and issues moving from one activity to the next. Epilepsy frequently co-occurs with both CDD and autism. Treatment of CDD and ASD are very similar, and CDD most resembles severe ASD in prognosis. Either way, CDD, which was reported in 2003 to occur in as few as 1.7 cases per 100,000, is listed in the DSM as part of ASD, which also includes regressive autism.

Childhood distinctive disorder was originally described by Heller, who noted that it occurred with an early sign or "prodromal" state (Westphal et al., 2012), in which children experienced night terrors, extreme agitations, tics, and other symptoms that many parents of children with regressive autism will recognize. Many parents describe head-banging, dragging the forehead across the floor and screaming fits, and regression after vaccination, as reported by a growing number of pediatricians. Although a single observation may be coincidental, when hundreds of thousands of people observe the same events after vaccination, their aggregate reports can hardly be called "anecdotal."

The erection of new clinical-level diagnostic classes can obfuscate or clarify the quest to understand disease etiology. This is true for any pair of clinical or subclinical "domains," which is why clinical researchers would do well to move toward the study of individual phenotypes in a manner that may appear independent of a specific diagnosis. Diagnoses of ASD and differential diagnosis within ASD are currently made on the basis of behavior (symptomology), not etiologies. These diagnoses will almost certainly change as more research continues to elucidate the genetic and environmental causes of ASD. *How* the field progresses with respect to the definition of clinical groups is important. Trying to place various subtypes of autism into neat categorical boxes had been compared to trying to "cleave meatloaf at the joints" (APA), leading to refinements in diagnosis in DSM-5.

A more in-depth study in 2013 (Kurita and Inoue, 2013) examined 19 variables, compared children with early-onset (younger than age 3) CDD and autistic disorder with speech loss (ADSL), and found very few differences between ADSL and CDD. The CDD group exhibited higher rates of noncore features such as psychosocial events before speech loss (SL), more fearfulness during speech loss, and a higher rate of epilepsy. The CDD group scored lower on a few technical autism measures on the first visit, but the researchers found no significant difference in the other 19 variables. The authors concluded that their results supported integrating CDD into autism spectrum disorder and called for further studying of CDD within that classification.

Barger et al. studied more than 30,000 people with ASD and found a loss of previously acquired skills in as many as 33 percent of all cases. Regression at age two or three years is traumatic to the individual and to family members. We cannot afford to play semantic games and to hide RA administratively.

Individuals with mutations in SHANK3 are described as having Rett syndrome–like phenotypes (Hara et al., 2015) and Heller syndrome-like regression (Philippe et al., 2015). Pediatricians would do well to look at symptoms as targets of treatment, consider genome scans, and confirm the gene/phenotype link with biochemical tests.

OVERALL CHANGES FROM DSM-IV TO DSM-5 IMPACT DEFINITION OF CLINICAL POPULATIONS

The largest change from DSM-IV to DSM-5 is the inclusion of four different clinical conditions into ASD. These include autism, Asperger syndrome, CDD, and PDD-NOS. These conditions differ from each other in degree of severity of symptoms in two core domains.

In DSM-5, three domains of ASD were recognized; in DSM, two have been combined, and thus DSM-5 identifies two domains, as shown in Table 2.

TABLE 2. DOMAINS OF AUTISM SPECTRUM DISORDER

DSM-IV	DSM-5
Social domain	Social/Communication domain
Communication domain	Restrictive, repetitive behaviors
Restrictive, repetitive behaviors	

Diagnosis of autism/ASD under DSM requires satisfaction of criteria A–D (from Kaufmann, WE. DSM-5: The New Diagnostic Criteria for Autism Spectrum Disorders. 2012 Symposium):

A. Persistent deficits in social communication and social interaction across contexts, not accounted for by general developmental delays and manifest by all three of the following:
   1. Deficits in social-emotional reciprocity
   2. Deficits in nonverbal communicative behaviors used for social interaction
   3. Deficits in developing and maintaining relationships

B. Restricted, repetitive patterns of behavior, interests, or activities as manifested by at least two of the following:
   1. Stereotyped or repetitive speech, motor movements, or use of objects.
   2. Excessive adherence to routines, ritualized patterns of verbal or nonverbal behavior, or excessive resistance to change.
   3. Highly restricted, fixated interests that are abnormal in intensity or focus.

4. Hyper- or hyporeactivity to sensory input or unusual interest in sensory aspects of environment.

C. Symptoms must be present in early childhood* but may not become fully manifest until social demands exceed limited capacities.
D. Symptoms together limit and impair everyday functioning.

*This condition is contradicted elsewhere within DSM-5.

Under DSM-5, if no restrictive, repetitive behaviors are present, social communication disorder may be diagnosed.

A major assumption was made in DSM-5 with a merger of social and communication phenotypes: that the bulk of a lack of social reciprocity is due to deficits in communication skills and not to a domain (of its own). Thus, the loss of speech is technically nudged toward CDD. Because the loss of speech after age two is no longer included as a core indicator of autism, some of those cases may end up diagnosed as social communication disorder. I asked a pediatrician, Dr. Anthony Kovatch, how he would diagnose a three-year-old who suddenly developed all core signs of autism. He said, "I would code that simply 'autism spectrum disorder' (F84.0)."

I asked Dr. Kovatch about two other cases:

- Three-year-old child, loss of speech, loss of social reciprocity, no restricted/repetitive behaviors.
- Three-year-old child, loss of speech, restricted/repetitive behaviors, social reciprocity intact.

He said: "Without further information, these cases would be PPD-NOS, which, under DSM-5, is a form of autism."

We will see that the overall core domains are only a start for understanding autism and that subgroups may exist within each domain. A focus on phenotype classes will help.

RETT SYNDROME, AUTISM, AND MOLECULAR SYNDROMICS

Rett syndrome is one of the conditions with symptoms that strongly overlap those with other forms of autism. Importantly, both can involve regression. It is little known that regressive autism is the type of autism most responsible for the rise in autism between the 1980s and the present. From 2000 to 2010, there was a

78 percent increase from RA in whites and 180 percent increase in RA in African Americans (Shenouda et al., 2015).

Some references report that Rett syndrome patients tend to be highly social (*Handbook of Autism and Pervasive Developmental Disorders, Fourth Edition*); others report that they tend to show autistic social characteristics (Nestler & McGinley, *Neurobiology of Mental Illness*). Another reports that social capabilities normalize at school age (Van Acker et al., 2005; *Handbook of Autism and Pervasive Developmental Disorders*). In Rett syndrome, head growth is initially normal (Van Acker et al., 2005), but then *slows* (as opposed to early rapid head growth seen in autism, followed by normalization). Clinical outcomes are more fixed (and worse) in Rett syndrome than in autism. Chronic microglial activation, typical of AD, may be absent in Rett syndrome. This is an important differential diagnosis marker and an important finding indicative of separate etiologies for Rett and other forms of ASD.

The attempted (but failed) rationale for removing Rett syndrome from ASD is that its molecular etiology is "known" and in many cases patients exhibit mutations in or differential methylation of the gene MeCP2. However, not all individuals diagnosed with Rett syndrome have MeCP2 mutations, and MeCP2 mutations play roles in ASD phenotypes.

Adding to the confusion, numerous genes other than MeCP2 have been thought to be a key diagnostic indicator of Rett syndrome, but many of those genes are important in autism as well. Rett syndrome shares a number of immunological signatures with ASD. Although Rett syndrome does not capture all of the phenotypes of autism, few causes of autism/ASD do. Millions of parents have witnessed their children regress quickly (hours or overnight) after suspected environmental exposures, and as the science cited in this book shows, the biological basis for a central role of environmental exposures is profoundly strong.

If Rett syndrome had been followed as a precedent for the fate of disease reclassification in development neurological disorder in and near the ASD, it would seem that any disease for which a molecular etiology is understood would lead to a reclassification outside of the broader category. As such a reclassification will clearly not happen, understanding which genes and proteins are involved in a specific case of breast cancer does not disqualify the disease as cancer, for example.

The role of environmental factors for Rett syndrome also cannot be ruled out. Fiumara et al. (2002) reported a case study in which a two-month-old girl developed "an acute encephalopathy with destructive brain damage twelve hours after acellular pertussis vaccination." They also reported: "Peripheral lymphocyte subset analysis revealed the existence of T lymphocytes double positive for CD4 and CD8 markers. This pattern normalized over the following 3 months.

Months later, the girl manifested a Rett syndrome phenotype. DNA screening of the MeCP2 gene was unrevealing in the child and her parents."

Landau-Kleffner syndrome, also known as acquired epileptic aphasia, is characterized by progressive receptive loss of speaking, accompanied by loss of vocabulary typically between ages four and seven years (Mantovani, 2000). EEG shifts occur that are helpful in diagnosis. Differential diagnosis from autism can be made difficult, as patients may exhibit avoidance of interpersonal contact, hyperactivity, and anger. Whereas patients with CDD exhibit autism symptoms, Landau-Kleffner patients retain nonverbal intelligence (Mantovani, 2000).

Due to an explosion of research in autism, powered in part by society's concern regarding the rapid increase in the rate of autism, we now understand that autism is clinically heterogeneous: partly neurological, partly gastrointestinal, and sometimes stemming from immunological conditions. Any of these origins or conditions can manifest at birth (infantile, a.k.a. natal, or congenital autism), or after a few years of essentially normal brain development (regressive autism). People with an autistic condition may exhibit all, some, or at times none of the stereotypical outward appearances that would cause one to recognize autism. Moreover, the degree (severity) and number of symptoms may increase or decrease over time. ASD is now generally considered to be a heterogeneous, overlapping group of neurological disorders with some inherited risk, caused primarily by myriad environmental factors. Significant steps in comprehension of causes are being made by advances in genetics studies. These advances have been made possible in part by a nondiagnostic category called *broader autism phenotype* (Piven et al., 1997), a concept extended beyond the diagnosis erected specifically to encompass parents of children in simplex autism families (families with an individual case of autism) who show autistic tendencies. The ASD phenotypes and impairments are found in 12.4 percent of siblings of ASD patients and in 10 to 45 percent of parents of children with ASD (Bailey et al., 1995; Freitag et al., 2007; Gottesman et al., 1996).

However, reclassification of conditions "outside" of ASD (e.g., Rett syndrome) is not universally accepted. This is important because, as we will see, defining a clinical population is important for establishing rigorous and meaningful study designs aimed at understanding the causes of autism. Rett syndrome also typically involves regression earlier (6 to 18 months) as opposed to regression later than age two years. Regression in Rett syndrome typically involves more severe regression, occurs mostly in females, and involves stereotypical behavior, including hand wringing. However, it shares core components of autism.

Asperger syndrome is similarly positioned and is now widely recognized to be on the ASD. A distinguishing feature of Asperger syndrome is the retention of verbal abilities, with reduced capacity for social interactions and weak motor skills. As originally described, AS patients also exhibit highly focused (circumscribed) interests, to the exclusion of focus on other areas, sometimes to the point of hindering learning. Some consider AS to be a form of high-functioning autism; it, too, is firmly planted on the autism spectrum.

Within ASD, PDD-NOS is a DSM-5 category in which individuals show relatively mild or an incomplete set of autistic symptoms and an absence of severe regression (Towbin, 2005). Such a catch-all category can be considered slight autism but not a tendency toward autism, because patients deserve a definitive diagnosis for proper care and access to services.

Future ASD research will likely include expansion of the spectrum. Addressing autism where it manifests is medically required to discern specificity of treatment when possible. A large study of patients with 16p11.2 deletions (Hanson et al., 2015) found that those who did not meet diagnostic criteria for ASD had a significantly higher prevalence of autism-related characteristics compared with a familial noncarrier control group. This indicates a continuum between ASD with 16p11.2 duplications and 16p11.2 deletions. Wider variation in expressivity of autistic traits is seen within people with 16p11.2 duplications than deletion, ranging from no symptoms to significant disability. Symptoms within patients with duplications include intellectual disability, motor delays, and attention deficit hyperactivity disorder (ADHD) in children and anxiety in adults, with ASD found in nearly 20 percent of child cases (Green-Snyder et al., 2016). Most duplication carriers showed no sign of social dysfunction. Hippolyte et al. (2016) found that CNVs at 16p11.2 influence specific cognitive traits, including language, verbal memory, and inhibition. The practical clinical significance of autism discovered in other syndromes is identification of specific phenotypic domains for the sake of routes to therapy and treatments.

MISDIAGNOSIS OF AUTISM AND AUTISM SPECTRUM DISORDER

Given the large number of autism symptoms and the semicompartmentalization of the molecular manifestation of disease phenotypes within ASD, misdiagnosis of autism seems likely. Some diagnoses are likely made to enable access to services. However, throughout this book, the complex overlay of autism and its heterogeneity reflect a better appreciation of the broad autism phenotype (Gerdts et al., 2013) in which subclinical autism-like traits may be evident in siblings without a full diagnosis of ASD. While early signs of developmental delay may or may not be evident prior to late-onset RA, and while we are born with our genetics, lifetime risk of disease due to environmental exposure of toxins is cumulative.

Deep and wide considerations of the published findings of gene associations and overlap among somewhat distinct clinical populations of autistics (e.g., family level, ethnic groups) are therefore needed to weigh the effects of every decision to erect or deconstruct any disease classification in autism, and the processes should be overt and open, science based, and not policy driven. The broad autism phenotype concept, with studies of autism phenotypes instead of hard-and-fast clinical categories, will likely prove most fruitful in aiding comprehension.

BIRTH ORDER AND GENDER BIAS

Older fathers with mothers older than thirty-five years of age have a larger number of de novo mutations, as well as change in methylation patterns in their sperm (Feinberg et al., 2015). The two-hit hypothesis could well explain part of the birth order risk and the risk due to having an older parent.

The aging parent theory may well also explain some of the gender bias. Male-to-male transmission does occur, suggesting X-linked inheritance, but it may not be as important as once thought. Many of the autism-related genes on the X chromosome are regulatory genes and control genes on other chromosomes. The effect of having a Y chromosome includes automated heterozygosity for some key loci.

Numerous reasons have been postulated for the existence of the four-to-one gender bias, including increased risk from testosterone and decreased risk due to estrogen (Baron-Cohen et al., 2014). Some genetic variants appear to be involved (Carayol et al., 2011). Specifically, variation in MARK1 and ITGB3 appear to be associated with males in ASD and variations in ATP2B2, PITX1 and HOXA1 with females (Carayol et al., 2011). Low penetrance of ASD in females has been seen in spite of mutations in SHANK1.

However, others have speculated that the dose of acetaminophen given to male babies following circumcision may be one of the synergistic environmental insults. In a very large retrospective study, circumcised males were in fact nearly 1.5 times more likely to be later diagnosed with ASD (Frisch et al., 2015). This link has been dismissed because the study was retrospective. Retrospective studies are often cited by the Centers for Disease Control and Prevention (CDC) to dismiss the link between autism and vaccines. However, the study by Frisch et al. (2015) involved analysis of data from more than 380,000 boys. The study also reported a twofold increase in risk for infantile autism before age five years. Circumcised boys in non-Muslim families were also 1.81 times more likely to develop hyperkinetic disorder. A possible association with asthma was also found.

The link between circumcision and ASD is likely mitochondrial damage and neuronal apoptosis (Bauer and Kriebel (2013) from depletion of glutathione due to acetaminophen use after the procedure. A country-level analysis by Bauer et al. (2013) found a high correlation between acetaminophen use and ASD diagnosis. Glutathione is supplied to microglia via astrocytes (Rodriguez and Kern, 2011).

The hypothesis of a role of nonsteroidal anti-inflammatory drugs (NSAIDs) as a causal factor in autism was postulated in 2003 by Torres (2003). Bauer and Kriebel (2013) provided an excellent discussion of numerous dimensions of biological plausibility of acetaminophen-autism link. The evidence of a role of acetaminophen is mounting (Avella-Garcia et al., 2016). Mitochondrial dysfunction is known from low doses of acetaminophen (Hu et al., 2016).

The fine details of excitotoxicity after mitochondrial stress are worked out (Barger et al., 2007). Glutathione, glutamate receptors, and neurotoxicity of microglial overactivation via aluminum and mercury are intimately linked. The effects of mercury neurotoxicity is mitigated by the cytokine CCL2, sparing the brain of decreases in glutathione levels induced by MeHg (Godefroy et al., 2012). In a population in which children are exposed to multiple toxins repeatedly, the utility of "either/or" thinking is severely limited. The focus, and concern, should be on pharmacodynamics, considering genetics, body weight, and nutritional status, and should always include a look at interactions.

Acetaminophen is not a process factor or proximate factor; it, like mercury and aluminum in vaccines, is one ultimate cause of ASD, and the Food and Drug Administration (FDA) should require a warning label on acetaminophen-containing products as a known cause of ASD. We cannot afford to wait for the FDA to take action.

References : see envgencauses.com

Chapter 3.

EVIDENCE OF GENETIC AND EPIGENETIC RISK COMPONENTS OF AUTISM AND AUTISM SPECTRUM DISORDER

Genetics and epigenetics interact with environmental factors to define large parts of an individual's entire set of phenotypes, and the same is true in autism/autism spectrum disorder (ASD). We know a great deal about the genetics of autism, but the evidence does not follow a simple Mendelian model of a major dominant or recessive single-allele trait. Further, "autism genes" do not all contribute to liability or risk, and many of those that do cannot contribute unless they are paired with specific environmental chemotoxic and biologically toxic challenges.

AUTISM AND ASD TRAITS INFLUENCED BY SINGLE AND MULTIPLE GENES

Some traits are simple and show a high correspondence with particular genetic variation. These traits tend to be expressed as discrete (categorical) traits, and their patterns of inheritance appear on pedigrees with remarkably predictable ratios. Many traits, however, are considered *complex traits.* They are also known as *multilocus traits*, because they involve more than one gene. The transmission of these traits from generation to generation is considered complex; that is, the traits may or may not appear in a given individual, even though they have the variation that encodes a given trait. This complexity is due to multiple layers of redundancy in much of the human genome. Each individual can be considered to have a chance (probability) of showing such traits. When the trait is a disease phenotype, we consider the chance to be the risk of having or developing the disease. Not all individuals with specific variants associated with a disease exhibit the disease traits. Thus, individuals with a specific mutation or variant are said to be *carriers*, and the variant or allele they carry is said to confer risk.

When geneticists observe that a species' trait can change over generations in response to environment but revert to its original manifestation if environmental conditions change back, they call it *phenotypic plasticity*. Phenotypic plasticity is best exemplified by a species of plant whose leaves are broad in a wet year but narrow and feathery in years with low precipitation. There are specific types of experiments one can do with plants to demonstrate that the distribution of traits among individuals supports a conclusion of a significant *gene × environment interaction* (or simply "*G × E*"). We will explore the evidence for phenotypic plasticity via evidence of a G × E effect on each of the well-known autism phenotypes in a later chapter. The fact that G × E interaction exists in autism is cause for real hope for highly focused clinical efforts toward individualized treatments, and that it is highly preventable.

Autism is widely recognized as a spectrum of phenotypes; however, unlike the electromagnetic spectrum, the characteristics at any location on the spectrum cannot be nailed down to a simple, single number. *Severe autism* is recognized by a larger number of, and strong degree of expression of, individual autistic phenotypes; however, beyond that, the rest of the spectrum, at this time, appears to be an overlapping patchwork quilt, obscuring clear routes to effective treatment. A myopic focus on only certain aspects of the available data on the genetics of autism has led some to suggest (incorrectly) that treatment and therapy may not even be necessary for people on the ASD spectrum; suggesting otherwise is to provide parents of autistic children with false hope.

Adding to the clinical complexity, many other medical conditions can co-occur within autism. It is just as valid to consider this co-occurrence from the alternate perspective: autism is found within many other medical conditions. The reasons for this co-occurrence include the need for a more completely defined model on how to think about disease co-occurrence with and involving autism. How we view this turns out to have profound effects on our attempts to understand autism via research studies by helping to define study populations. For now, it is sufficient to introduce the idea that *autism exists where it is found regardless of other diseases that may also be present*. This perspective is critically important, as studies sometimes exclude individuals with other conditions. It is correct to stratify by other diseases or conditions (i.e., studies of autism versus no autism in Down syndrome), just as it makes sense to stratify phenotypes within autism. However, it makes little sense to try to tease autism phenotypes away from other neurological diseases when they may share the same underlying disrupted molecular pathways. Similarly, autism may be noted in children with other serious clinical conditions because they are under closer clinical scrutiny. It is also important to recognize that, at the same time, some conditions may be confused with autism; thus, knowing when differential diagnosis vs. ascertainment of comorbidity of conditions that share root causes with autism is important.

AUTISM SPECTRUM DISORDER GENE RISK CATEGORIES

Much work has been done to demonstrate that autism has a genetic component. However, the studies to date do not support the idea that autism is primarily a genetic disease. An ever-growing number of genes involved in autism have been identified. Since that time, the roles of various types of genes contributing to autism risk have been at least partly elucidated. Although most clinicians and researchers may not yet be aware of them, the differences between various risk categories of genes, such as *autism risk genes, environmental susceptibility genes,* and *autism phenotype intensity modifier genes* have also been elucidated by the ongoing research. Although not formalized as yet into these categories, the pattern is clear in most studies, and recognizing them requires deep and broad knowledge of molecular biology. The only genes that would make ASD a classically genetic disease are autism risk genes. Studies should focus on, and seek to establish and maintain, a distinction when defining the role of genes associated with autism in these terms.

Although autism is highly heritable within families, the genes and mutations contributing autism risk differ widely across families. Genes with mutations associated with ASD do not always associate with autism-like traits in the general population (Jonsson et al., 2014). This suggests a great deal of individual personality and environmental influences on these traits in the general population, and this diversity has also been seen in abundance in the autistic population. Many factors—including the entire rest of the genome, environment, and individuality—diffuse the contribution of genetics to ASD-related characteristics. Many of the mutations point to reductions in the capacity of the mammalian, including human, brains (and other organs) to defend themselves against toxic effects. Other mutations appear to compromise synaptic function, whereas others impact mitochondrial function. The sum of this knowledge positions us to better understand the role of specific mutations on phenotype, and to better understand routes by which environmental factors can intrude on neurodevelopmental programming in utero, and in specific infants, toddlers, teens, adults, and families, and in the general population.

EARLY HINTS AT GENETIC COMPONENT OF AUTISM PHENOTYPES

The earliest indications that autism phenotypes may have a genetic component included observations that other neurological disorders and chromosomal abnormalities were associated with autism (Gillberg and Wahlstrom, 1985; Wahlstrom et al., 1986).

It was not initially obvious that the risk of developing autism had a genetic component. However, observations that other conditions tended to run in families with autistic children spurred research. This is the role of observations in science: it begins with someone noticing a potential pattern or trend. This allows us to formulate a hypothesis and begin studies of the problem more objectively. Bolton et al. (1994) reported that 12.4 to 20 percent of siblings of autistic patients also had symptoms of autism.

Children with ASD and depression are at least three times more likely to have a history of family depression than neurotypicals (Bolton, 1994). This strongly indicates that segregation of the genes for depression is independent of segregation of those involved in ASD. In fact, a much larger study confirmed that autism risk is correlated with bipolar disorder and schizophrenia, but not ASD (Cross-Disorder Group, 2013). There appears, however, to be a slightly increased prevalence of bipolar disorder in ASD (Vannucchi et al., 2014).

Observations have also included patterns of inheritance observed for motor tics, epilepsy, obsessive-compulsive disorder, and anxiety disorders with autism. These traits appear to run in families with one or more autistic family members and are often found is studies of the effects of vaccines. However, as is true for all initial observations, sometimes they are only partly confirmed.

The occurrence of these diverse conditions within a family, alongside autism, suggests that a fairly large number of genes contribute to the risk of autism. In studies of the concordance of autism in siblings (co-occurrence of autism in siblings), the results indicated a weak genetic component (low concordance). Studies show a wide range of concordance, supporting a large role for environmental factors (environments vary widely). The co-occurrence of a condition among siblings is not a direct measure of the heritability of a condition. Siblings share much in their environment, most often including the same uterus, the same prenatal care, and the same medical care in the earliest stage of life. Teasing apart how much of the concordance is due to genetics versus due to shared environments calls for high-quality, objective, and challenging research.

In the late 2000s, after heritability was established, the accumulated evidence for a role of many genes became apparent. The kinds of mutations identified were quite varied. Microscopically visible chromosomal anomalies had already been seen in 1 to 2 percent of cases of autism through classical and molecular cytogenetics. Array-based gene hybridization studies refined cytogenetics and led to the identification of many copy number variations (CNVs), which are submicroscopic deletions and duplications of stretches of DNA; they occur in many genes, in 10 percent or more of sporadic cases, and in less than 30 percent at most of inherited risk cases (Krumm et al., 2013).

CONCORDANCE PATTERNS IN TWINS INITIALLY HINTED AT HIGH HERITABILITY

Autism, like other semiheritable traits, is often studied using measures of the degree of co-occurrence in families. Concordance rates of autism (the rate of appearance of autism in siblings) typically range from 40 to 90 percent in identical twins but is much lower (0 to 10 percent) in fraternal twins (Folstein and Rosen-Sheidley, 2001; Folstein and Rutter, 1977; Rutter, 2000; Steffenburg et al., 1989; Veenstra-Vanderweele et al., 2003). Bailey et al. (1995), for example, found 92 percent of monozygotic pairs of twins concordant for a broad spectrum of related cognitive and social abnormalities, versus only 10 percent of dizygotic pairs.

Due to this large difference in reported concordance rates between identical and fraternal twins, autism was initially considered one of most heritable of neurodevelopmental disorders. This facet of autism genetics, if taken at face value, would seem to justify a cessation of focused research on environmental factors. However, the advent of next-generation sequencing has unleashed a torrent of findings of mutations in genes that appear to be associated with autism in different families. There are many inherited and de novo mutations in genes that also have high biological plausibility as being causal factors in autism, but the precise genes vary across families.

Iossifov et al. (2014) found that de novo mutations contribute to 21 percent of the 2,500 individual-case (simplex) families. Interestingly, they found two sets of de novo mutations: a set of 400 that appear to contribute to ASD in females and low IQ males, and a semi-private set of de novo mutations found in high-functioning ASD.

This certainly suggests a significant role for chance in the question of risk of ASD. In this complex context, finding a way forward (Eapen, 2011) for meaningfully designed population-based research studies on prevention and individualized diagnosis and treatments is challenging. One could ask "Is the incidence of ASD higher than expected given just genetics?", and since it is increasing exponentially, the answer will, of course, be "yes," pointing to environmental factors. The future of autism research must also go beyond cataloging variation and move to identify effective protein networks and pathways, which would be highly valuable for identifying putative drug targets. Creating a translational research path forward when so many diverse causes are at play, in a manner that keeps the pharmaceutical industry interested, will be doubly challenging.

A large study comparing more than 3,000 monozygotic and dizygotic twin pairs at ages 7 and 8 years (Twins Early Development Study Institute of Psychiatry; Ronald et al., 2006) found that each core of the autism domain triad is highly heritable, with heritability in individual differences observed at the extremes (Ronald et al., 2006a, 2006b). The genes that contribute to heritability in one domain, however, are largely independent of those involved in the other two; at least half of the genes that contribute to variation are independent across domains (Ronald et al., 2005, 2006a).

Direct measures of heritability and concordance, however, do not consider that some of the unique variation shared between twins and siblings is from shared environment (same womb environment, similar diets, similar parenting, exposure to similar repertoire of environmental exposures). Until environmental factors are studied directly, it is only correct to infer that autism traits show "family aggregation." This is true for all apparently heritable traits for which environmental factors have not yet been fully elucidated. Twin studies often find differences in estimates of heritability for twins that share a placenta, compared to those who do not. Examples include studies in cognitive ability (including intelligence; Derom et al., 2002; Sokol et al., 1995), schizophrenia (Davis, 1995), and brain structure (corpus callosum; Reed et al., 2002).

A number of published studies reported 0 percent concordance, which seems too low given the range of reported concordance among sibling studies (reported as high as 14 percent). For this reason, Hallmayer et al. (2011) examined concordance in autism families considering "strict autism" (i.e., autistic disorder) and ASD. Their more recent study found a large amount of room for and evidence of environmental influences, in contrast to previous studies.

A breakdown of concordance rate by gender in the study also indicates room for environmental factors. Male identical twins showed 77 percent concordance, whereas female identical twins showed 50 percent. The rates among fraternal twins were 31 percent for male pairs and 36 percent for female pairs (Hallmayer et al., 2011). The difference between twin types is usually taken to indicate the degree of direct genetic heritability. However, considering that ASD has a congenital component strongly influenced by maternal exposure, events unique to an identical twinning gestation may also contribute to the higher identical twin concordance.

GENETIC AND ENVIRONMENTAL INFLUENCES OF AUTISM

Compared to the proportion of liability explained by genetics for strict autism (37 percent) and for ASD (38 percent), a much larger proportion of causal influences was found for shared environmental factors (55 percent for autism and 58 percent for ASD).

A much larger study involving 2,049,973 Swedish children (born 1982 through 2006) included 37,570 twin pairs, 2,642,064 full sibling pairs, 432,281 maternal and 445,531 paternal half-sibling pairs, estimated heritability of autism at 50 percent and ASD at 54 percent (Sandin et al., 2014). They found that individuals with an autistic sibling have a cumulative probability of an ASD diagnosis at age 20 of 13 percent, compared with 1.2 percent for individuals without an ASD sibling. Concordance (estimated by a tetrachoric model) was found to be 54 percent for identical twins, 25 percent for fraternal twins, 11 percent for siblings.

Considering the full population, which included a term for shared environment, contribution from shared environmental factors was estimated to be 4 percent. Overall, nonshared environmental factors were more important (54 percent variance explained) than heritability (42 percent). Using all twins, heritability (or, more accurately, family aggregation) was estimated to 52 percent; some of this may be due to hidden shared and nonshared environmental factors.

Compared to other conditions with familial genetic risks (BRCA-mediated risk with > 90 percent lifetime risk of breast cancer), the risk of autism before age 20 is relatively low. Among developmental disorders, it is among the highest.

This Swedish study is an excellent example of epidemiological assessment of disease risk. It has a number of important characteristics that bolster its validity, beyond the obvious power from the sample size. The first of these is that they used time-to-event measures to accommodate different enrollment lengths; they calculated cumulative instead of relative risks. They also avoided biases that have plagued other studies of autism, including those that result from self-reporting, by following all participants from birth using clinical registers (Sandin et al., 2014).

The preponderance of evidence supports the need for a renewed focus on environmental factors. Political messages that state autism is genetic *rather than* environmental are not supported by these studies and are founded on a fundamentally incorrect interpretation of genetic and environmental diseases. In fact, available studies suggest that as much research is needed on environmental causes in the context of genetic factors as there are studies of genetics in the context of environmental factors. Because they interact, neither genetics nor environmental factors has primacy.

Although the evidence for a genetic component to the risk of autism is clear, the specific risk is also highly heterogeneous. Estimates that mutations at any individual single gene or mutation type accounts for no more than 1 to 2 percent of all cases of autism (monogenic) were presented by Abrahams and Geschwind

(2008). A large Swedish study (Sandin et al., 2014) also found that only additive genetic terms were explanatory, suggesting multiple independent pathways impacted across families that are otherwise unlinked. This reveals extremely high within-disease heterogeneity. CNVs are more common in sporadic cases of autism than in families in which there is a pattern of inheritance (Sebat et al., 2007). Many variants that confer familial risk are single-gene mutations.

In 2011, there were more than a hundred genes with variation thought to potentially contribute to autism and ASD (Betancur et al., 2011). Current estimates are higher, with approximately eight hundred genes contributing either risk or causing *syndromic autism* (Butler et al., 2015).

Each individual gene and pathway that contributes to autism risk will therefore have, considering the entire population, a weak effect, even though the effect on the individual is large. In fact, this is precisely what was found (Anney et al., 2012). One of the greatest mysteries of the genetics of autism is the fact that many people with the same genetic variants that are associated with autism do not express autistic phenotypes. In general, this is called *incomplete penetrance,* and it belies a complex causal network that leaves the field wide open for the study of potential environmental triggers that may interact with one or more genotypes to cause ASD.

HUNTING ASD GENES

Initial studies in the search for genes associated with autism used linkage analysis. In linkage analysis, differences in the frequencies of anonymous markers (nonfunctional, common variations called *single nucleotide polymorphisms [SNPs]*) located along the lengths of all chromosomes are studied. The most reproducible linkage findings zeroed in on regions on chromosomes 7q, 2q, and 15q. Studies then focused on sequencing the DNA in these regions in many individuals with autism and those without, in search of mutations (nucleotide base substitutions), gene CNVs, or other indications of genetic or genomic differences between the groups in specific candidate genes. The positive associations from candidate gene studies were hard to reproduce, although some seemed more robustly involved than others (examples are GABRB3 and serotonin transporter genes). Additional candidate ASD risk genes were found by linkage mapping studies and direct sequencing. The resulting list of genes in which substitutions and insertions or deletions of small stretches of DNA (indels) is immense and varies across individuals. Although no individual gene is implicated in the majority of cases of autism, the functional categories of variation match the specific constellation of phenotypes in individual cases very well. This indicates a high likelihood of success in individualized treatment guided by whole-genome sequencing. Functional losses or changes of function in these genes are also often associated with other neurological disorders, and compounded diagnosis is not uncommon. Again, here we see the importance of focusing on specific phenotypes, as opposed to being distracted by a search for perfectly hierarchical disease classifications.

Most recently, exome and whole genome sequencing have led to an explosion of candidate genes, sometimes matching the cytogenetic and linkage studies and sometimes not. Although both a diversity and large numbers of rates of de novo or recent mutation are seen in each gene in autism and ASD, individually any one gene contributes causally to only a tiny percentage of autism cases. Initially, these factors complicated genetic linkage studies, as the results for any given locus appeared largely irreproducible. Any time an individual factor is important in a tiny subset of patients, the statistical power of most studies at the population level will be too low to detect significant association. This is true, importantly, for genetic and nongenetic factors. Studies with very large population sizes have therefore been undertaken, all indicating strong support for immense genetic heterogeneity in autism and in ASD.

Only between 5 and 15 percent of autistics are found to have previously known chromosomal rearrangements or single nucleotide variations. These differences are sometimes used to suggest syndromic autism, a concept that we will revisit. Germline de novo mutations are much more rare, being found in only 5 to 10 percent of idiopathic cases (Devlin and Scherer, 2012). The false discovery rate from pure genetic studies is not known, and not every mutation found in a study is a true *risk gene* that would have led to autism without environmental toxins, or second or third molecular hits. Efron and Zhang (2011) provided methods for estimating false discovery rates in CNV.

Some genes influence severity (*modifier genes*); some may be *environmental susceptibility genes.* Others may, in fact, be *neutral variants* that either do not change a protein sequence, or that change a protein sequence, but not necessarily its shape or function. Furthermore, some high-frequency mutations in some genes may be *compensatory* for others in ASD-related genes.

The specific examples of genes chosen for further discussion in this book are selected on the basis of their role during development, as currently understood by molecular biologists (biological plausibility). By virtue of the heterogeneity of the genetics of autism, they cannot be thought of as common autism genes. They do, however, represent the classes and types of mutations in specific functional categories and biological compartments and pathways. Most of cellular biology is arranged into regulatory and signaling pathways. Thus, when we see different genes, or functional categories of genes, found with mutations across independent studies, our confidence in their contribution to risk increases. When we see different genes in the same pathway, our confidence in a role for that pathway also increases.

PENETRANCE AND EXPRESSIVITY IN SIMPLEX AND MULTIPLEX FAMILIES

Families with more than one case of austim are considered "multiplex families." Families with female autistic members have higher expressivity (more severe ASD) or a greater penetrance (higher risk of recurrence) than families with only male cases (Frazier et al., 2015). Multiplex families have lower expressivity than simplex families, but non-ASD family members have more severe autism-like traits in multiplex families than in simplex families. Although the severity of autistic phenotypes can be quantified for many traits, studies of the levels of exposure to environemental toxins and the study of severity of autism traits are rare. Social trait variation (language) in females is attributed to "early environmental exposure" (teaching) rather than genetics (Constantino, 2003, 2011).

IGNORING FAMILIAL CLUSTERING LEADS TO MISSED ASSOCIATIONS

Álvarez-Iglesias et al. (2011) found no association between mtDNA mutations and rates of autism. The biological expression of loss-of-function (LoF) mutation-sourced mitochondrial dysfunction varies both with mutation type and which mitochondrial gene is functionally disrupted. This negative result is most likely due to the widespread problem of seeking association with low-prevalence (relatively rare) and heterogeneous mutations in a general population with small sample numbers. This agnosticity of population substructure poses problems for building genetic classifiers in general (Belgard et al., 2014) and is not restricted to mtDNA variations nor to ASD.

The Álvarez-Iglesias study had 148 ASD patients, which means they relied on the alleles of approximately seven or eight patients to drive the result to significant association. They had 753 unaffected individuals as controls. Perhaps one patient in the unaffected population could be expected to have mtDNA mutations. The study hinged on finding a significant difference between allelic population frequencies of 5 percent and 0.01 percent. Although this may seem reasonable, extreme value statistics require more power (larger sample sizes). This flaw is typical of retrospective epidemiological studies such as those relied upon the CDC to stand firm on their claim that no association exists between autism and vaccines. They are the weakest type of study that could be used in this context. The most meaningful type of study that could be imagined would be to compare autism rates in a cohort of individuals with mutations in ASD-related genes with those in individuals without such mutations—considering individuals of both genotype classes in vaccinated and unvaccinated groups.

The study also examined only twenty-five mtDNA variants previously suspected of being pathological. The mitochondrial genome contains thirty-five genes, many of which work in concert with nuclear-encoded genes on processes including respiration and oxidative phosphorylation.

The existence of mutations in either the mitochondrial genome or the nuclear genome can lead to precisely the same phenotype: mitochondrial dysfunction. This is known as phenomimicry. The specific nutraceutical, dietary, or pharmacologic targets of the genes, however, may be very different, and thus these details are important.

EXAMPLES OF DIRECT-RISK GENES IN AUTISM

Risk genes can involve CNVs, LoF mutations, protein change, or promoter mutations (if confirmed to be pathogenic), or they can be differentially methylated (epigenetic). In autism, the primary categories that mostly likely have true risk alleles are synaptic genes, neurotransmitter genes, mitochondrial genes, neuronal migration/axon guidance genes, glutamate receptors, and receptors of products of all of the above.

NEURONAL MIGRATION (REELIN GENE)

During development, neurons make connections between brain regions, sometimes at a remarkable distance. They follow a development program. Reelin is a large secreted protein that regulates neuronal migration during development. It also serves as a signal for the growth of extensions of dendrites and axons, maintains synaptic plasticity, and influences neurotransmitter function. Some variants in RELN show very strong likelihood of contributing to autism in some cases (see Wang et al., 2013, for a meta-analysis). Variants are known to contribute to schizophrenia, bipolar disorder, major depression, and migration defects associated with temporal lobe epilepsy.

Many other genes involved in neuronal migration are candidate genes for natal autism. These are reviewed by Reiner et al. (2015) and include: Astrotactin 2 (ASTN2), ASD, autism susceptibility candidate 2 (AUTS2), contactin associated protein–like 2 (CNTNAP2), distal-less homeobox 1/2 (DLX1/2), NudE nuclear distribution E homolog 1 (NDE1), T-Brain-1 (TBR1), and WD repeat and FYVE domain containing 3 WDFY3.

AUT2 is a regulatory gene that is found, in combination with a polycomb repressor complex gene, PRC1, as a PRC1-AUTS2 complex (Gao et al., 2014). The genes that PRC1-AUTS2 regulates in turn regulate genes in the central nervous system (CNS) through promoter association (e.g., H3K4me3). As such, AUTS2 has a high likelihood of having a large effect on phenotype. Indeed, AUTS is thought to have an effect on a large number of neurological disorders (Oksenberg and Ahituv, 2013).

SYNAPTIC GENES

There are a bewildering number of molecules and processes within nerve cells and on the proteins expressed on the surface between the dendritic spine and axon. There many ways to break a synapse, and there are many ways to alter and disrupt the complex, highly regulated developmental pathways in synaptic and circuit assembly and the consequences for brain development and function.

There are additional within-cell transport systems involved in nerve impulse transmission, including Golgi apparatus, endoplasmic reticulum in the dendrite, endosomes, and synaptic vesicles, in the axon and invaginations in the axon, any of which can be rendered dysfunctional by mutations. Synapses are complex signaling stations between nerves involving numerous proteins. At the synapse, an axonal CASK/VELI/MINT/CAMK complex communicates via both calcium channels and exocytosing vesicles at the axon surface, with AMPA-type glutamate receptors at the synaptic cleft, with internal uptake by the GUK/GKAP/SHANK complex. Each of these entities represents at least one protein-coding gene that may be disrupted by any number of mutations; therefore, consideration of synaptic mutations is extremely complex and can rapidly overwhelm. It is tempting to write a catalog of human variation in synaptic genes, and this type of work is available in a number of readily available reviews. However, it must be kept in mind that even these dysfunctional genes may contribute to the ASD phenotype either as cause or modifier in type or degree, and that their relative dysfunction may be problematic without neurotoxin-induced chronic microglial activation (environmental injury).

NEUROTRANSMITTER GENES

Clearly, individuals born with aberrant neurotransmitter proteins are likely to have difficulties with proper cell-cell connectivity and communication. These include mutations that influence acetylcholine (Ach) and γ-aminobutyric acid (GABA) neurotransmission. Polymorphisms within genes that encode GABR, including GABRγ1 located on 15q11-13, are associated with autism (Vincent et al., 2006; Ashley-Koch et al., 2006). Interactions (epistasis) between GABRα4 and GABRβ1 genes are found in some autistic probands (Ma et al., 2005).

SHANK1, SHANK2, SHANK3

SHANK genes combine in various forms with each other, forming large complexes at excitatory synapses. The SHANK3 protein plays a dual role at excitatory synapses, anchoring glutamate to the cell surface. It is also involved in the formation and maturation of dendritic spines. SHANK3 genes belong to the ANKRD (ankyrin repeat domain containing) family of genes. Mutations in each of these genes have been found in some cases of autism with severe intellectual disability (Durand et al., 2007, 2012; LeBlond et al., 2014; Sato et al., 2012).

Mice lacking SHANK2 genes showed brain-region-specific upregulation of ionotropic glutamate receptors at the synapse, increased levels of SHANK3, fewer dendritic spines, and reduced basal synaptic transmission. They were extremely hyperactive and displayed repetitive grooming and abnormalities in vocal and social behaviors (Schmeisser et al., 2012). Autism-related mutations in SHANK3 induce, or help induce, channelopathy (specifically, impaired hyperpolarization-activated cation, or Ih, channels; Yi et al., 2016). Thus, channelopathy is not necessarily an alternative diagnosis to autism.

Individuals with Phelan-McDermid syndrome (22q13.3 deletion syndrome, or PMS) often have profoundly autistic features, including absent or delayed speech and moderate to profound intellectual disability. The deletion includes SHANK3. Leblond et al. (2014) provides a full account of the research on the SHANK genes in ASD and call for genetic screening for SHANK3, especially given its relatively high prevalence (more than one in fifty). Frye et al. (2015) hypothesize that mitochondrial complex activity abnormalities due to mutations in nuclear genomic region 22q13 may explain phenotypic variation in PMS symptoms, finding mitochondrial dysfunction in 59 percent of Phelan-McDermid syndrome patients. The abnormalities involved Complex I (43 percent) and IV (16 percent), but did not involve Complex II+III and II activity. This shows that much of the genetic risk leading to other types of cellular dysfunction may be married to mitochondrial dysfunction in autism. A critical question for ASD studies overall is how many of each of the two-hits or multiple-hits involve common, nonpenetrant variants, de novo variants caused by exposure, or direct damage caused by environmental hits in either nuclear or mitochondrial genes? A full accounting of these categories will add substantially to our understanding of the nature of genetic contributions to autism.

Truly syndromic autism involving mutations specifically and only in synaptic genes alone, uninfluenced by environment, is likely rare. They would require homozygote genotypes, or potentially differently weakened or altered proteins expressed by both copies of genes. Two mutations in different synaptic genes, coupled with mutations—for example, in Toll-like receptor (TLR) molecules—causing microglia to become and stay activated (say, misinterpreting normal cytokine signals as activators), could occur. Mutations in mitochondria or metabolic pathways paired with synaptic mutations might also occur. Pairs of mutations that co-occur in the key pathways are conceivable but are rarely reported because they are already independently rare events.

NEUROLIGNINS AND MDGA

Mutations in Neurolignin 3 have been found in ASD (Fuccillo et al., 2014). Functionally, the mutation causes a specific synaptic dysfunction that leads to repetitive motion with impaired striatal circuits in the nucleus accumbens/ventral striatum (Fuccillo et al., 2014). This impairment may not reflect a core causal factor of AD but may contribute to a diagnosis by increasing the severity of stereotypic motor behaviors.

MDGA (MAM domain containing glycosylphosphatidylinositol anchor) genes encode proteins that interact with neuroligins in inhibitory synapse development. MDGA-2 is found in some autistics (Bucan et al., 2009).

MIRNAS AND AUTISM

Some genes implicated in ASD are regulated by microRNAs (miRNAs). These are a type of noncoding RNAs ~22 nucleotides in length that suppress translation by annealing to miRNA recognition elements (MREs) found in the 3′ untranslated region (3′UTR) of target mRNAs. Variation in miRNAs, or in MREs, could alter the efficiency of miRNA:DNA annealing. Vaishnavi et al. (2014) studied single nucleotide variations present in the 3′UTRs of mRNAs and found a number of 3′UTR mutations that might affect MREs (Vaishnavi et al., 2014) for the following genes:

- DISC1 (disrupted in schizophrenia 1)
- EPHB2 (an ephrin gene)
- HEPACAM (hepatic and glial cell adhesion molecule)
- HLA-DRB1 (major histocompatibility complex, class II)
- PCDHA1 (Protocadherin alpha 1)
- PIK3CG (phosphoinositide-3-kinase, catalytic, gamma)
- RGS7 (regulator of G protein signaling 7)
- SCFD2 (Sec1 family domain-containing protein 2)

- TNIP2 (A20-Binding Inhibitor of NF-Kappa-B Activation 2)
- XIRP1 (xin actin-binding repeat containing 1)

The biological functions of these genes make them likely candidates for involvement in ASD in a variety of ways.

A second study of miRNA variation in ASD found numerous miRNAs with variation, but considered that many of the miRNAs they found are also found in the general population, they considered many of them nonpathogenic, at least without environmental exposure (Marrale et al., 2014).

Marrale et al. (2014) found eight miRNAs in common with the previous study by Vaishnavi et al. (2014). They also found one (hsa-miR-185) that had previously been found to display upregulation in lymphoblastoid cell lines from autistic patients. Marrale found three copies of the hsa-mir-185 gene in the two ASD patients from our APL data set.

Each of the miRNAs can have thousands of experimentally predicted target genes, so it is difficult to know downstream effects of miRNA and MET. Assigning specific functional and clinical significance to variation in miRNA genes is more challenging than finding mutations in their target sequences at ASD-related loci.

MITOCHONDRIAL DYSFUNCTION AND AUTISM

Mitochondria are cellular organelles, the powerhouses of our cells, with their own genome. Mitochondrial dysfunctions occur in a variety of human inherited disorders, including autism (Giuliv et al., 2010) and other neurodegenerative disorders (Nunnari and Suomalainen, 2012). Mitochondrial electron transfer chains function in the production of adenosine triphosphate (ATP). They contribute to response to stress at the cellular level via management of reactive oxidative stress (ROS) and are involved in processes such as autophagy and apoptosis.

Evidence for mitochondrial dysfunction in ASD is very strong (e.g., Rossignol and Frye, 2012). The mitochondrial dysfunction in the brain can be severe in ASD. Alterations in protein levels in mitochondria respiratory chain protein complexes, decreased Complex I and IV and mitochondrial antioxidant enzyme SOD2, and increased oxidative DNA damage were all found postmortem in the temporal cortex of early childhood ASD patients compared to controls (Tang et al., 2013).

Gu et al. (2013) found disruption of electron transport chain Complexes I-V and pyruvate dehydrogenase in frontal cortex tissues of 14 percent of ASD patients. Compared to age-matched controls, they also found elevated mitochondrial DNA (mtDNA) CNV in autistics as well as mutations in the mitochondrial genes ND4 and CytB (44 and 33 percent, respectively). Elevated mtDNA copy number has also been found in peripheral blood cells of autistic children (Chen et al., 2015).

Mitochondrial dysfunction is found in 5 percent of patients with ASD, compared to 0.01 percent in neurotypicals. This may be an underestimate, however. Mitochondrial dysfunction is detected by looking for elevated markers of mitochondrial energy metabolism dysfunction, including elevated lactate, pyruvate, alanine levels in blood, and urine and/or cerebrospinal fluid. Weissman et al. (2008) found elevated blood lactate (76 percent), plasma alanine (36 percent), and mitochondrial electron transport chain dysfunction (52 percent) in ASD patients. The mitchondrial dysfunctions involved deficiencies in Complex I (64 percent) and Complex II (20 percent). Only 8 percent of patients had mtDNA mutations likely to cause LoF. Other markers of mitochondrial dysfunction include serum carnitine deficiency (Frye et al., 2013) and measures of enhanced oxidative stress.

Between mtDNA and genomic mutations, mutation-based mitochondrial dysfunction may be as high as 8 percent (Haas, 2010). Although evidence of mitochondrial disorder involvement in ASD is strong, with deficiencies in energy and electron transport in the brain, the findings of actual mtDNA mutations are few and far between. In disorders other than ASD, the specific mutations involved in mitochondrial dysfunction vary and include individual mutations and small DNA deletions/duplications that may be involved in energy and respiration functions. One study found alleles associated with autism in noncoding regions near tRNA genes in the mitochondrial genome (Mousavizadeh et al., 2013). Other studies have reported mtDNA mutations in autistics including two patients in Bulgaria (Avdjieva-Tzavella et al., 2012) involving amino-acid altering mutations in the MTCO1 and MTCO2 genes.

Pons et al. (2004) found a 3243A>G mutation in two patients. Another study reported the same mutation in two out of 810 ASD patients (Serajee et al., 2006). This mutation is the most common mtDNA mutation that causes disease in adult patients, which includes risk of complications during pregnancy (de Laat et al., 2015), migraine headaches (Guo et al., 2015), and epilepsy (Whittaker et al., 2015), among other problems. Neurological conditions were found to be the most common source of mortality in an analysis of pedigrees with the 3243A>G mutation (Majamaa-Voltti et al., 2008).

Graf et al. (2000) reported the mutation in a family with neurological disorders associated with the mtDNA 8363G>A mutation; at least one family member had ASD symptoms, described as follows: "During his second year of life, he lost previously acquired language skills and developed marked hyperactivity with toe-walking, abnormal reciprocal social interaction, stereotyped mannerisms, restricted interests, self-injurious behavior and seizures."

Pathogenic mutations in the mitochondrial genes are common in the general population (Elliott et al., 2008). It is worth noting that mitochondria are maternally inherited, which means that the effective population size of any study of patterns of inheritance is one-half that for genomic studies. Some accommodation to study design should be made (either larger sample sizes for power of association or relaxing the stringency of statistical tests for significance of association).

Dysfunction of mitochondria due to aberrant nuclear-gene encoded signals may be much more common than mtDNA mutation-based pathologies. As much as 70 percent of ASD that show signs of mitochondrial dysfunction had no mutations in the mitochondrial genome, indicating that nuclear-gene encoded dysfunction may cause secondary mitochondrial dysfunction (many proteins' nuclear genes regulate mitochondrial function). The CNVs found in areas that encode genes for bioenergetics and ionic metabolism were found in autistics (Smith et al., 2012).

One example of how this could occur is by calcium channel disruption due to mutations in the mitochondrial aspartate-glutamate carrier gene SLC23A12, which has very strong replicated evidence of having LoF mutations associated with ASD (Ramoz et al., 2004; Segurado et al., 2005; Silverman et al., 2008. Dhillon et al. (2011) reviewed numerous studies reporting mitochondrial mutations contributing to autism available at the time. The two largest of these, Ramoz et al. (2004) ($N = 411$) and Sequrado et al. (2005), found the single nucleotide polymorphisms (SNPs) rs2056202 and rs2292813 in the SLC25A12 gene. Mutations in the SLC23A12 gene may compromise or enhance the delivery of glutamate.

Biomarkers indicating mitochondrial dysfunction are even more prevalent, and some markers correlate with autism severity. Rossignol and Frye (2012) also reported that in ASD with mitochondrial dysfunction, the prevalence of developmental regression (52 percent), seizures (41 percent), motor delay (51 percent), gastrointestinal abnormalities (74 percent), female gender (39 percent), and elevated lactate (78 percent) and pyruvate (45 percent) levels were all significantly higher than in the ASD population without evidence of mitochondrial dysfunction. This suggests that much of mitochondrial dysfunction in ASD is acquired (environmental) rather than inherited.

Experimental and observational evidence supports this very well. In a study of mitochondrial respiration in lymphoblastoid cell lines from individuals with autism and unaffected controls, Rose et al. (2015) found that environmental mercury exposure and the resulting increased risk of developing autism may be mediated through mitochondrial dysfunction and that a subset of individuals with autism may be vulnerable to environmental influences, with detrimental effects on development through mitochondrial dysfunction. Autistic children with mitochondrial dysfunction had lower communication and daily living skill scores than those without, even though language and ASD symptom levels were similar (Frye et al., 2013). Mitochondrial dysfunction appears to also be associated with higher use of dietary supplements, perhaps contributing to the evenness of the scores and symptoms.

The idea of an increased capacity or "reserve" of oxidative tolerance in autistic children with mitochondrial dysfunction may explain how a cohort study by Rose et al. (2014) found that ASD lymphoblastoid cell lines exhibited a higher reserve capacity at baseline and a more rapid depletion of reserve capacity when ROS exposure is increased relative to control lymphoblastoid cell lines. The decreased ability to tolerate oxidative stress in ASD overall points again to nuclear-gene mediated mitochondrial function, an element of the genetics and environmental aspects of autism that should be kept in mind during mutational analysis and interpretation.

Mitochondrial dysfunction is seen in a percentage of cases of regressive autism as well. A connection between infectious/inflammatory triggers with ASD and mitochondrial dysfunction was found in a study of 28 children with ASD and metabolic disorder. Shoffner et al. (2010) found that 71 percent of the children who regressed into ASD did so within 2 weeks of an episode of fever greater than 101°F. In 33 percent of these cases, the fever occurred after routine childhood vaccinations. Serum of young autistic children have been observed to show antimitochondrial antibodies (Zhang et al. 2010).

Variations in these genes carried by autistics are very likely to contribute either to specific risk of autism and ASD diagnosis or the degree and severity of AD and ASD symptoms, or, in some cases, both. van Daalen et al. (2011) found, in a cohort study of multiplex and simplex families, CNVs that contain genes that participate in the phosphoinositol signaling pathway (PIK3CA, GIRDIN), of the contactin-based networks of cell communication (CNTN5, CNTN6), and CNVs encompassing genes such as IMMP2L, MCPH1, and HOXA. Their study also confirmed the finding of Ozgen et al. (2009) for a role for microcephalin 1.

IMMUNOLOGICAL AGGRAVATION OF MITOCHONDRIA WITHOUT MTDNA DAMAGE?

The postmortem study of autistics by Palmieri et al. (2010) found that with no mitochondrial dysfunction (i.e., no mutations), excessive Ca^{2+} levels were responsible for boosting aspartate-glutamate carrier activity, mitochondrial metabolism, and, to some extent, oxidative stress in autistic brains by producing an unbalanced Ca^{2+} homeostasis. They concluded that mitochondrial dysfunction in autistics without mtDNA mutations was likely due to downstream combined consequences of dysreactive immunity and altered calcium (Ca^{2+}) signaling (Palmieri and Persico, 2010). These conclusions are supported by other studies. For example, decreased lymphocyte bioenergetics is accompanied by variance in immune markers (monocytes, T cells, and NK cells) in ASD (Giulivi et al., 2013). In mice, maternal immune activation during early gestation has been shown to cause long-lasting effects in the mitochondrial bioenergetics of splenocytes of offspring into adulthood (Giulivi et al., 2013).

For the subset of ASD with mitochondrial dysfunction, acetyl-carnitine profiles may be useful specifier markers, and treatment with carnitine supplementation or drugs that target mitochondrial dysfunction are prospective (Frye et al., 2013).

EPIGENETICS AND DRUG INTERACTIONS WITH MITOCHONDRIAL DYSFUNCTION

Changes in methylation observed in autistics are associated with oxidative stress and impaired methylation functions (James et al., 2004). Mitochondria can also cause changes in the methylation status of nuclear genes (Naviaux et al., 2008), including those involved in inflammation (Atilano et al., 2015). Mitochondrial dysfunction causes a number of changes in microglial function, including failure to express the inflammation-attenuation signaling cytokine, IL-4 (Ferger et al., 2010). Failure to downregulate microglia is a key indicator of autism at the cellular level.

Children of older mothers show increase rates of mutation in their mitochondria, leading to a greater amount of heteroplasmy (Rebolledo-Jaramillo et al., 2014); this could contribute to familial factors of risk such as parental age and birth order.

GENES THAT MAY CONFER BOTH DIRECT RISK AND ENVIRONMENTAL SUSCEPTIBILITY

GLUTAMATE RECEPTORS

Measurements of AMPA-type glutamate receptors and transporters are increased in the cerebellum of autistics (Purcell et al., 2001). Glutamate acts as excitatory signal for microglial activation and is damaging to neurons via glutamate neurotoxicity (GNT). GNT occurs when glutamate binds to the *N*-methyl-D-aspartic acid (NMDA) receptor. Glutamate increases have been observed to result from pro-inflammatory signaling from the mTOR pathway via glutamate receptor 5 (mGluR5) (Auerbach et al., 2011). Involvement of the innate immune system points to a compound effect of repeated or chronic excess glutamate called immunoneuroexcitotoxicity (Figure 5).

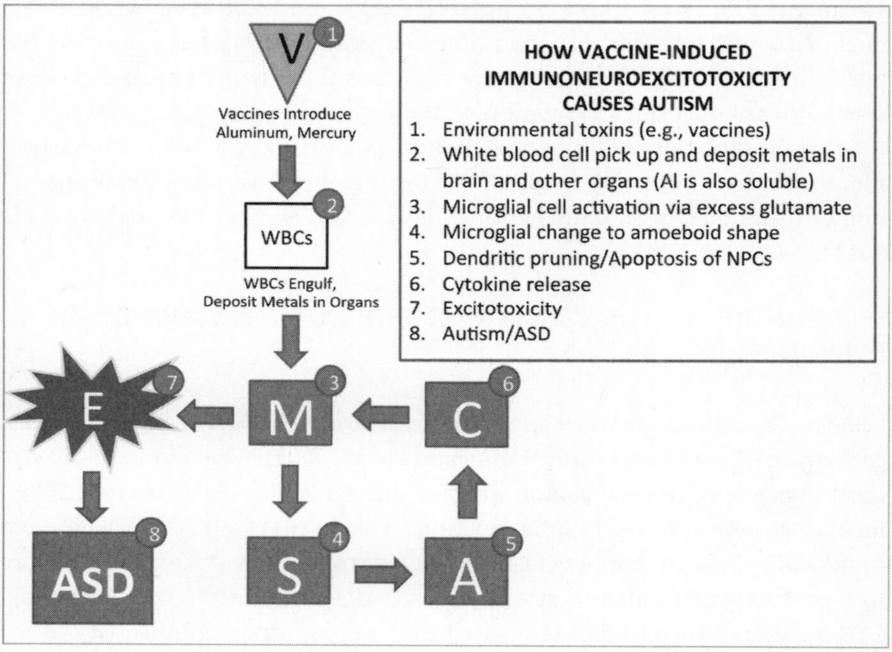

Figure 5. Immunoneuroexcitotoxicity can lead to chronic microglial activation, which results in autism due to damages to neurites, dendrites, and neural precursor cells. Normal cytokine signaling is disrupted by toxic substances that interfere with astrocytic uptake of glutamate between steps 2 and 3. The sources of immunoneuroexcitoxicity are numerous. Dr. Russell Blaylock worked to formalize these concepts, and the entire process has been demonstrated as fact by numerous studies.

The effects of glutamate-induced immunoneuroexcitoxicity are not limited to astroglial cells. The process leads to damage of cell components, including mitochondria (Atlante et al., 2001). Excesses of glutamate combined with hypoxia induce morphological changes in mitochondria, reduction in ATP, and increase in reactive oxygen species (ROS) in mixed cultures of NT2/N neurons and NT2/A astrocytes derived from human NT2/D1 cells (Sandhu et al., 2003).

In the mGluR gene network, involving more than 270 genes, CNVs occur more frequently in children with ASD than in controls (Hadley et al., 2014). A recent study also found that second hits in the mGluR gene network are associated with increased risk of ASD in 22q11.2 deletion syndrome (Wenger et al., 2016). Genes identified as second hits associated with ASD in 22q11.2 deletion syndrome included GRM3, HRAS, NRXN1, GNB2L1, and MKNK2.

Excess glutamate, binding to its receptors NMDA and AMPA, activated enzymes that damage cellular structure, membrane permeability, and electrochemical gradients (Atlante et al., 2001). It also caused mitochondrial hyperpolarization, increased ROS production, and enhanced oxygen consumption (Kumari, et al., 2012). The same authors found that glutamate increased the levels of mitochondrial fission protein markers pDrp1 and Fis1, leading to increase in mitochondrial fragmentation, and also activated autophagy markers Beclin 1 and LC3-II.

As we will see throughout the book, intercellular glutamate signaling is key to understanding autism caused by chronically activated microglia. The balance of glutamate, mediated by astrocytes, plays a critical role in both the normally developing and functioning brain. Within glial cells, glutamate regulates both transcription and translation initiation and elongation. As the brain grows, the number of connections grows. Rising glutamate levels increase microglial activation, which in turn induces cytokine release soliciting microglial hyperactivation, weakening synaptic connections. The concentration of glutamate in the brain is much lower than that in plasma. To maintain this homeostasis, the blood-brain barrier transfer is mediated via a high affinity transport system (Smith, 2000).

Glutamate receptor dysfunction is apparent in numerous cognitive disorders (Volk et al., 2015). Perhaps the most comprehensive and detailed review of mutations in glutamate receptor genes in ASD is by Uzunova et al. (2014). Their review is valuable in part because it brings forward studies showing alterations in the expression of ionotropic glutamate receptors (iGluRs) and their regulatory proteins in several brain regions, adding to the previously observed shifts in metabotropic glutamate receptors. Aberrant glutamate receptors caused by mutation would prevent astrocytes from clearing out glutamate. They point out that the mutations "account" for less than 1 percent of ASD cases and cite case studies of observed mutations in the kainate glutamate receptor 6 (GluR6 or GRIK2). Kainate receptors are ionotropic receptors that respond to the neurotransmitter glutamate. Variation in GluK2 gene also shows cosegregation (shared patterns of inheritance on pedigrees) with ASD.

Another major review of mutations involved in autism, schizophrenia, and addiction was presented by Yuan et al. (2015). The authors reported: "A new and unexpected outcome from sequencing efforts has been the surprising number of mutations found in glutamate receptor subunits, with the GRIN2A gene encoding the GluN2A N-methyl-d-aspartate receptor subunit being most often affected."

In 2011, Tarabeux found that mutations in one class of genes for glutamate receptors, which they call NMDAR (for *N*-methyl-D-aspartate glutamate receptors), were associated with autism. Mutations in these two genes, GRIN2 and GRIN2B, also is associated with intellectual disability. Two other studies had already found association of CNV in four NMDAR genes with autism (Gai et al., 2011; GRIN2A, GRIN2C, and GRM7; O'Roak et al., 2011; GRIN2B). Gai et al. also found CNVs in previously known autism candidate genes CTNND2, CNTN4, NRXN1, and PARK2; and O'Roak et al. found mutations in FOXP1, SCN1A, and LAMC3.

CTNND2 is essential for synaptic formation, and it forms stable complexes with glutamate receptors (mGluRs). CNTN4 interacts with glutamate receptors. NRXN1 (neuronexin 1) is involved in building the glutamate synapse. Specifically, it initiates the differentiation of GABA and glutamate postsynaptic specializations via neuroligins (Graf et al., 2004). PARK2 mutations increase kainate receptor expression via interactions with ionotropic GluK1 receptors (Maraschi et al., 2014). NRXN1 protein-altering mutations are found in ASD families (Matsunami et al., 2013).

Numerous additional studies had previously reported mutations in either glutamate receptors or in genes that regulate glutamate receptor expression associated with autism (Jamain et al., 2002). A good review is that by Choudhury et al. (2012). Some mutations include those in glutamate receptor GluR6 6q21 and kainate family receptors, both of which are important in brain development; those in the 11p11-13 region linked to glutatmate transport proteins; genes that regulate metabotropic GluR8; and variation (hemizygosity) in genes that regulate AMPAr (GluR2), as well as GLRA3 and GLRAB (Ramanathan et al., 2004).

Whether the mutations are inherited or de novo does not matter for the individual patient; however, knowledge of whether a given mutation is inherited can be important in terms of assessing familial risk.

COMORBID GENES MAY BE PLEIOTROPIC

Some genes found in the association studies are not specific to autism. SCN1A mutations, for example, are found in autism (D'Gama et al., 2015), in 88 percent of individuals with Dravet syndrome (Rosander et al., 2015), and in epilepsy. Finding a variant does not necessarily mean that they contribute causally; importantly, exclusive specificity is not a criterion for a causal genetic, nor environmental factors, for that matter. And of course, synaptic dysfunction is known as a basis of schizophrenia and bipolar disorder, which often co-occur with ASD. Thus, multiple phenotypes, perhaps differing only by severity, can be expected from the same molecular pathologies (pleiotropy). Variants at the same locus can have different phenotypic effects within the same disorder. Fry et al. (2016) identified specific copy number variants thought to be pathogenic at the SCN1A locus for both intellectual disability and epilepsy. At the chromosome region or gene "locus" level, "variation" can be said to have pleiotropic effects; however, this should be reexamined for individual mutations, which can be difficult because most are idiomorphic. The low penetrance of the majority of autism genes makes studying these relationships challenging. Studying high-penetrance genes, Casanova et al. (2016) reported that genes related to highly comorbid autism tend to be expressed in the nucleus, whereas genes related to more variable autism tend to involve CNS patterning. Intellectual disability without autism epilepsy tend to involve the Golgi transport system.

An examination of environmental factors can mimic molecular pathologies as well; this is known as "phenomimicry." Either/or generalizations about causes of autism are premature and unscientific. Similarly, mutations in different genes can render the same phenotype; thus, focus on the impact of mutations on pathways is more productive. Three other genes identified as potentially causal (Fmr1, Shank2, and Cntn5) were used to create knockout mice; these mice showed alterations in glutamate receptors (Poot, 2013). Double knockout Shank2$^{-/-}$ mice also carrying an ASD-associated microdeletion (CNV) showed a significant decrease in NMDA glutamate receptor (NMDAR) function (Won et al., 2012).

A study of adults with ASD (both narrowly and broadly defined) showed significant differences in brain glutamate and/or glutamine metabolism, and variation in glutamate levels was found to be correlated with intensity of ASD-associated behavior; that is, specially, reduced basal ganglia combined glutamate, and glutamine signal was significantly correlated with increased impairment in social communication (Horder et al., 2013).

Finally, mutations in apolipoprotein E (APOE) genes have been widely associated with schizophrenia and Alzheimer's disease. APOE is well known for having numerous isoforms that result from alternative splicing caused by mutations. Mutations in APOE are associated with autism (Giunco et al., 2009). Excess APOE causes a reduction in glutamate receptor function and results in lowered synaptic plasticity (Chen et al., 2010).

The fact that genetic variation may lead to diverse diagnoses in complex ways means that they are not likely to be useful for differential diagnosis and that the causal overlap between, for example, seizures and autism may not be easily teased apart. Therefore, studies should be designed that keep these functional linkages in mind.

DATA FROM VARIOUS TYPES OF STUDIES

TARGETED SEQUENCE STUDIES

D'Gama et al. (2015) reported that postmortem DNA sequencing of brain tissue revealed increased numbers of protein-changing and LoF mutations, as well as recurrent mutations in ARID1B, SCN1A, SCN2A, and SETD2.

EPIGENETICS

Gene expression control is mediated via methylation patterns. Epigenetic silencing occurs via methylation; enhanced expression occurs via demethylation. For example, differential methylation of CGG repeated nucleotide sequences on the first exon of Fmr1 gene causes loss of its protein product FMRP, leading to Fragile X syndrome.

Methylation is a normal process by which genes are deactivated (caused to not be expressed). Demethylation activates gene expression. The process involves the addition of a methyl group to cytosine-phosphate-guanine (CpG) sites, converting the cytosine to 5-methylcytosine, reducing promoter-binding genes that activate transcription.

Changes can also occur via chromatin modifications and by histone post-translational modifications. These are intermediate endpoints, molecular injuries that can mimic inherited disease.

In addition to finding genes involved in synaptic processes and functions, DeReis et al. (2014) found histone-modifying enzymes and chromatin remodelers in autistics, notably among those that mediate post-translational lysine methylation/demethylation modifications of histones.

Specific mutations have been found that influence methylation in autism genes. The genetic studies to date show function-altering genes in abundance in genes involved in methylation. Lasalle (2013) reviewed the autism genetic association literature and found reports of genes encoding nuclear factors involved in chromatin remodeling, histone demethylation, histone variants, and in the recognition of DNA methylation.

Among these was CHD7, which is essential for neural crest cell migration and patterning during early brain development. It has long been observed that early exposure to neurotoxins such as thalidomide and valproaic acid, prior to neural crest development, led to autism-like features in animal models. We know that methylation repatterning due to environmental toxins is responsible.

In a scan comparing 465,000 functionally relevant CpG areas between ASD and neurotypicals, only four regions were found. The study involved forty postmortem brain samples, including nineteen cases and twenty-one controls, across three brain regions. The study found four regions that were differentially methylated using fold-change ratio; the nearest genes tended to be regulatory genes.

CHROMODOMAIN HELICASE DNA BINDING PROTEINS

Remarkably, in one of the most important finds in epigenetics of *natal* autism, Hill et al. (2015) found that the chromodomain helicase DNA binding protein 7 (CHD7) gene, essential for neural crest cell migration and patterning, was found to be hypomethylated in animals exposed to the anticonvulsant and mood stabilizer valproaic acid. CHD7, like CHD8, reads H3K4me methylation landmarks. CHD8 (not to be confused with CDH8, cadherin 8) is among the most frequently mutated genes in autism (O'Roak et al., 2012; Zaidi et al., 2013). CHD7 is regulated by STAT3 and Oct4. During inflammation, STAT3 is mediated by interleukin (IL)-6 (Parker et al., 2010). IL-6 has both proinflammatory and anti-inflammatory effects (Scheller et al., 2011). In the presence of epidermal growth factor, as in cancer, the effects of IL-6 are sustained inflammation via chronic STAT3 activation. This is seen in neurological disorders involving chronic brain inflammation, such as Alzheimer's disease.

Wei et al. (2011) found an excess of IL-6 in the cerebellum of patients with ASD and that its upregulation caused an excess of granule cell excitatory synapses. Mice with elevated IL-6 in the brain displayed impaired cognitive abilities, deficits in learning, anxiety traits, and decreased social interactions. In addition to causing changes in excitatory and inhibitory synaptic formation and disruption of the balance of excitatory/inhibitory synaptic transmissions, elevated IL-6 elevation caused autism-like change in the shape, length, and distributing pattern of dendritic spines are observed (Wei et al., 2012). These autism-like behaviors are therefore mediated by IL-6 via neuronal circuitry imbalances (Wei et al., 2013).

GENES POINT TO MICROGLIAL ACTIVATION, AN ENVIRONMENTALLY INDUCED PROCESS

Why are the findings cited in the previous paragraphs so important? The process described leads to the same outcome as has been reported as a lifelong pathological process in autism: immunoexcitotoxicity. The accompanying increase in proinflammatory cytokine activity brought out by chronic STAT3 activation causes persistent inflammatory conditions not found in normal physiological conditions, including corresponding cellular morphological changes and activity in microglia (Parker-Athilla and Tana, 2010).

Remarkably, IL-6 signaling during maternal immune activation (MIA) also causes changes in the placenta, including activation of decidual macrophages, granulocytes, and uterine NK cells, indicating elevated early immune activation. IL-6 also disrupts the growth hormone-insulin-like growth factors (Hsiao and Patterson, 2011). Disruption of these placenta-expressed factors can influence birth weight (Coutant et al., 2001). Low birth weight is associated with increased risk of autism. In fact, preterm babies tend to show signs of autism (Ure et al., 2015; Eryigit-Madzwamuse et al., 2015). Gestational environmental risk factors may be a common root cause.

Association of high aluminum in the blood of preterm babies has been incorrectly interpreted by Dr. Paul Offit as a sign of aluminum levels reducing during the course of a pregnancy, as if preterm babies were a random sample of pregnancies. He published on the CHOP website in 2013: "Aluminum is considered to be an essential metal with quantities fluctuating naturally during normal cellular activity. It is found in all tissues and is also believed to play an important role in the development of a healthy fetus."

There is no scientific or medical evidence that supports this claim; it is absolutely dangerously misleading. Neonates fed more than 4 to 5 μg of aluminum a day showed significant neurodegeneration. This prompted a small study of neonates 24 h after injection with 1,200 mg of aluminum that found no increase in aluminum in the serum (Bishop et al., 1997); however, the concern is long-term, repeated exposures leading to chronic toxicity. Also, the study did not measure aluminum deposition in the organs, where sequestration and neuroexcitotoxicity occur.

A 2002 CDC study concluded that total body burden of aluminum from vaccines on the CDC schedule was higher than that from diet in neonates, but that it was low enough to be considered safe. A follow-up study by the FDA in 2011 concluded the same (Mitkus et al., 2011). However, these studies have a number of fatal flaws. First, the majority of aluminum in the blood is bound to plasma proteins, not serum. Second, serum preparations exclude proteins including fibrinogen, to which aluminum binds. Another flaw is that aluminum tends to bind to any tissue it comes into contact with. It is taken up especially by macrophages (white blood cells), which are excluded from serum preparations. These cells deposit the poorly soluble aluminum in the brain. Clearance studies did not bother to study localization of aluminum, nor did they examine long-term total body cumulative exposure and retention. Future studies of the toxicity of chemicals and compounds should examine total body deposition, retention, and turnover.

Because of macrophagic uptake and membrane affinity of aluminum, findings of excess aluminum in the serum would involve megadoses of aluminum. Its very long-term persistence in the body (weeks) and its chronic bioreactivity is the source of its utility as an adjuvant and its toxicity. Aluminum aggregates in the brain, away from serum, remain for weeks or months. In individuals with impaired detoxification pathways, such as malfunctioning endoplasmic reticuli or dysregulated glutathione pathways, biopersistence could be years. Thus, theoretically, most people may be "genetically tolerant" of aluminum toxicity at vaccine-schedule exposures, without overt signs of neurological damage, at least in the short term. However, that is a very low bar to pass. Risk of neurological damage due to environmental exposures from all sources is cumulative during the lifetime of the individual. Other reported short-term signs of aluminum toxicity include confusion, "brain fog," problems with memory retention, and loss of motor coordination. Long-term exposure is strongly linked to Alzheimer's disease.

Aluminum causes inflammation at nanomolar concentrations. Aluminum in the first year (approximately 4,000 μg) is much higher than mercury (approximately 25 μg), and the elimination kinetics of aluminum are far slower, so it is reasonable to expect aluminum to be more likely to cause brain inflammation than mercury. However, cumulative lifetime risk of neurological damage is due to cumulative lifetime exposure, and additivity and synergy are important.

In mice, even moderate doses of aluminum can cause changes to brain function, including the dopaminergic system, with attendant deficits in motor reflexes, memory, learning, and neurotransmitter functions; the timing of exposure in the postnatal period is related to different deficits, reinforcing evidence that aluminum impacts neurodevelopment (Abu-Taweel et al., 2012).

Adults absorb less than 0.1 to 0.3 percent of dietary aluminum; amounts absorbed by infants vary, but reducing aluminum exposure to neonates is a large concern. Studies showed that babies who are fed breastmilk instead of formula have a decreased risk of developing autism; formula contains a great deal of aluminum. Chuchu et al. (2013) found the amount ranged from 100 to 430 μg/L and concluded that these amounts were "too high."

A more realistic interpretation compared to Offit's is that high aluminum concentrations may have contributed to ill health of the fetus, the placenta, and/or the mother, and premature birth. This is supported by many studies. Given that dose is determined by route of delivery, it is remarkable that even exposure to airborne particles of aluminum increases the risk of low birth weight by 4.9 percent (Ebisu et al., 2012). Aluminum from roadside dust also increases the risk of low birth weight (Bell et al., 2010).

After birth, newborns especially are at risk of aluminum toxicity due to their body weight and immaturity (Chuchu et al., 2013; Fanni et al., 2014). Aluminum from formula may be part of the increased risk caused by bottle versus breastfeeding (Gallup et al., 2011). Some think the effect may be due to a lack of growth factor (insulin-like growth factor) present in breast milk (Steinman and Mankuta, 2013). Even if that effect is real, there is less aluminum in breast milk than in formula (67 μg/dL vs. 210.5 μg/dL; NRDC et al., 2015). Thus, aluminum exposure baseline is higher for bottle-fed versus breastfed babies.

According to Tomljenovic and Shaw (2011), an infant of typical body weight that receives 1 Hep B injection at birth receives the aluminum dosage equivalent of ten adult Hep B doses. Furthermore, infants that receive Hep B booster injections at two months on the US schedule receive the same exposure to aluminum as an adult receiving 34 Hep B doses. In neonates, of course, the problem is even worse. In total, Tomljenovic and Shaw estimated that newborns, infants, and children to six months of age in the United States (and other developed countries) receive 14.7 to 49 times more aluminum than the Food and Drug Administration (FDA) safety limits of aluminum in vaccination programs.

The changes leading to microglial activation can be modified with the flavonoid luteolin both during pregnancy and in adults, conferring protection against environmental toxin-induced IL-6 mediated gliosis (Parker-Athilla et al., 2009). Luteolin is available in chamomile tea, carrots, celery, olive oil, oregano, peppers, peppermint, rosemary, and thyme. Many other routes to reducing gliosis exist (see Chapter 12). Fenugreek prevents aluminum-induced damage to astroglial cells in Wistar rats (Belaïd-Nouira et al., 2013). The drug deferoxamine induces excretion of aluminum.

Aluminum, of course, does not act in an isolated manner. Interactions with other metals and toxins may be very important. Dickerson et al. (2016) found, in a study of over four thousand individuals, that increased total ambient lead, arsenic, and mercury was a risk factor for autism.

Changes to the epigenome may be inherited because they are circulating in the population or may occur anew during gamete formation (de novo). These changes may be caused directly by environmental exposures. More recent results have shown that they may also occur secondary to, and as a result of, inherited or de novo mutations in the germ line or be impacted by other cellular factors (Berko and Greally, 2015). A number of studies point to mutations in genes that regulate methylation. One example is the gene H3K4me3, which provides landmarks on chromatin for active gene promotors.

Methylation patterns can influence behavior, and vice versa (Zeisel, 2009). Therefore, dietary preferences impacted by methylation patterns can lead to deficiencies in key nutrients that can further alter methylation patterns. Adopting healthy dietary choices can be challenging in cases of autism where the patient has a narrow band of dietary preferences and habits.

AUTISM IS ONLY SOMETIMES PRIMARILY DEVELOPMENTAL

It is tempting to think primarily about development when considering synaptic genes. However, brain maintenance and functioning are lifelong processes built on layers of development. The processes involved in establishing and maintaining synapses involve more than synaptic structural proteins and neurotransmitters. Microglial cells maintain, facilitate, monitor, and prune synaptic structures, and their state is highly influenced by environmental factors such as diet and exposure to toxins. Brain development and function is a lifelong process. Exposure to toxins at any time can cause injuries that can then cause the epistatic effects of previously nonproblematic mutations to become manifest.

In older populations, ASD would not be diagnosed. In the original considerations, it was called *natal Alzheimer's.* Microglia phagocytose Aβ filaments and any failure on the part of microglial cells to cellular debris may be involved in the beta amyloid deposits. Thus, we see risk of autism-like features at any age.

Genetic studies do not typically assess vaccination × gene interactions. As a result, large-sample population-wide studies by design cannot even begin to address the question of whether individuals with certain genotypes are highly sensitive to ill effects of environmental factors, including vaccines. Such research would appear to be high priority, given the massive knowledge base pointing to chronic microglial activation, which could be a useful intermediate outcome measure. These unknowns represent pathways to increased understanding—science is, after all, a human endeavor that involves asking questions.

In a very important study, Boggess et al (2016) examined the serum of thirty children, aged 2-9, who had ASD diagnoses, and thirty age, sex, and socioeconomically matched control children. They reported detection of 17 common organic pollutants, and found that the mean of the concentrations of most of the pollutants (combined into a single variable called mean xenobiotic burden) was significantly correlated with the Autism Diagnostic Observation Schedule (ADOS) total score within the ASD group, but not the control group (Fig 6A). The ADOS total score measures communication and socialization difficulties and increases in score represent larger deficits in these areas. As the mean burden of chemical toxicants rose in children with autism they had greater difficulties in the core features of autism. No individual pollutant had a significant correlation with total ADOS score alone. They also noted that the group with ASD retained a larger range of concentration of environmental toxins, with significantly higher within-group variability than the control group. Polybrominated diphenyl ethers (PDBE) and PCB's (polychlorinated biphenyls) were present in more children with ASD compared to neurotypicals (Fig 6B). Specifically, PCB-101, PBDE-47 and PBDE-99 were detected in the ASD group, but not in the control group. The investigators found many other common organic pollutants in the serum of both groups (Fig 6B).

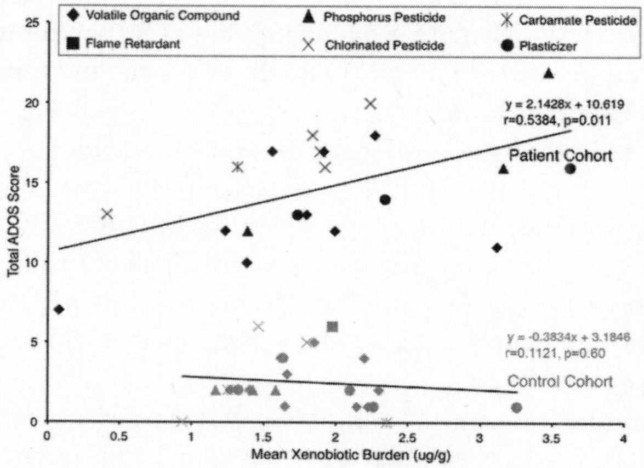

Correlation of total organic pollutant serum concentrations and ADOS behavioral score.

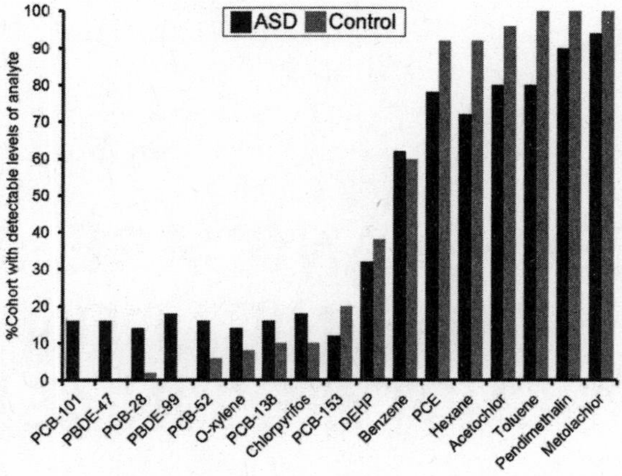

The percent of each group (ASD and Control) with detectable levels of each pollutant. Both Fig 6A and 6B reproduced from Boggess et al (2016) with permission.

A good review on synaptic genes in ASD is provided by McGee et al. (2014).

References : see envgencauses.com

Chapter 4.

SPEECH, LANGUAGE, AND COMMUNICATION PHENOTYPES IN ASD

To clinicians, most autism-related phenotypes are synonymous with symptoms. To educators and other caregivers, the phenotypes are individual traits. These traits are not fixed but can respond to conditions in the environment. To those who know and love autistic people, their symptoms are easily seen as characteristics that contribute to personality. However, to examine the genetics of autism in the context of symptoms alone would risk creating a static and therefore incomplete picture. Symptoms are the outcome of processes, while genetics can provide views into the specific molecular mechanisms of both biological and environmental causes. Therefore, it is useful to examine the genetics of each of the phenotypes independently, examine how they are used in diagnosis, and then see which phenotypes might be related to each other via shared molecular pathways. It is interesting to note the overlap and discordance between findings in different phenotypic areas, with respect to the apparent degree of influence of genetics and environmental factors.

It is too easy to become clinical about these phenotypes. Autism is also a human experience that influences the input and interpretation of sensory information for millions. We learn via our senses. Some autistics experience altered multisensory integration—where sounds can be transformed in the mind into lights. In one study, autistics tested with series of lights and beeps reported lower perceptual fusion between visual and auditory stimulation compared to typically developing children (Stevenson et al., 2014).

The rates of development of social skills and language are inextricably linked to both perceptual and cognitive abilities inside and outside ASD. Imagine trying to learn about your family members, your world and yourself through a maze of confusing, cross-linked signals. This is not the universal autism experience (it is doubtful there is such a singular thing). Even as clinicians and scientists, it is best to remember that those characteristics of autistics that we are now able to study are much more than topics for high-minded scientific inquiry and debate. They are someone's—many someones'—reality. While their human experience varies from that of neurotypicals, it is still profoundly and eternally human.

Nevertheless, science seeks to understand. It is easy to accept and love autistics. We do not have to accept and love neurotoxicity. Learning is the basis of social behavior; perception is required for learning. Questions such as "Do people with autism disorder or ASD perceive the world differently?" are important for many reasons, not the least of which is to inform and empower parents and teachers to do a good job as life skill trainers and educators. A better question is "How does *this* person perceive the world?"

Data from various types of studies (neuroimaging, eye tracking, and electrophysiology studies) support the hypothesis that given a particular start at birth, ASD phenotypes emerge via developmental cascades influenced by abilities to perceive stimuli. Deficits in perception can lead to impaired interactions with primary caregivers. The neurocircuitry differences extend beyond perception to include social cognition, which in time can lead to behavioral and functional differences in a manner that is dependent on early developmental processes, such as language and communication development (Eapen et al., 2013).

With a high level of compassion, then, for all of these phenotypic areas, we will examine the evidence for, and effects of, genetic components of risk and review some likely candidate genetic suspects found for each domain. Although there are many suspected and biologically plausible genes that may contribute to an individual's autism risk and to the specific constellation of symptoms and their severity in individuals with autism, a few are especially noteworthy. They provide opportunities to learn of the nature of autism from genetic and environmental studies, including results limitations thereof. For each of the phenotypic areas, a number of important gene suspects are explored for the various dimensions of speech, language, and communication (SLC) phenotypes.

SLC DOMAIN PHENOTYPES

Most of us take our ability to perform speech tasks, such as forming words we intend to use and speaking full, intelligible sentences, for granted. But our everyday experiences belie the stunning complexity of speech behavior. Our spoken communication begins with a verbal, but still symbolic, representation of thought, which is a complex process in itself. A thought, or stream of thoughts, is sent via our motor cortex, which commands a symphony of actions that involve our vocal chords, jaws, lips, tongue, and breathing patterns (articulation). Speech is a complex trait that not only involves numerous skills, but also a wide portion of the left hemisphere of the brain and Broca's area, a region linked to speech function.

Learning speech, language, and nonverbal communication also requires the ability to assign meaning to abstractions of thought. This aspect involves perceptions of sounds, sights, and motion. Interestingly, a study has shown that the ability of people with ASD to perceive nonbiological motion is similar to that of non-ASD individuals. In contrast, biological motion (walking, talking, hand gestures) seems to be less well developed among the ASD population (Freitag et al., 2008). Blockage of perception is a large component of autism, and understanding the physical (neurological) mechanisms involved is key to understanding causes, etiologies, and manifestations.

The earliest descriptions of autism by Kanner (1943) and Asperger (1944) noted delayed speech development. Specific speech development and social/communication skill traits were also seen in relatives of patients with autism, suggesting one or more genetic components.

Impaired language and social and communication traits that are characteristic of autism include:

- Delay or lack of spoken language that cannot be compensated for by other means of communication,
- Difficulties in initiation and maintenance of conversation,
- Repetitive and stereotypic language patterns and expressions (Pisula and Ziegart-Sadowska, 2015; World Health Organization, 2002), including echoalia (repetition of other's words or phrases), and
- Minimal use of gesturing to accommodate lack of speech ability (Tager-Flusberg et al., 2001).

MEASUREMENTS

A variety of formal measurements of dimensions of speech and communication are examined in the assessment of patients for a variety of conditions indicative of ASD. Formal measurements are available for some dimensions, including verbal intelligence quotient (VIQ) and repetitive speech patterns, of which there are at least two, more likely four, and perhaps six phenotypic subtypes (Bishop et al., 2013).

Typically, developed speech patterns begin by one to one-and-a-half years of age. These patterns involve an intuitive acquisition of language-specific rules of grammar and word categorization. Atypical autism/ASD problems include the stereotypical aspects and, for many, pronoun reversal.

Verbal intelligence quotient is a measure that reflects an individual's ability to use various components of language to analyze and solve problems. The components include one's ability to listen to, analyze, remember, and understand information that is communicated to them verbally or in written form. Other components reflected in VIQ include processes such as reasoning, logic, and abstractions used in language to represent concepts and perform comparisons. These mental operations are typically used in a variety of settings, and thus the measure is thought to reflect one's ability to operate well in logical, scholarly, and social settings.

EVIDENCE FOR HERITABILITY OF SPEECH AND COMMUNICATION ABILITIES

The evidence for a genetic component in speech traits that characterize autism was thoroughly reviewed by Pisula and Ziegart-Sadowska (2015), who tabulated 42 peer-reviewed studies that reported significantly higher co-occurrence of autism-like language and communication traits in first-degree relatives (i.e., parents and siblings) of autistic patients compared to control groups.

A large number of studies are consistent with speech abilities having a genetic component in autism. Studies included comparisons of the rates of speech pathologies in first-degree relatives of autistic individuals, comparisons of the occurrence of autism-like traits in family members with a single autistic member versus two or more members, and comparisons of the number of autistic children in families where one versus both parents show autism-like traits in speech and communication.

The types of traits in the studies reviewed by Pisula and Ziegart-Sadowska (2015) included receiving and expressing communication, language deficits, verbal fluency (i.e., VIQ), reading abilities, delay in language development, and difficulties in conversational skill and syntax (i.e., ability to form or comprehend phrases, clauses, and sentences). However, this does not imply that all aspects of speech and communication show higher concordance in first-degree relatives. Traits found to be similarly correlated between families with autistic patients and control families included language development history, verbal fluency, reading abilities, spelling abilities, phonological processing (Wilson et al., 2013), structural language (Pisula and Ziegart-Sadowska, 2015), pragmatic language processing (Sucksmith et al., 2011), and prosody (i.e, tone; Paul et al., 2005).

There is as yet no specific amalgam of language and speech phenotypes that exhibit identical heritability. One study by Ben-Yizhak et al. (2011) found that a subset of siblings of children with autism had reduced linguistic abilities, but their school performance and reading practices were not affected. Compared to controls, the heritable variation in activated cortices appears to be related to deficits in phonological processing (Wilson et al., 2013). Although parents of autistic patients showed the same variations in cortical activation in functional magnetic resonance imaging (fMRI) scans as their offspring, they did not exhibit the same behavioral evidence of phonological processing deficits (Wilson et al., 2013). Importantly, this suggests that these ASD children experienced environmental triggers or additional genetic variants not shared by their non-ASD parents.

The abilities to interpret nonverbal cues and to properly interpret emotional expressions are clearly part of social communication functions that are impacted in autistic individuals with speech and language deficits. There is some evidence of a degree of heritability in nonverbal communication—and that intensity is related to the degree of heritability (likely a genetic dose effect). Gerdts and Bernier (2011) found that parents and siblings from ASD families with multiple autistic members (multiplex) were less expressive in their nonverbal communication compared to parents and siblings from families with only one autistic member (simplex). Fathers in simplex families had better communication skills than fathers in multiplex families.

Not all differences in the concordance of traits shared between identical twins has to be genetic; importantly, a component of increased concordance may be due to the increased similarities in monozygotic twins' physical and temporal environments compared with those shared by fraternal twins, and this includes exercise of health care options, diet, home setting, and incidental environmental exposures that diverge over time, as can the experience and habits of parents.

PENETRANCE STUDIES IN SPEECH AND LANGUAGE

The degree to which a genetic trait appears in a population or a family is called *penetrance.* A family that has one member with a phenotype of interest is called a *simplex* family; a family with two or more members is called a *multiplex* family. Severity of autism seems related to penetrance. In classically severe cases of autism, communication is nil; that is, loss of speech is not supplanted by attempts at communication using gestures. Various studies based on the numbers of family members have found a consistent pattern—the larger the number of autistic people in a family, the more likely other, nonautistic family members will be found to have difficulties with social communication and language skills. Losh et al. (2012) reported that in families with the most pronounced autism in children, both parents tended to have autism-like speech problems; Schmidt et al. (2008) found phonological processing deficits in parents of children with severe autism. Families with less severely pronounced autism tend to have only one parent with autism-like speech and language traits. Further, these traits tend to be more pronounced in the autistic children. The preponderance of published studies have also found that families with larger numbers of autistic members (multiplex vs. simplex) also have not only higher penetrance but also higher expressivity of social, speech, and language traits (Gerdts et al., 2013; Schwichtenberg et al., 2010). Expressivity is the number of or degree of severity of symptoms. Language ability is a highly plastic trait, malleable to many environmental influences. This may explain why variation in gene copy number has been found to make only modest, specific contributions to variation in language and communication abilities in autistics (Gialluisi et al., 2016).

SIBLING CONCORDANCE VERBAL INTELLIGENCE QUOTIENT STUDIES

Studies of VIP heritability show inconsistent results. However, Goin-Kochel et al. (2008) found higher concordance in VIQ in related autistics than in unrelated autistics. Some interesting and important variations on VIP concordance exist. For example, among subgroups of children with autism or ASD, some children are completely nonverbal, whereas others show no language deficit. After controlling for age and VIQ, such differences were lost (Sucksmith et al., 2011). These findings indicate that the environment can influence rate of development within autism or ASD.

ENVIRONMENTAL FACTORS THAT CAUSE DELAYED SPEECH AND COMMUNICATION DISORDERS

A variety of environmental factors can cause speech disorders. Traumatic brain injuries (TBIs) are known to cause a loss of ability to perform well at speech and communication tasks. Aphasia, in which one's ability to understand and express language is lost or limited, is usually caused by damage to a specialized area in the left side the brain (such as Broca's region). The most common causes of TBIs are stroke, brain tumor, epilepsy, Alzheimer's disease, migraine headache, and head injury. There are various clinical subtypes of aphasia, depending on the extent and exact location of injury.

Other non-ASD causes of aphasia include encephalitis, seizures, and neurosurgery. Acute stress and anxiety can influence word choice, including difficulty in finding the "right" word. Aphasia is a potential side effect for as many as 75 drugs (SIDER 4.1, 2016). For example, aphasia is listed as a frequent side effect of galantamine (Razadyne, Reminyl), a drug used to treat Alzheimer's disease. Another example is fentanyl; its use to treat chronic pain has caused aphasia in a number of cases.

Aphasia affects more than the ability to generate speech. For example, it can also involve losses in the ability to understand spoken and written language. Thus, aphasia involves failed conductance of information from one region of the brain to another. Furthermore, generative brain functioning is effected as well. This tells us that aphasia can result from a number of causes. The primary causes are brain injury, due to either mechanical physical injury or to chemical exposure, and hindered development of brain structures in the young.

POST-MARKETING SURVEILLANCE RESEARCH OF VACCINES HINDERS STUDIES OF LANGUAGE AND OTHER TRAITS IN ASD

Post-marketing surveillance of vaccines is conducted, in part, by the Centers for Disease Control and Prevention (CDC) with the use of the passive Vaccine Adverse Event Reporting System (VAERS). In spite of the high rate of ASD reported by parents after vaccination, a grand total of 46 instances of "autism" were reported after vaccination in VAERS 2014. Aphasia after vaccination is reported in 115 instances. Critics of the citation of adverse events from VAERS must keep in mind that the CDC has published studies using VAERS data. Numerous other serious neurological conditions are sometime observed, via central nervous system demyelination. Demyelination is the removal of the protective covering myelin sheath that surrounds nerve fibers in the brain and spinal cord. The sheath acts as an insulator, ensuring proper nerve (ion) impulse propagation along the length of the nerve cell. The degradation of the sheath is a cause of multiple sclerosis. There is strong evidence throughout the autism research literature that suggests neurotoxin-induced autoimmunological damage. However, adverse events to VAERS are drastically underreported.

VAERS 2014 reported 323 instance of central nervous system (CNS) injury after vaccination and 198 instances of post-vaccination paralysis. In their review, Huynh et al. (2008) examined acute disseminated encephalomyelitis (ADEM), which often involves demyelination. They write:

> *Post-infectious and postimmunisation encephalomyelitis make up about three-quarters of cases, where the timing of a febrile event is associated with the onset of neurological disease. Although the two syndromes are distinguished by their precipitant, clinically and pathologically they are very similar. ADEM forms one of several categories of primary inflammatory demyelinating disorders of the CNS.*

Huynh et al. (2008) also reported a long history of ADEM due to vaccinations:

> *The initially termed "neuroparalytic accidents" gained recognition in 1853 after the widespread introduction of Jenner's smallpox (actually cowpox) vaccine and in 1885 with Pasteur's rabies vaccine. Post-vaccination ADEM is associated with several vaccines including those for rabies, diphtheria-tetanus-polio, smallpox, measles, mumps, rubella, Japanese B encephalitis, pertussis, influenza, hepatitis B and the Hog vaccine. For most vaccines, incidence rates are as low as 0.1 to 0.2 per 100,000 vaccinated individuals. ADEM following immunisation seems to occur significantly more frequently after primary vaccination as compared to revaccination. Post-vaccination encephalomyelitis accounts for less than 5% of present cases of ADEM. It should be emphasized to parents, patients, health care providers and all others concerned with immunization safety, that encephalomyelitis or ADEM—or any other adverse event—that follows administration of an inactivated component or live vaccine may be temporally associated with, but is not necessarily the result of, administration of a vaccine.*

Of course, parents, patients, health care providers, and all others concerned with immunization safety should also note that encephalomyelitis or acute disseminated encephalomyelitis (ADEM)—or any other adverse event—that follows administration of an inactivated component or live vaccine *may indeed be the result of an administered vaccine.* In fact, ADEM leading to autism (pervasive developmental disorder not otherwise specified [PPD-NOS]) was found to be caused by vaccination in a case leading to a settlement of more than $800,000 (*Bailey Banks vs. US Health and Human Services*). Temporal association is an important level of evidence used by epidemiologists to infer causality, and coincidental occurrences are the initial observations on which a hypothesis of causality is based. To dismiss temporal association as level of evidence is to abort the logical process of science just after conception. The occurrence of CNS inflammation post-vaccination is another indicator of potential causality, as it adds to biological plausibility.

The review continues with a second tier of evidence—reversibility:

> *Initially, post-vaccination ADEM was thought to be caused by the vaccine's viral*

component but it was later recognised that it could also be related to contamination with CNS tissue in which the vaccine was propagated. For example, the anti-rabies vaccine had been cultured from rabbit, sheep or goat brain and the Japanese encephalitis vaccine from murine brain. This theory has been highlighted by a significant drop in post-vaccination ADEM incidence rates after the development of vaccines based on recombinant proteins rather than from in-vivo infected tissue. . . . However, this does not explain the origin and cause of post-vaccination ADEM due to smallpox and several other vaccines that are prepared without the involvement of neural tissues.

GENETIC SUSPECTS (LANGUAGE)

Among the numerous genetic suspects for autism risk, two in particular, ADNP and FoxP1, stand out as biologically plausible in their relation to speech.

THE ACTIVITY-DEPENDENT NEUROPROTECTIVE PROTEIN (ADNP) GENE

The activity-dependent neuroprotective protein (ADNP) is a protein essential for brain development. It protects the brain against injury; specifically and remarkably, a single dose of the protein from ADNP in mice protects against the long-term effects of traumatic brain injury (Romano et al., 2002). Activity-dependent neuroprotective protein also allows the neural crest in the brain to develop normally.

ADNP is considered a culprit in the genetics of speech pathologies in autism for a number of reasons. First, mutations in ADNP gene have been found in numerous individuals with autism with speech and language processing disorders (Vandeweyer et al., 2014). Second is the ADNP(+/–) mouse model. Mice without ADNP should have incomplete rostral neuropore closure in the homozygote state (lethal). The ADNP(+/–) mouse is heterozygotic for a normal (ADNP+) gene and has one defective copy (ADNP–). The mouse is therefore a haploinsufficient model. The behavioral characteristics of these mice are extremely autism-like (deficiencies in object recognition and social memory; Malishkevich et al., 2015). The final reason stems from evidence derived from a large, next-generation (exome) sequencing project (Simons Simplex Collection autism data set; O'Roak et al., 2011; 2012). These studies identified ADNP as a candidate autism gene. The studies found ten autism individuals with mutations in exome 5; of these, five were able to be determined to be de novo mutations. A more recent study found mutations in the last exon of ADNP (Helsmoortel et al., 2014) in ten autistic individuals (out of 5,776). Nine of these individuals' parents provided genetic material to the study, and the mutations were found in those cases to be de novo. Mutations in ADNP are estimated at a rate of 0.17 percent, which is tiny as a percentage of autistic cases, but still the largest percentage of genetic contribution: most individual genes contribute less than 1 percent.

Pescosolido et al. (2014) reported a case of a girl with moderate to severe expressive and receptive language delays; fine, gross, and oral motor delays; attention deficit hyperactivity disorder (ADHD); and episodic mood disorder not otherwise specified. A pathway analysis and a recurrent function-altering ADNP mutation with *visual* impairment led them to conclude that "genes highly coexpressed with ADNP show interesting and novel biological processes for future research, particularly in strongly anticorrelated processes like myelination. This suggests a role for ADNP involvement in neuronal/glial cell differentiation."

The distribution and types of mutations present in autistic cases with ADNP mutations studied to date also provides a good example of the challenge of deriving a *mutational mechanism* that captures a general understanding of molecular pathology derived from function-altering mutations. Most of the loss-of-function (LoF) mutations are acquired "stop codons," which cause a termination of a protein product before the full length of the protein is transcribed. This can result in a defective protein or, in rare cases, a protein with a new, albeit aberrant, function. The presence of the mutation in an individual can render the phenotype in the heterozygote condition (different alleles from each parent). However, it must be remembered that when the effects of these mutations are not completely penetrant, dominance of the disease trait has not been established. The effect of a single mutation could be dominant in a healthy individual; in the presence of a second mutation, the effect could be deleterious. This effect is true whether its initial effect is negative (downregulation of another protein, binding of a protein to a copy of itself to form a dimer) or positive (facilitating expression or acting as a coenzyme toward a given phenotype). Traits involving multiple genes are referred to as *complex traits* for good reason.

THE FOXP2 GENE

The Forkhead box protein P2 (FOXP2) is a protein encoded by the FOXP2 gene. FOXP2 resides on the human 7q31 and is very well known as a gene essential for speech development. Mutations in FOXP2 cause developmental verbal dyspraxia with profound speech and language deficits. Studies of Neanderthal genome FOXP2 sequences revealed that Neanderthals had the derived, not the ancestral, form of FOXP2 and thus are likely to have had the capacity for speech development.

A linkage study initially pointed to FOXP2 as a potential major susceptibility locus for autism. However, Newbury et al. (2002) showed a lack of linkage between FOXP2 and the AUTS1 locus, leading the authors to conclude that FOXP2 was "not a major susceptibility locus for autism" (or specific language impairment). In retrospect, that study is not evidence that FOXP2 does not play a role; it appears that no genes are major susceptibility loci for autism. Reproducibility of genomewide association studies is low (Torrico et al., 2016), and this is not unexpected for a condition with hetereogeneous genetic and environmental causes. There may be no "major susceptibility" loci for autism. However, if one gene has a function-altering variant, a potential major risk exists for the carrier of that rare allele. It is also possible for variation at one locus to influence numerous clinically relevant features of ASD without being a "major susceptibility" locus (e.g., OXT locus; Francis et al., 2016).

Studies on association of mutations in FOXP2 are inconsistent; one study failed to find any association in a Spanish population (Toma et al., 2013). A study of a Korean population (Park et al., 2014) revealed importance of interaction between FOXP2 mutations and mutations in the monoamine oxidase A (MAO-A) gene, which encodes an enzyme related to monoamine neurotransmitters metabolism, including serotonin, but found FOXP2 mutations alone did not show association. This is to be expected for rare but real genotype/phenotype associations.

Further studies of variation in FOXP2 have indeed revealed association of mutations in FOXP2 with autism—but only in a small percentage of cases of autism (Wang et al., 2015). Deletion of FOXP2 was observed in idiopathic intellectual disability (Le Fevre et al., 2013; Utine et al., 2014).

Generally speaking, FOXP2 has a dose effect; in fact, it is typically expressed higher in women than in men. One study found mutations in FOXP2 within specific language impairment (SLI), a neurodevelopmental deficit in acquisition of spoken language in which intelligence is unaffected. Thus SLI exists in some patients who are otherwise neurotypical, and autism may involve impaired speech development with, and without mutations that cause SLI. Here, we see the failure of the expectation of a purely hierarchical, dichotomous classification not just for autism, but for neurological development disorder overall. These issues are explored by simulation by Bishop (2010) and tend to be nearly existentialist in nature; however, the field has developed a framework of simple genetics, etiology, liability traits, and endophenotypes within which concepts can be navigated. The complexity of making the distinction between endophenotype and other liability traits is also exemplified by the limited and varied role of FOXP2 in autism. The weak effect of the gene is expected due to the rarity of mutations; however, the role of the environment is made more clear due to more recent studies.

FOXP2 has been shown to undergo a process called random monoallelic expression (RMAE; Adegbola et al., 2015). In RMAE, through histone modification, some neurological genes can express the phenotype of neither, one, or both parental alleles, which makes studies of the genotype x environment association even more challenging. Here, environment (histone modification) meets genetics (mutation) and interacts with it.

The story of FOXP2 does not stop with association with disease, however. A study in transgenic mice with human FOXP2 sequences (Enard, 2011) reported alterations in dopamine levels, striatal synaptic plasticity, and neuronal morphology. Mice with only one functional FOXP2 showed additional and partly opposite effects, and the authors concluded FOXP2 may have contributed to tuning cortico-basal ganglia circuits during the evolution of language acquisition or vocal learning in human evolution. Other genes regulated by FOXP2 are very likely important in ASD (Vernes et al., 2011; Spiteri et al., 2007; Vernes and et al., 2007). FOXP2 partly directs neurite outgrowth in primary neurons and modulates neuronal network formation, via regulation of mRNAs involved in the development and plasticity of neuronal connections (Vernes et al., 2011). The current trend to map genes and mutations must be followed by an era of functional studies.

FOXP1, which forms a heterodimer with FOXP2, is a protein that was observed to the upregulated (overexpressed) in the brains of ASD males (Chien, 2013).

CONTACTIN ASSOCIATED PROTEIN-LIKE 2 (CNTNAP2)

Contactin associated protein-like 2 variants, identified as risk factors for ASD and related neurodevelopmental disorders (Alarcon et al., 2008; Arking et al., 2008; Bakkaloglu et al., 2008), show a specific association with language development. The CNTNAP2 genotype impacts language-learning task as well as connectivity patterns and differential frontostriatal activity and increased gene expression. CNTNAP2-mice exhibit low sociality, infrequent vocalizations, and behavioral preserevation, as well as delayed learning (Rendall et al., 2016), and are a good model for studying treatments including risperidone, which alleviates repetitive behaviors (Jeste and Geschwind, 2014). The best overall review of CNTNAP2 is by Poot (2015).

Valencia et al. (2012) found an association and evidence of epistasis (gene-gene interaction) between the serotonin transporter gene SLC6A4 and the serotonin receptor gene HTR2A in autism.

TBR1

Gene-gene interactions help highlight the importance of genes that have a weak overall population effect. FOXP2 interacts with and shows strong coexpression with another gene, TBR1, within which de novo mutations have also been found in a small percentage of cases of ASD. TBR1 is important during early neurogenesis and cortical development, defining the functional identities of neurons. TBR1 targets six genes, three of which are known to cause autism when disrupted: RELN, GRIN2B, and AUTS2; this link with autism led Deriziotis et al. (2014) to hypothesize a molecular network involving these genes. When disrupted, this network contributes to speech pathologies in autism and other neurological disorders. Deriziotis et al. (2014) also characterized the biological nature of the interactions between TBR1 and FOXP2 as likely influencing axonogenesis.

The functional considerations of mutations must include overall pathways. As I have said for years in the classes I teach, there are many ways for mutations to break a gene; there are many more ways for mutations to disrupt pathways. TBR1 appears to be regulatory gene that may influence the expression of up to 24 genes involved in autism in the developing neocortex (Notwell et al., 2016).

DEVELOPMENTAL TRAJECTORY STUDIES

The development trajectory for language skills is complex in autism, especially given that initial deficits are sometimes overcome later in life. In terms of language outcomes, autistics appear to fall into two groups. One group, which involves 15 percent of autistics, remain nonverbal throughout life. In the second group, which represents 40 percent of autistics, language skills progress and individuals become fluent and use complex speech (Lord et al., 2006). Nonverbal individuals also tend to have more severe symptoms of ASD, oral-motor difficulties (Gernsbacher et al., 2008), and intellectual disabilities (Luyster et al., 2008).

It appears that language-sensitive superior temporal cortices are hypoactive in ASD toddlers with poor language development outcome compared with those with good outcome (Lombardo et al., 2015). Two developmental trajectory groups were also seen in a longitudinal study using quantitative measures (Tek et al., 2014). In this study, nearly all measures remained flat for children with poor language development outcomes compared with those with better outcomes. In both studies, indicators existed early, which suggested at least two subgroups of language development delay within autism and ASD. Where these have a genetic or environmental basis is unknown. fRMI scans may prove useful in predicting eventual language development in children with autism; such predictions may be useful in constructing alternative pathways to teaching language and communication skills. Studies of the genetic basis—and the potential role of shifts in environmental exposures—in these two clinical groups are necessary.

ARE LANGUAGE FOCUS AND MOTION FOCUS SWITCHES REVERSED IN AUTISM?

The Lombardo et al. (2015) study also revealed a striking finding. When typically developing and mildly autistic children listened to and processed spoken language, a trade-off was observed between activity in two large-scale brain systems, one for language focus, and one for motion focus. Specifically, the sensory input caused a dampening of the somatomotor areas and primary visual areas, while the areas governing reward, emotion, and memory became more engaged. When severely afflicted autistic children processed language, the opposite occurred: their primary visual areas and motor areas engaged, but their reward, emotion, and memory regions showed little activity. Understanding what governs this focus switching may be critically important to helping autistics acquire the desire to learn (social reward and reinforcement learning theory).

Better oral and motor skills at a young age predicts later verbal fluency (Gernsbacher et al., 2008). This prediction makes sense given that if the motor skill activation and language activation are "cross-wired" or "miswired" (Fan et al., 2015) in autistics, intact motor skill processing networks would be necessary for proper language articulation. A potentially related interesting finding is that mothers of babies at high risk of autism spectrum disorder (ASD) use more hand gestures (Talbott et al., 2015). The behavior may be learned or there may be a genetic aspect of this preferred mode of communication (parental coping). The subset of ASD children with speech language difficulties differs from non-ASD patients, with specific language impairment in the low-level information domain of language (specifically, nonword repetitions, but not visual memory or processing speed; Hill et al., 2015). This difference suggests that language impairment in autism is a core symptom, not one that can be removed and replaced by a diagnosis of SLI for children with ASD and language impairment. Language impairment in autism, which for some involves the inability to perform the abstraction necessary to connect objects to works, and for others involve the ability to memorize words, may be a *phenomimic* (Bishop et al., 2010) of that in SLI after all.

Language abilities and autistic traits show high heritability and are negatively correlated, but genetic overlap between these two traits is low at the extremes, indicating unique sources of extreme autistic traits (Taylor et al., 2014). Deficits in language in autism are almost certainly partly due to deficits in learning. In advanced stages, most knowledge is deductive (from general cases to specific); however, learning is experimentally inductive (specific cases leading to attempts to generalize). Here, we see the link with observations in the classroom, that autistic children have difficulties with abstractions and generalizations. The repeated reports of an absence of low-level information processing means that inroads for learning may have to be built via high-level information channels (particulars, specifics, and details) and that learning how to make connections and generalizations is not intuitive for many with autism.

NEUROBIOLOGY/NEUROPATHOLOGY

A wide diversity of pathological malformations accompanied by measured dysfunctions, usually by fRMI scan, has been observed. Rodier et al. (1996) reported variation "from case to case" in which brain regions structural and functional anomalies appear. Abnormalities in minicolumnar structures are seen postmortem in the frontal and temporal lobes (Casanova et al., 2002). The authors wrote, "Specifically, cell columns in brains of autistic patients were more numerous, smaller and less compact in their cellular configuration with reduced neurophil space in the periphery." The minicolumn cores were wider in Brodmann 44 (BA44) region in neurotypicals, which includes Broca's area; loss of minicolumn architecture is likely involved in language impairment in ASD.

Minicolumn differences appear to be a macroscale representation of functionally related to neuronal cell shape changes and two major microfeatures: excitatory-inhibitory synapse numerical imbalance in ASD (Uzunova et al., 2015) and glial fibrillary acid protein glial fibrillary acid protein (GFAP) accumulation at the surface of the cell. Excitatory-inhibitory balance in ASD is reflected and measured as abnormal glutamatergic and GABAergic neurotransmission across numerous brain regions such as amygdala, cerebellum, hippocampus, and the neocortex in ASD. It is now known that aluminum causes excesses of GFAP filaments near the cell nucleus (Theiss et al., 2002). Rare risk CNV alleles have been reported involving $GABA_A$ receptor genes (Matsunami et al., 2013). Various lines of evidence also support that α5GABAA receptor deficiency can bring about behaviors seen in autism (Zurek et al., 2016).

Imaging studies of autism have provided key insights into developmental structural differences. We now understand that the aberrant trajectory of growth during early childhood is present in the whole brain, but is exaggerated in specific structures (including the amygdala and Broca's area.). Local and regional hyper- and hypoconnectivity are both seen, but a paucity of inhibitory synapses is by far the most generally seen form. Inhibitory synapses develop at the site of predecessor axon-dendrite contacts without any protrusive activity from axons and dendrites (Wierenga et al., 2008). This is in keeping with microglia both failing to foster reinforcement of GABAergic inhibitory synapses and instead devouring dendritic shafts and axon initial segments (early buds) while in their activated forms.

Specific regional dysmorphism and dysfunction (altered activity levels compared to a neurotypical state) vary with specific pronounced autism phenotypes. Mapping specific ASD phenotypes to specific regions has not been universally successful in language, speech, and communication deficient AD and ASD. For example, accelerated neocortical maturation (Courchesne et al., 2003) is seen in early AD, with laminar disorganization in the temporal cortex (Jacot-Descombes et al., 2012). There, auditory and language micro- and macrocircuits development is seen to be disrupted (Eyler et al., 2012; Williams et al., 2013). Variations on these themes abound; for the most part, it has proven difficult to nail down specific phenotypes to specific regions, reflecting another dimension of the complexity of ASD.

Variations in neuropathology have been sought for specific speech delay and language and communication pathologies in ASD, with some success, but with inconsistent results across studies. This is not unexpected given the genetic heterogeneity of AD and ASD. However, some results make good sense. Using verb challenge tests under fMRI scan, a study of ASD with language impairment found that modulatory control and automation function by the cerebellum is hampered by a loss of functional connectivity between the right cerebellar region and the supratentorial regulatory language areas and decreased connectivity between the interhemispheric Broca's region and modulatory control dorsolateral prefrontal region (Verly et al., 2014).

Abnormalities observed in the cerebellum of autistic individuals include reduction in Purkinje cell number, cytoarchitectonic abnormalities, and cytoplasmic inclusions in the deep cerebellar nuclei and vermal hypoplasia (Fatemi et al., 2012). White matter differences between SLI and autism indicate that specific microstructural properties may differentiate the two conditions. Specifically, autism was found to have axial diffusivity as a main indicator of damage, whereas SLI showed radial diffusivity as the primary effect on white matter microstructural properties. Axial diffusivity, indicative of autism white matter differences, is also a primary correlate of axonal injury due to autoimmune encephalomyelitis (Budde et al., 2009). Thus, the neurobiological signatures appear to specific microstructural damage, not large macrostructural differences, indicating persistent autoimmunological injury as a penultimate cause of autism, furthering the case for environmentally triggered autoimmune damages.

The ability of the brain of autistics to perceive secondary channels of information in spoken language is also a phenotype of interest. Impairment in the attribution of emotion or mental state within a voice (Rutherford et al., 2002) will impact learning meaning from context, and a low score on preference for their mother's voice (Klin, 1991) is an early indicator. Autism and ASD social deficits may be a partial product of a lack of perception of a highly significant portion of human speech.

RELATIONSHIP TO OTHER PHENOTYPES

Difficulty in learning categories by persons with autism has been attributed to executive dysfunction. A great deal of mastering language is learning categories of words and the relationships among the words (syntax and grammar). Chapter 6 contains more information on executive function phenotypes and learning categories.

Difficulties in language and communication are the first half of the story. Impairment in communication will also lead to delay in the acquisition of social skills (see Chapter 5).

SPEECH AND LANGUAGE SUMMARY

The genetic contributors to speech and language pathologies in autism can be distinct from those for SLI. They appear to involve comprehensive disruption of low-level information processing, possibly caused by hypoconnectivity. This leads to lack of developmental functional specialization among brain regions, or confusion by the brain in terms of when to switch modalities from motion processing to language processing. This finding suggests that modalities of learning language may exist in autistic children that are counterintuitive; that is, existing models of teaching language may not apply. For all sensory input, it seems that high-level information (detail) is absorbed, but its fundamental and functional low-level functions and interrelationships do not appear to register. Social reinforcement may be lacking in some with autism and ASD, hindering the development of a comprehension that one *should* want to learn language processing skills. Biomarkers are under development to discern patients with low probability of good language skill development. Attempts to use the available knowledge focused on use of high-level inputs to help the autistic child construct a mental picture of low-level relationships (details leading to generalizations) may prove fruitful. There are multiple molecular bases for these phenotypes, some of which are genetic in origin.

There are numerous lessons for genetic studies of autism from consideration of speech and language alone. If genetics and environment interact, the layered deficits may lead to the more obvious phenotypes, which themselves may not require further factors for cause, only modulators. The knowledge that histone modification can alter allele expression provides one likely mechanism for environmental exposure and the effects of aging on autism phenotypes. Studies of genes in autism may miss important associations if genes are studied independently. As we will see, studies of environmental factors may also be missed if they are studied for the whole population and not studied in the population of those individuals likely to be at higher risk due to inherited and de novo mutations. Studies of the mechanisms of genes and their expanded network of relationships may reveal one-off functional associations not seen in the consideration of the main, or best-known function of a gene, and thus molecular pathology should be studied in patients at the level of biological pathway.

References : see envgencauses.com

Chapter 5.

GENETIC AND ENVIRONMENTAL FACTORS THAT INFLUENCE SOCIAL COGNITIVE SKILLS IN ASD

In this chapter, the evidence for both genetic and environmental factors in determining social skills is explored. We have seen that, independent of any consideration of genetic data, the medical field has made decisions on disease classification based on the presence, absence, and degree of severity of specific phenotypes. It is now well established that autism is a multigenic condition that can be caused by environmental triggers interpreted against a given genetic background. After consideration of individual phenotype groups, or medical domains, that are found in varying degrees in individuals with autism, the next logical step is to explore how genetic variation contributes to the overall groups of phenotypes within autism, their occurrence in specific cases, and how they may modulate the degree of severity of manifestation. In this chapter, the literature on the genetic and environmental contributions to the social-affective phenotype are explored.

In most primate species and in many other social species, the meaning of actions or the assessment of the context of a situation is communicated by facial expressions, body movements, and vocalizations. The ability of individuals to engage as a member of a social species is dependent on their ability to receive signals sent via both visual and auditory cues, including facial expressions, body stances (threat), and vocalization. Intention of conspecifics is determined via a combination of these signals and by assessment of movement; for example, direction and speed of body motion can signal threat. Mating signals involve color, dances, and songs. The animal world is alive with perception.

Humans, of course, communicate a great deal of information using facial expressions. Some expressions are nearly universal across cultures, suggesting both a cultural and genetic basis of the meaning of specific facial expressions. Some of the social characteristics that indicate autism include decreased levels of smiling (Cassel et al., 2007), lower eye-to-eye gaze with mothers (Merin et al., 2007), limited ability for simultaneous teacher-subject matter focus, and preferential use of gestures (Cassel et al., 2007; Goldberg et al., 2005; Mitchell et al., 2006; Presmanes et al., 2007; Stone et al., 2007; Yirmiya et al., 2006). The absence of the use of pointing to elicit another person's attention to something or someone (joint attention) is an early indicator of autism (Sullivan et al., 2007). Such differences have a profound neurological basis in numerous areas of the brain (Engel et al. 2014), detectable by formal measures such as Reading the Mind in the Eyes tests (Baron-Cohen et al., 1997; Baron-Cohen et al., 2001).

HERITABILITY AND SEMI-INDEPENDENCE OF DOMAINS

Teasing apart genetic and environmental factors influencing personality is challenging because social skills are influenced both by genes and environment. Heritability of social cognitive skills has long been demonstrated (Scourfield et al., 1999). Social disabilities are often found among nonautistic siblings of autistics (Le Couteur et al., 1996). Based on the observations that half of genes responsible for heritability in each of the three main domains of autistic disorder (AD; social skills, repetitive movements, and communication difficulties) were domain specific, Happé et al. (2006) argued that autism might be fractionable and that no single gene or single treatment for autism would likely prove universally informative of a singular, coherent medical condition. They noted low correlations in autism-related behaviors within each of the domains in families. When viewed at the level of population, low correlations of behavior reflect high heterogeneity of the disease and diversity of genes contributing to autism and autism spectrum disorder (ASD).

Heterogeneity exists within social skills as well. Various heritable cognitive components of the social affective phenotype are variously manifest across the ASD population (Brunsdon et al., 2014).

We all recognize heritability of certain social characteristics and traits, and, of course, children learn society norms regarding social behaviors at a young age. The study of the heritability of social skills has been made semiquantitative via available scores and checklists, making assessment more objective.

Social Reciprocity Scale scores showed concordance of 0.73 for monozygotic twins and 0.37 for dizygotic twins (Constantino et al., 2000). Numerous others studies have been published demonstrating heritability of social cognitive abilities. Both the Social Responsiveness Scale (Constantino and Gruber 2005) and the Social and Communication Disorders Checklist (Skuse et al., 2005) scores show high heritability (Bölte et al., 2011). One of the best general reviews on sociality in autism to date is by Misra (2014).

RECOGNIZING EMOTION

Studies aimed at understanding the heritability of recognizing emotion have found indications of a genetic component. Neves et al. (2011) compared 40 parents of children with autism to 41 parents of healthy controls and found that parents of children with autism scored lower in a facial emotion recognition test than controls. Similarly, Oerlemans et al. (2014) studied 90 children with ASD, 79 unaffected siblings of ASD patients, and 139 controls (six to thirteen years) and found lower performance of unaffected siblings of ASD patients at recognition of facial emotion tasks compared to the controls. Partial heritability of these traits was apparent in 2008, when "bubbles" face-testing was used. Nonautistic parents of autistic children have reduced processing of the eye region and enhanced processing of the mouth compared to neurotypical controls (Adolphs, 2008). Some infants (four to seven months) at high-risk for ASD show atypical neural responses to human voices with and without emotion, compared to age-matched infants at low risk (Blasi et al., 2015). Early deficits may be apparent in some autistic children, but those differences can change with time (Pisula and Ziegart-Sadowska, 2015).

LOSS OF A THEORY OF MIND

Another interesting aspect of language skill deficits in children with autism is a dearth of words referencing mental state (Baron-Cohen, 1994). This may be related to concepts of failure to develop self-versus-other concepts of identity in the severely autistic, due to a failure to develop a theory of mind (ability to hold the perspective of another's mind). This is more than a deficit in empathy; the question is whether an individual knows the difference between one's own and another's mind. This may be caused in part by inability to perceive other people's feeling and thoughts, and thus to learn to distinguish "self" from "other." The combination of cognitive and perception deficits may lead to reduced capacity in growth and learning trajectories.

Empathy plays a key role in the social affect phenotype. The demonstration of awareness and consideration of another mind's perspective and the ability to demonstrate empathy denote the presence and therefore the ability to form a theory of mind (Baron-Cohen et al., 1985). As we have discussed, this ability may be hampered by perceptual limits and by the loss of ability of an individual to biochemically "enjoy" the rewards of social interaction, thus preventing reinforcement. Within the domain of social skills, additional genes may play a role in the ability to form a model of another's mind. ASD individuals with Prader-Willi syndrome have an especially reduced social cognitive functioning.

GENETICS OF EMPATHY AND SOCIALITY

Large-scale gene mapping studies show that heritable genetic variation across the human genome is responsible for approximately 20 percent of variation in social communication traits (e.g., Hopkins et al., 2014). This is notably much lower than the measures derived from behavioral measures. One reason is that the measure of genetic heritability and heritability of phenotype are distinct measures (Thapar and Harold, 2014). Mazina et al. (2015) found that CNVs interacted with maternal infection and brought about deficits in social communicative impairments and repetitive/restricted behaviors but not in cognitive and adaptive functioning.

The more important reason, however, is genetic heterogeneity of highly expressed traits. That is, most of the heritable genetic variation is unique to families, or at least represents mutations that have recently emerged. These are rare, low-frequency alleles. Under these circumstances, that same phenotypic effect of deleterious mutations scattered among different genes will appear, at the phenotypic level, to show high heritability, which it does from parent to child. However, different variants are responsible for the phenotypic heritability in different families. When all of the families are combined into very large mapping studies, very few of the genes will appear to be associated with the disease overall, and thus the population-wide heritability will appear low. This artifact will emerge more strongly when the environment has a major effect, and even more so when a gene × environment interaction exists.

Initial genome-wide association studies of social responsiveness found multiple loci distributed among many chromosomes (e.g., Duvall et al., 2007). Some single nucleotide variants with unknown function are included among the results. For example, a variant at SNO rs53576 with an AA genotype was associated with better social ability compared to the AG genotype, and a variant at SNP rs13316193 was associated with TT genotype associated with better social ability than the CC genotype. No variation was found significantly associated with autism diagnosis itself.

OXYTOCIN RECEPTOR (OXTR)

The neuropeptide oxytocin has a large influence on social and emotional behavior. It provides a type of "reward" feeling and is considered a strong bonding hormone. Present in breast milk, it helps babies form a strong bond with their mothers. It is also produced in the brains of lactating mothers, helping to produce the maternal bond.

Perception may be altered by oxytocin. Variation in face processing and genetic variation in the oxytocin receptor (OXTR) gene have been associated with social cognitive deficits and ASD traits in diverse ethnic and demographic populations (Wu et al., 2005; Ylisaukko-oja et al., 2006; Jacob et al., 2007; Lerer et al., 2008; Liu et al., 2010; Wermter et al., 2010).

Park et al. (2010) found that variation in the OXTR gene influences social cognition in ADHD probands. Specifically, two variants were found to be significantly different in frequency between more and less social ADHD patients. Oxytocin receptor variation interacts with social support to reduce measured stress levels (salivary cortisol levels; Chen et al., 2011).

Because previous studies had used small sample sizes with inconsistent results, Campbell et al. (2015) studied 25 markers in the OXTR locus using 1,238 pedigrees including 2,333 individuals with ASD. They found three variants to associated autism risk. LoParo and Waldman (2015) performed a meta-analysis and found association at both the gene level and four single-nucleotide variations. Association of variants in OXTR has been corroborated in multiple meta-analyses (Kranz et al., 2016). Measurements of the plasma oxytocin concentration and variations in the OXTR gene were found by Parker et al. (2014) to be useful in predicting social impairments in children, both with and without AD.

Some variation in the processing of emotion in the population is due to differential methylation (epigenetics) at the OXTR locus. Puglia et al. (2015) found that higher methylation at the OXTR locus was associated with decreased functional coupling of the amygdala with regions involved in affect appraisal and emotion regulation, and with face and emotion processing including the amygdala, fusiform, and insula. Elagoz-Yuksel et al. (2016) found evidence of differences in methylation at the OXTR locus in autistics compared to neurotypicals.

The epigenetic link points to environmental factors. The lack of genetic association does not mean that oxytocin will not be an effective treatment in many or even most cases. Plasma oxytocin levels are decreased in AD children (Modahl et al.,1998), and there is an excess of a truncated, prehormone form (Green et al., 2001). Studies support that oxytocin can lead to improvements in other domains as well. It has been shown to reduce repetitive behavior

(Hollander et al., 2003), with no serious adverse effects. Anagnostou et al. (2012) found medium-term (six weeks) treatment with oxytocin led to improvements in the Reading the Mind in the Eyes test and in the World Health Organization Quality of Life Questionnaire on emotion.

Oxytocin was administered via nasal spray in these studies, which also found that the duration of the benefit is short-lived. Dr. Bonnie Auyeung of the University of Edinborough is studying adjuvant treatments that might prolong the efficacy of oxytocin. Even if the treatment opens a window of time in which learning may be enhanced for autism and ASD patients, oxytocin could make a big difference in the ability of people on the spectrum to more fully participate in life. Dr. Auyeung is currently designing studies to look at the effects of oxytocin treatment on rates of learning sign language, spoken language vocabulary acquisition, and other measures of cognitive function, with the goal of defining clear translational end points that are relevant to the lives of children—now adults—with autism. Initially, there was some concern whether oxytocin administered via the intranasal route could cross the blood-brain barrier; however, numerous studies have now shown it to be found in higher amount both in blood and in cerebrospinal fluid after administration (e.g., Dal Monte et al., 2014).

It is not clear why, but Jansen et al. (2006) found higher levels of oxytocin in the plasma of adults with ASD. Hammock et al. (2012) pointed out that individual profiles in neuropeptides such as oxytocin and serotonin may prove to be useful in tailoring individualized approaches to treatment. A process of failed oxytocin update may also be at work.

It is important to recognize that genetic variants at the OXTR and other receptors do not *determine* behavior per se. However, studies of two emotional characteristics in neurotypicals, the speed of reactions to violations of trust and expressed satisfaction after betrayal (Takak et al., 2014), were each found to be associated with different variants within the OXTR locus. This degree of granularity of influence is surprising.

SEROTONIN, SEROTONIN RECEPTORS, SEROTONIN TRANSPORTERS, AND MICROGLIA

Serotonin (5-HT) is a synaptic neurotransmitter that is found in the CNS, blood platelets, and the gastrointestinal (GI) tract. In the GI tract, it helps regulates GI motility—the smooth muscle phasic contractions that effect waste transit through the gut. In platelets, it appears to aid in wound healing. In the CNS, upon release at the synapse, serotonin is taken up by 5-HT receptors. Serotonin is important in neural development, mediating synaptogenesis, neurite outgrowth, and neuronal migration. It has influences on many emotional phenotypes, including memory, cognition, learning, sleep, mood, anxiety, and aggression and appetite.

The serotonin transporter (or 5-HTT, also known as sodium-dependent serotonin transporter and also as solute carrier family 6 member 4, or SERT) is a protein that in humans is encoded by the SLC6A4 gene. Serotonin transporter is a type of monoamine transporter protein that transports serotonin from the synaptic cleft to the presynaptic neuron.

Serotonin encoding genes and those for its receptors and transporters have long been plausible candidates for autism genes due to observations that serotonin is increased in the blood of autistics. And indeed, studies of serotonin, serotonin receptors, and serotonin transporters have all borne fruit.

Serotonin receptor genes may also be autism phenotype modifier genes. This hypothesis is supported by the observation that autistics with the Lg allele of the 5HTTLPR promoter region were more likely to exhibit self-injurious behavior than those with the La allele (Kolevzon et al., 2014). Rare variants in adenosine A3, a serotonin 5HT regulator, are more prevalent in ASD cases than in controls (Campbell et al., 2013). Shirley et al. (2016) report variants in ZEB2, a transcription factor, and in HTR2C, a serotonin receptor, associated with self-injurious behavior.

Sometimes, the mechanism of disease is not absence of gene product. MOA-B is one of the proteins responsible for 5-HT degradation. A recent study found that variation around the MOA-B gene was associated with increased levels of platelet serotonin aggregation, and more pronounced autism, in males (Chakraborti et al., 2016).

MICROGLIA REGULATE SEROTONIN PRODUCTION

The glycogen synthase kinase 3β (GSK-3β) pathway is responsible for dendrite/axon ratio balance (Yoshimura et al., 2005). Microglia provide a physiological link between the serotonin system and the glycogen synthase kinase 3β-Wnt pathway through innate immune-system mediated neuroinflammation (Watkins et al., 2014). So where is the link to serotonin?

Remarkably, microglia have been shown to control the expression of serotonin in the brainstem (MacFarlane et al., 2015). The mechanism is likely through reduced serotonin synthesis from tryptophan via the kynurenine pathway (Lim et al., 2015). The kynurenine pathway, which is an intermediate step in the degradation of tryptophan to serotonin, is expressed in both macrophages and microglia (Guillemin et al., 2003). Microglial activation is also accompanied by kynurenine pathway activation in ALS (Chen et al., 2010).

Lim et al. (2015) directly observed dysregulated kynurenine pathway in ASD. Importantly, they established a link between inflammation, glutamatergic activity, and the kynurenine pathway. They also found a downstream metabolite, quinolinic acid, which enhances glutamatergic neurotransmission. Elevated levels of glutamatergic compounds are measurable with magnetic resonance imaging in ASD (Bejjani et al., 2012).

Microglia attack bacteria and other unwanted entities that express complement proteins. Microglia are also found near immature, postnatal synapses in response to the presence of the complement C1q, expressed by immature neuronal cells (Stevens et al., 2007), required for canonical brain development (Paolicelli et al., 2011). Dendrites and axons express complement protein C3, opsonizing the cell surface (making the cell surface more susceptible to phagocytosis by macrophages). Microglia express C3R/cd11b on their surface and recognize which extensions and buds to prune, engulfing C3-tagged processes (Schafer 2012; Tyler and Boulanger, 2012).

A definitive causal link has been established between neurotoxins, glutamate, and microglial activity in exquisitely fine detail. Mutations in any of the genes in these pathways will modulate brain functions in diseases and condition, including the maintenance of the balance between dendritic extension growth and pruning via microglia. Maternal induced immunity also introduces interleukin (IL)-6, which has been shown to also disrupt kynurenine pathway metabolite production (Brown et al., 2014).

SEROTONIN RECEPTOR GENE (HTR2A)

Reduced levels of binding of the 5-HT2RA serotonin receptor were seen in patients with Asperger syndrome, compared to controls (Murphy et al., 2006), in a variety of brain regions, including the total, anterior, and posterior cingulate; bilaterally in the frontal and superior temporal lobes; and in the left parietal lobe. Murphy et al. also found that receptor binding levels were significantly related to abnormal social communication.

Smith et al. (2014) confirmed their earlier studies that the GG variation at rs6311, located within the serotonin 2A receptor gene (HTR2A) locus, was associated with ASD in families, likely with increased expression of a long 5′UTR mRNA serotonin isoform. This variant was shown to modulate expression of HTR2A mRNA in the dorsolateral prefrontal cortex, via an alternative transcription start site, resulting in a longer 5′UTR with increased protein translation efficiency (Smith et al., 2013). Hranilovic et al. (2010) found association of the same allele (GG) in a Croatian population with AD. The variant also influences Alzheimer's disease and anorexia (Smith et al., 2014).

Depression in autistics and in first-degree relatives of ASD patients is common. There is strong evidence of microglial-mediated neuroinflammation associated with depression in manner involving serotonin. As in motor behaviors and seizures, serotonin is a key neurotransmitter. Specifically, glutamate-mediated excitotoxicity in depression was described by Dantzer and Walker (2014) as follows:

> *Kynurenine produced from tryptophan in a reaction catabolized by indoleamine 2,3 dioxygenase is transported into the brain where it is metabolized by microglial enzymes into a number of neurotropic compounds including quinolinic acid, an agonist of* N*-methyl-d-aspartate receptors. Quinolinic acid can synergize with glutamate released by activated microglia.*

Gadow et al. (2014) found the variation at the rs6311 locus was associated with the severity of depression in children with ASD. Abdelrahman et al. (2014) found that the G allele and the GG genotype at rs6311 (also known as 1438A/G polymorphism) of the 5-HT2A receptor gene were observed more frequently in children with autism than control. They also found a significant increase of homozygote A allele of the –1438A/G and CC genotype of the 102T/C polymorphism in ASD children with gastrointestinal disorders (GIDs) in autism.

Other variants in HTR2A are found to be associated with IQ, intellectual disability (ID), and language onset delay within ASD (Hervás et al., 2014).

A class of drugs called 5-HT2a antagonist have shown efficacy in treating bipolar disorder in Asperger syndrome patients (Vannucchi et al., 2014). The benefits included improved psychotic and behavioral symptoms and reduced social withdrawal. Mestre et al. (2013) reviewed the literature on the efficacy of 5-HT2a antagonists and reported little clinical impact on schizophrenia, depression, anxiety, obsessive compulsive disorder, and psychosis in Parkinson's disease or Alzheimer's disease. Biomarker-directed treatment may improve efficacy. Indiscriminate use of drugs on an entire population with high genetic and etiologic heterogeneity is not likely to be fruitful.

SEROTONIN TRANSPORTERS

The role of serotonin receptors in autism has been well studied. Studies have found association of variation with autism (e.g., Kim et al., 2002). Serotonin transporters modulate serotonin levels and localization. Event-related potentials (the reaction of the brain to stimuli) have been shown to be different in adults with ASD than neurotypicals when shown emotional facial expressions, and, interestingly, a specific variant in the serotonin transporter was also found to have a distinct neurological response (Faja et al., 2016). The serotonin transporter genotype of autistics determines (in part) the degree and rate of amygdala habituation to sad faces (Wiggins et al., 2014). Variants in serotonin transporter gene promoters have been found to be associated with self-injury in ASD (Kolevzon et al., 2014). Variation in serotonin in the blood of autistics can be caused by genes that regulate serotonin, transporters, and receptors (Hranilović et al., 2009).

ALUMINUM AND SEROTONIN

Cumulative exposure to aluminum in vaccines is a serious concern. Laabbar et al. (2014) found that aluminum caused increased serotonin levels in the dorsal raphe nucleus; however, they did not check the isoform produced. Given that mutations leading to the long isoform are associated with autism, future studies should measure isoform levels, not overall serotonin.

Lithium may be a neuroprotectant against oral aluminum neurotoxicity (Laabbar et al. 2014), although it can have some serious side effects.

SELECTIVE SEROTONIN UPTAKE INHIBITORS

In a study of prenatal exposure to selective serotonin uptake inhibitors, El Marroun et al. (2012) found that the use of selective serotonin uptake inhibitors is associated with autism, a number of autistic traits, and affective (social) phenotypes measured by the Social Responsiveness Scale. They also found that exposure to prenatal maternal depression was associated with PDD symptoms, but to a lesser degree. Numerous other studies have confirmed this observation (e.g., Gidaya et al., 2014). Gentile (2015) cautioned against jumping to conclusions; however, six of the eight studies confirmed the association, and Gurnot et al. (2015) found that gestational exposure to selective serotonin reuptake inhibitors (SSRIs) induced methylation changes in neonates.

We know that serotonin pathway genes carry risk alleles for autism; it is possible that the association is a correlation between the genetic risk of depression and of ASD. Gene enrichment or molecular allocation studies are needed; however, trials restricting mothers from exposure with follow-up on autism rates would be useful for fully characterizing the role of SSRIs and other gestational exposures.

Mercury in thimerosal causes downregulation of both the serotonin 2A receptor (5-HT2AR) and the dopamine D4 receptor (DRD4) in rats (Chen et al., 2013). Mercury also generates ROS in cells, and ROS inhibits Janus kinase (JaK) and its downstream STAT transcription pathways. Jak and STAT are involved in cytokine signaling leading to the activation of glial cells (Garrecht and Austin, 2011). Serum from autistic children injected into mice leads to autistic features, reversible by a peptide P6, which has been shown to provide a neuroprotective effect by modulating the CNTF/JAK/STAT pathway and LIF signaling and by enhancing brain-derived neurotrophic factor (BDNF; Kazim et al., 2015).

DOPAMINE D4 RECEPTOR (DD4R)

As in most heritable traits, variation in social abilities exist in the human population. There are differences among genders and a large environmental component. Ben-Israel et al. (2015) found that mutations in the dopamine D4 receptor interact with gender in their influence on a child's affective knowledge. Specifically, they found that boys with a 7R DD4R allele had higher affective knowledge scores than girls. Among children without the 7R allele, no significant effect of gender on affective knowledge was found.

A previous study had indicated that variation at the DD4R locus interacted with gender in their combined influence on cognitive empathy among adults in an opposite manner (Uzefovsky et al., 2014). Theory-of-mind abilities appear to have a similar genetic basis; Lackner et al. (2012) found that dopamine patients' receptor D4 status could predict preschoolers' abilities to express ideas related to theory-of-mind representation.

ARGININE VASOPRESSIN AVPR1A

Multiple studies have shown that mutations in arginine vasopressin V1a receptor gene (*AVPR1A*) are associated with degree of sociality in autism and variation in *AVPR1A* is related to social cognition in both neurotypical humans and chimpanzees (Hopkins et al., 2014; Yirmiya et al., 2006; Kim et al., 2002; Israel et al., in press). AVRP1A is a seven-transmembrane domain-containing G-protein coupled receptor (GPCR) related to oxytocin receptor. Variants in AVPR1A have been shown to be related to social attitudes (Knafo et al., 2007). Vasopressin in the plasma has been twice shown to be a robust biomarker for autism (Carson et al., 2015; Parker et al., 2015). In both studies, low blood vasopressin was strongly associated with low theory-of-mind ability, an aspect of social ability.

GFRA2, LNCRNAS, AND AN AUDITORY SIGNAL PROCESSING PROTEIN CODING GENE

Lowe et al. (2015) found two regions on chromosome 8 associated with social responsiveness variation in autism. One region, chr8p21.3, lies next to the GFRA2 receptor, which is part of the glial cell line-derived neurotrophic factor family (GDNF) involved in neuron survival and differentiation. In fact, the association was strongest in this region for an intronic variant in the gene GFRA2.

The other region includes some long, noncoding RNAs (lncRNAs, PVT1, RP11-47304.5 and RP11-62901.2) and the KIAA0143 protein, which reprograms auditory brainstem neurons. Specifically, mice with hearing deficits showed lowered expression of the KIAA0143 protein in the lateral superior olive compared to those with normal hearing ability. This may point to evidence of auditory processing variation in autism related to social skills.

Copy number variation in zinc finger protein 804A (ZNF804A) is associated with verbal deficiency in autism (Anitha et al., 2014).

NEUROBIOLOGY OF SOCIAL COGNITION

The regions of the brain considered to be involved in social cognition include the prefrontal cortex, anterior cingulate, medial parietal cortex, supramarginal gyrus, and middle and inferior temporal cortex.

Each of these regions involved in social cognition show chronic, sustained microglial activation in individuals with autism. Morgan et al. (2012) found microglial and neuronal variation in the prefrontal cortex of individuals with autism. Specifically, both microglial activation and increased microglial density in the dorsolateral prefrontal cortex of the autistic brain. Di Martino et al. (2011) found that children with ASD show abnormal functional connectivity between nearly all striatal subregions, including the right superior temporal gyrus. Chauhan et al. (2012) found reduction in glutathione GSH and increased amounts of oxidized glutathione GSSG in the cerebellum and frontal, temporal, parietal, and occipital cortex of postmortem brains of autistic patients, compared to age-matched neurotypical controls. Low levels of GSH play a significant role in microglial activation, contributing to the self-sustaining feedback loop of immunoneuroexcitotoxicity.

Brain scans of autistic individuals showed that highly idiosyncratic brain responses to passive observation of social situational comedy was associated with poor social comprehension of a character's motives (Byrge et al., 2015). The study found a great deal of heterogeneity in the types of patterns associated with watching NBC's sitcom *The Office*. Such findings have been reported in the past, but with inconsistency (Gallese et al., 2011).

INTRINSIC SENSORY PERCEPTION IN AUTISM: ROADBLOCKS TO LEARNING SOCIALITY?

Tannan et al. (2008) used a novel test to determine that neuronal disinhibition may underlie some outwardly antisocial behavior in autism. They used a vibratostimulatory device with and without a period of adaptive learning on autistic individuals and controls. The control individuals could autonomously and adaptively learn to modulate their response to the vibratostimulatory device, whereas autistic individuals could not. Excitatory/inhibitory imbalance in ASD, associated with abnormal glutamate or GABA signaling (Coghlan et al., 2012; Horder et al., 2013; Mendez et al., 2012), may in part explain the disinhibition. This implies a neurological basis of disinhibition-based behavioral traits. Such traits can include speaking too loudly without being aware of volume, not being aware of personal space norms, saying inappropriate things, and speaking at inappropriate times. Aggression and self-injurious behaviors are sometimes seen in severe AD. Specific measures are also consistent with at least part of the damage as the loss of inhibitory synapses, a known outcome of chronic microglial activation, which results from glutamate signaling.

DIFFERENCES IN AND LOSS OF PERCEPTION SKILLS

Sufficient attentiveness is essential for learning. As in learning language, perceptual attentiveness is required for learning certain social skills. Social skills are then also required in a learning setting. Autistic infants given stress stimuli tend to avoid looking at the source of the stimulation (e.g., sustaining focus on a toy) compared to neurotypical controls (Dawson et al., 2001), and thus stress avoidance behavior. This behavior may cause some with ASD to fail to learn critical social cues, especially in the area of conveyance of emotion.

Disruption of inhibitory signaling is evident in a study of binocular rivalry (Robertson et al., 2015, 2016). Binocular rivalry is a basic visual function that requires a balance of excitation and inhibition in the visual cortex. Neurotypical participants in the study showed correlation between binocular rivalry ability and both GABA and glutamate levels in the visual cortex. The correlation between GABA and binocular rivalry dynamics was completely missing in the autistic participants. The ability of autistics to learn to interpret social signaling certainly contributes to delays in learning social skills.

BIOMARKERS OF SOCIALITY

Parker et al. (2014) found that OXTR variation and its oxytocin concentration could predict social skills scores both independent of autism diagnosis and within those diagnosed with autism. Therefore, rather than a biomarker for autism and ASD, the work to date linking neural circuitry differences in socially able and less able individuals with autism may also reflect normal variation imposed on the autistic condition. This would imply that at least some of the genetic variation that modulates one of the main domains of autism may in fact be more of an interaction with deficits in cognitive communication abilities. If so, the DSM-5 combination of social and communication autism domains may ultimately be found useful for diagnosis but may be misleading for establishing well-defined (homogeneous) clinical populations for studies of biomarkers and etiology. For example, the degree of sociality present in an autistic individual may be more apparent than in others who may be better able to use inhibition routines to camouflage their lack of sociality (i.e., social masking). In these individuals, the neocortex would be seen to be involved in thinking about how to "appear" to be more social, whereas in instinctually social individuals, the regions are unable to provide that function. Other proposed biomarkers include measures of serotonin uptake (discussed in detail by Veenstra-VanderWeele and Blakely, 2012).

MEASURES

Social perception and abilities are measured clinically via Social Responsiveness Scale. Social Responsiveness Scale scores include social awareness, social cognition, social communication, social motivation, mannerism, and an overall T score. Studies on social perception indicate that it can be improved via education.

In some autistic individuals, the ability to pick up on social cues is hindered. In some severe cases, the ability appears to be completely missing. The causes of this have been studied from various angles. The differences in perception abilities may involve problems with sensory input such as low-level vision (Pei et al., 2014), hearing, and tactile sensations. Sensory processing deficits are also indicated (Pei et al., 2014).

Response to sensory stimuli in ASD was initially compared to and found to be similar to that in deaf-blind children (Kanner, 1943; Wing, 1969). Parent-reported sensory abnormalities showed high rates (Baranek et al., 2006; Klintwall et al., 2011) and are found across a variety of senses (Marco et al., 2011). More than 90 percent of individuals with ASD have some form of tactile, auditory, or visual hypersensitivity or hyposensitivity (Leekam et al., 2007). Studies of higher-level processing have reported less consistent results (as reviewed by Pei et al., 2014). High-level visual processing is thought to be exceptional in some autistics, as would be consistent with a propensity for paying attention to minute detail. As with many aspects of autism, a high degree of variation exists in the anticorrelation between low- and high-level spatial acuity. This is likely due to temporal divergence driven by diverse environment, initial differences, and heterogeneity in the underlying genetic and genomic variation. It is clear from other research, however, that both low-level and high-level spatial frequencies are used in the sensory processing of human faces (Cheung et al., 2008).

STUDIES ON RECOGNIZING EMOTION

Studies aimed at understanding the heritability of recognizing emotion and other social affective phenotypes have found indications of a genetic component. Neves et al. (2011) compared 40 parents of children with autism to 41 parents of healthy controls and found that parents of children with autism scored lower in a facial emotion recognition test than controls. Similarly, Oerlemans et al. (2014) studied 90 children with ASD, 79 unaffected siblings of ASD patients, and 139 controls (6 to 13 years) and found lower performance of unaffected siblings of ASD patients in their ability to recognize facial emotion tasks compared to controls. Partial heritability of these traits was also seen in 2008 with "bubbles" face testing. Nonautistic parents of autistic children have been found to have reduced processing of the eye region and enhanced processing of the mouth compared to neurotypical controls (Adolphs, 2008). The findings of Blasi et al. (2015) that high-risk infants can respond differently to human voices suggest that these differences are present in early life. Early deficits may be apparent in some autistic children, but those differences can change with time (Pisula and Ziegart-Sadowska, 2015).

The effect of autism on emotion and the presentation of emotion in autistics can be profound. The most thorough review of the role of emotion in the autism experience to date is by Lartseva et al. (2015), who conducted an unbiased literature review and concluded that sociological, perceptual narrowing (sensory alteration) and basic neurological factors influence the emotional impairments in ASD in light of altered development of sociality.

THE SOCIAL PARADOX OF SEVERITY

Autistics with severe symptoms often have fewer social contacts (including friends) and live in a relatively simplified social context. A study of anxiety (Mazurek et al., 2010) found that more severe AD symptoms were associated with fewer symptoms of anxiety and depression and poorer quality and fewer reciprocal friendships than study participants with existing, but limited, friendships. This does not mean that it is better for autistics to be socially isolated; however, depending on the child and the degree of severity exhibited, the result is important because anxiety and depression can influence retention in learning.

ANIMAL STUDIES

Along with a decrease in NMDA glutamate receptor (NMDAR) function, double knockout Shank2$^{-/-}$ mice carrying an ASD-associated microdeletion (copy number variation [CNV]) have reduced social interaction, perform less frequent social communication by ultrasonic vocalizations, and exhibit repetitive jumping (Won et al., 2012).

ARE EXPERIENCE-SEEKING BEHAVIORS INVERSELY RELATED TO GENETIC AUTISTIC TRAITS?

Autistic individuals experience two significant challenges socially. One challenge stems from a negative environment (e.g., risk of bullying, isolation), which induces preferences for isolation. This preference leads to restricted experiences and a dearth of opportunities to develop social skills. The second challenge results from a genetic basis of preferences that also leads to limited social exposure. A heritable component to preference in experience-seeking was found in a study of the distribution of that trait related to autistic traits (Romero-Martínez et al., 2015). Like everyone, choices, decisions, and preferences of AD and ASD individuals help determine their social environment. However, as we have seen, the biological/neurological basis of social preferences may be largely plastic to environmental influences. Caregivers, teachers, guidance counselors, and peers should consider whether they are contributing to a social environment for AD and ASD individuals that is different from the general population. Absent any risk of harm (aggression behaviors), such bias must be overcome via education and awareness.

MIRRORING, EMPATHY, AND IMPULSES

Autistic individuals sometime imitate the movements and speech of others. Studies that show a trade-off in language and motor skill abilities (Lambardo et al., 2015) imply that motor neural circuits and the language and speech circuits appear to be "cross-wired" during development. Visual inputs on body movements are encoded in the sensorimotor (motor cortex) area of the brain (Orgs et al., 2016). Control of one's movement in anticipation of a stimulus involves completely different areas (inferior frontal gyrus, anterior insula, and intraparietal cortex; Di Russo et al., 2015). The story of automimicking may lie in the lack of inhibition in these areas, combined with a confusion of input from the motor cortex by the anterior insula.

MIRROR NEURONS

We all may experience empathy with body movement as a way of "knowing" where another person or animal will likely be as we project their path in the immediate future. In that case, the lack of inhibition alone may suffice to induce imitative behaviors. Anytime you have experienced a "jolt" watching another person fall, you are feeling this innate form of autonomous empathy. A body of evidence exists that suggests that we empathically register the experiences of others by, in part, coexperiencing them in a type of internal simulation.

The concept of *mirror neurons* emerged approximately 20 years ago, when macaque monkeys showed signs of firing a set of neurons while observing hand movements in other monkeys. A response identical to those fired when they moved their hands themselves. In humans, empathic excitability of the motor cortex occurs while seeing and hearing speech (Watkins et al., 2003). It is thought that activity in the ventral premotor cortex and inferior frontal gyrus that occurs in response to watching biological movement represents mirror neuron activity.

However, empathy for pain involves neither the posterior insula and secondary somatosensory cortex nor the sensorimotor cortex under experimental conditions (Singer et al., 2004), although the uncontrolled jolt typically experienced by seeing someone fall would imply an evoked motor response. Mirror neurons have been proposed as being involved in the arousal of emotion by music (Gridley and Hoff, 2006; Molnar-Szackacs and Overy, 2006).

Interpretation of the many studies that attempt to identify mirror neurons in humans has been controversial due to lack of reproducibility (Gallese et al., 2011). At the root of the question is not so much whether mirror neurons exist, but rather whether their activation is required for action understanding. The fields that study autism have seen a schism on whether autistics are aware of intentions of others. From the beginning, Kanner reported that autistic individuals showed fear of a needle upon being pricked, but not of the person holding the needle. Observations like this and the tendency of autistics to imitate others' movements, but to be apparently unaware of others' imitation of their movements, are potentially reconciled via a shift in the focus of the functional role in a mirror neuron circuit that involves the sensory motor cortex in the first place.

The human mind experiencing cognition understands information via different modes. When we read or are spoken to, the sensorimotor cortex is not necessarily involved. When we watch motion, however, especially biological motion, the information is apparently passed through motor cortex circuits. It is unlikely that we need this to cognitively understand motion, or intention. However, animals evolved in a setting in which motion either meant *food* or *you're about to be eaten;* thus, the ability to build up potential for rapid reaction is highly advantageous.

The lack of inhibition is clearly evident in the excitatory/inhibitory E/I neuronal imbalance in autism, and therefore the dampening of signals that occurs in neurotypicals may merely reveal a lower trigger of neurological discharge. The theory-of-mind ideas of failure to comprehend intention (action understanding) are not as well supported (see the exchange in 2011 by the Mirror Neuron Forum in Gallese et al., 2011).

Alternatively, combined with a lack of inhibition, the imitation may be the result of another example of cross-wiring. When combined with a lack of inhibition, the autistic brain may confuse input visual signals as actionable impulses and express imitation not as a form of emotive empathy, which implies reaction, but as reactionary motor actions. Research in this area with fMRI indicates differences that support these possibilities (Iacoboni, 2011). Developmentally, unusual maturation processes appear to be at play, leading to variations in roles in which different regions of the brain are utilized to perform and/or control. Autistics also appear to process motion, rather than emotional signals, when processing facial expression (Han et al., 2015). These differences in processing do not mean that autistics live in an emotionless, sterile world. In fact, it could mean quite the opposite. Cross-wiring means that they may route emotional impulses through any number of pathways not usually activated in neurotypicals. Research on the alternative processing of affective information without biological movement could be instructive.

UTILITY FOR EARLY DETECTION/RISK PREDICTION?

Lloyd-Fox et al. (2012), using functional near-infrared spectroscopy, found that temporal lobe specialization for processing visual and auditory social stimuli during infancy differs between infants at risk and those not at risk. Infants aged four to six months at risk for autism showed less selective neural responses to social stimuli (auditory and visual) than low-risk controls.

IMPLICATIONS FOR TREATMENT

The existence of a genetic contribution to social ability in autism must not be used (or abused) as an excuse to not provide educational and enrichment opportunities. That is, genetics do not always determine one's fate. Here is an example: in a study of the ability to develop empathy and a theory of mind, individuals with autism were given the chance to control external representations of themself and others (de Guzman et al., 2016). The exercises helped these children progress in their scores for social skills. Another way to think about this is that variation in social skill of non-ASD individuals should not be used as an excuse to not educate or train unaffected people. Instead, biomarkers of sociality, genetic or otherwise, may inform one more or less effective means of educating autistics and ASD individuals. We must never forget that brain plasticity is strongly impacted by our environment (i.e., our experiences).

If a mixed-marker risk prediction model could be developed that utilizes familial information, such as presence of first-degree relative with autism and ASD, age of parent, presence of one or two genetic markers, followed by functional near-infrared spectroscopy under social and auditory stimuli, early intervention could be more frequent. The genetic markers could also point to specific routes to therapy and dietary changes to reduce toxic load.

Also, given that cross-wiring and different-purposing of brain regions appear to play significant roles in the rendering of classic autistic phenotypes, reinterpretation of stereotypical autistic behavior is needed. Nadel (2015) points out that imitation may be a route for learning by individuals with neurological conditions and may not be something that should necessarily be corrected or discouraged. He cites a coupling between perception and action resulting in imitation in autism.

References : see envgencauses.com

Chapter 6.

COGNITIVE PHENOTYPES IN ASD

Intellectual disability is seen in some autistics and is therefore not included as core autistic spectrum disorder (ASD) symptom. Executive functioning deficits are seen in many autistics. However, one of the most important focal areas for understanding autism—and for understanding our species—is the study of cognitive development and ability. What factors establish the range of intelligence quotient (IQ) and executive function abilities in autistics? The need to answer this question is shedding light on how the human brain works. Perhaps it is not unexpected, given the multitude of ways in which biological pathways can be disrupted in autism, that multiple ways exist by which the brain itself may become dysfunctional. The ability of individuals to plan, stay focused on a task, use working memory, and control immediate responses has utility in terms of raw survival skills and the ability to fit into social networks.

Much of the same genetic variation that contributes to intellectual variation in autism also contributes to variation in cognitive functioning in the general population. Notable rare exceptions to this include potential variants that contribute to reversible oxidation pathway deficiencies due to mitochondrial dysfunction, which can also be caused primarily by environmental exposures. Individual rare genetic mutations that contribute to intellectual disability may also be found in autistics individuals, and these tend to involve fundamental cellular processes such as transcription and translation, cell-cycle control, energy metabolism, and fatty-acid synthesis.

INTELLIGENCE (INTELLECTUAL ABILITY)

Intelligence is bimodal in ASD, polygenic, and multifactorial in origin and a topic of great interest. In the general population, approximately 66 percent of heritable genetic variation is explained by ancient, common variants (Plomin et al., 2013). A study by

Davies et al. (2011) estimated that 40 percent of the variation in crystallized-type intelligence and 51 percent of the variation in fluid-type intelligence are accounted for by unknown genetic variants among individuals in the general population.

Approximately 70 percent of individuals with autistic disorder (AD) show general cognitive ability impairment (that is, intellectual disability [ID]; Fombonne et al., 2006). A much smaller percentage of individuals with ASD show ID. Intelligence in autism may be underestimated (Dawson et al., 2007), but that depends on how one measures intelligence (Bölte et al., 2009). Children with autism can exhibit superior math skills with a neurobiological basis. Iuculano et al. (2014) found that children with ASD had better numerical problem solving abilities in general. They clearly think differently: the children were observed to rely on sophisticated decomposition strategies for single-digit addition problems more frequently than neurotypical peers. Differences were seen in ventral temporal-occipital cortex, posterior parietal cortex, and medial temporal lobe activity when solving more complex math problems. Patterns in ventral temporal-occipital cortical areas predicted individual numerical problem solving abilities in ASD, but not in neurotypical, children. Those areas were previously known to be involved in face processing.

Another study (Turi et al., 2015) found that the same type of sensory perception variation present in AD: low flexibility in how to perform math operations (adaptation in numerosity) is seen. Autistics may be less likely to use prior information in solving problems, leading to faulty general reasoning, with less ability to transfer knowledge from one situation to the next. This may be traced to inefficiencies in the adaptive interpretation of sensory signals, with difference in processing in both parietal and temporal functions (Turi et al., 2015). If one varies a stimulus for a person with AD, one may expect variation in responses. Autistics tend to show low predictive ability in multiple cognitive tasks (Sinha et al., 2014). Compassion and patience, without pity, is the best prescription for parents, caregivers, and educators.

How can these two perspectives be reconciled? In a highly controlled and simplified environment, autistics will likely excel at a given task when it is presented in a manner suitable to their sensory perception, that is, a narrow focus. Transfer of knowledge may have to be explained in concrete terms. Autistics do not always perform generalization tasks without all of the intermediate steps being laid down for them. Similar explanations exist for discordant findings of superior peripheral vision in AD.

GENES ASSOCIATED WITH VARIATION IN GENERAL COGNITION IN ASD

Because some variants in the human population associated with variation in intelligence are common, any genes associated with intelligence impairment or enhancement in ASD may be expected to be associated with variation in intelligence in neurotypicals, and vice versa. A cross-sectional study of polygenic-based risk-allele markers for AD was found to be associated with higher intelligence in neurotypicals, provided they do not have AD. The cross-sectional study examined genetic variation in more than ten thousand individuals from Scotland and Australia and found a slight edge in intelligence, measured by a battery of instruments.

Intelligence in humans is largely polygenic, although a few standout genes are interesting to consider. The gene FNBP1L is associated with general cognitive ability. Its function in the nerve cell is to enhance the transfer of signals from the cell surface to the actin cytoskeleton by promoting CDC42-induced actin polymerization, increasing the speed at which nerve cells can change shape in response to external stimuli. Three studies have found strong gene-level association of variation in FNBP1L with measures of cognitive ability in humans (Hill et al., 2014). However, to date, no variation in FNBP1L has been found to influence cognitive differences between ASD and neurotypical humans. Other genes found by Hill et al. (2014) to be associated with general cognitive ability include BCAR3, RFFL, OR4P4, and EIF5A2. To date, no studies have been published that attribute intellectual impairment in ASD to variation in any of these genes.

Approximately 50 percent of the heritability of cognitive ability in the general population is explained by common variants in the population. Compared with the genetic heritability of general cognitive ability (approximately 80 percent at adolescence), the increase in cognitive ability afforded by AD risk alleles is tiny (approximately 0.05 percent). This means that in addition to heritable variation, much of the genetic determination of intelligence will be determined by environment and by de novo genetic variation. Severe impairment will almost certainly be found in specific cases to be due to acute toxicity, or to de novo variation, such as CNVs. Sander et al. (2015) found that ASD individuals at the low end of cognitive ability had more CNVs, and Iossifov et al. (2015) found, in severe autistics, a surprising number of rare loss-of-function (LoF) deleterious mutations in genes involved in brain development, with biased transmission from mothers.

Rare genetic variants tend to lead to recessive genetic traits; that is, those that only appear to manifest themselves when both parents contribute the same allele. Najmabadi et al. (2011) examined deep sequencing results across numerous cognitive disorders and found that rare variants that may contribute general risk of ID genes tend to be involved in cellular operations such as transcription and translation, cell-cycle control, energy metabolism, and fatty-acid synthesis. There did not appear to be, across various conditions with ID, specific sets of neurological genes shared across conditions in which ID is found.

Some of the better-studied genetic variants, with positive findings of association with intelligence differences and cognitive ability in ASD and closely related conditions, are included here. Sporadic de novo mutations associated with severe AD, which is typified by extreme intellectual impairment, are reported by O'Roak et al. (2011) and include FOXP1, GRIN2B, SCN1A, and LAMC3. Of these, SCN1A is particularly associated with sensitivity to vaccine-induced encephalopathy. In the FOXP1 mutation carrier, they also reported an inherited, but rare, variant of CNTNAP2, providing evidence for the multiple-hit hypothesis. Contactin-associated protein-like 2 is a neurexin neuronal-adhesion molecule and receptor. Mutations in both FOXP2 and CNTNAP2 are linked in numerous studies to speech and language disorders and ASD (Chien et al., 2013). For a review that emphasized causality of de novo mutations, see Ronemus et al. (2014).

MONOAMINE OXIDASE A

Monoamine oxidase A (MAO-A) is an important enzyme that catalyzes the oxidative degradation of serotonin (5-hydroxytryptamine, 5-HT). Recalling that microglial cells modulate serotonin production (MacFarlane et al., 2015), the effects of mutations in MAO-A can present phenomimicry in which different causal factors of fundamentally distinct nature can render the same effects on phenotype.

A functional MAO-A promoter region polymorphism was found to be associated with IQ (Yirmiya et al., 2002). Variation in MAO-A is known to be associated with antisocial, aggressive, and preservative behaviors in humans and mice (Bortolato et al., 2013), and mouse models display autism-like phenotypes (Bortolato et al., 2013). Morphological similarities include reduced thickness of the corpus callosum, dendritic complexity of pyramidal neurons in the prefrontal cortex, and disrupted microarchitecture of the cerebellum (Bortolato et al., 2013). Ameis et al. (2016) found disruption in interhemispheric circuitry in the corpus callosum shared by ASD, attention deficit hyperactivity disorder (ADHD), and, to a lesser extent, obsessive-compulsive disorder (OCD) patients. Variation in a MAO-A promoter confers increased risk of autism, with an apparently maternal inheritance pattern (Tassone et al., 2011), with cortical enlargement and low activity in autism and with ADHD and anxiety in autism (Roohi et al., 2009).

The genetic contributors to autistic traits and intelligence appear to be largely independent (Hoekstra et al., 2010). This matches previous work that showed that approximately 60 percent of ASD individuals have nonverbal IQs similar to typically developing children, while many others exhibit intellectual disability (Fombonne, 2005; Tidmarsh & Volkmar, 2003).

BRAIN-DERIVED NEUROTROPHIC FACTOR

Many genes important in autism also contribute to measurable variation in the unaffected population. For example, variation in the brain-derived neurotrophic factor (BDNF) and 5-HT2A serotonin receptor influences performance on standardized cognitive tests (Cirulli et al., 2010). BDNF is a key neurotrophin that regulates synaptic plasticity, neuronal differentiation, and survival. Low levels of BDNF are reported in a number of neurodegenerative and psychiatric disorders.

Tsai (1995) posited that autism may be caused by hyperactivity of BDNF. A study of 48 ASD and 29 age-matched controls found higher levels of BDNF in the serum of ASD patients compared to controls (Kasarpalkar et al., 2014). Similar results were found by Bryn et al. (2015) in plasma from 65 ASD patients compared to 30 neurotypicals, with difference in BDNF in autistics with ID, but no pro-BNDF differences. Wang et al (2015) compared 75 autistics with 75 neurotypicals and found elevated BDNF in the autistics. Many studies have replicated this finding in humans. Valproaic acid, a known cause of autism, increases BDNF in early brain development of mice (Almeida et al., 2014). Brain-derived neurotrophic factor is trophic for serotonergic neurons (promotes the survival and differentiation of 5-HT neurons) and a lack of a functional serotonin transporter reduces BDNF expression in early postnatal development (Calabrese et al., 2013).

The most common polymorphism in BDNF is G196A. This variant changes the amino acid at the 66th position from a valine to a methionine. Brain-derived neurotrophic factor may be regulated by MeCP2 (Schanen, 2006), again reflecting the overlap with Rett syndrome involving the product of the gene used for diagnosis.

Levels of BDNF in serum and mutations in the gene are just some of the ways in which BDNF varies in autism and among autistic families. Various isoforms of the protein exist, presumably due to alternative splicing (Halepoto et al., 2014). Variations of this type result from different combinations and orders of exons in messenger RNA, and can result from mutations in upstream regulatory regions. There is no doubt that as more investigations in alternative splicing are undertaken, variation in amounts of proteins in serum may be found to reflect variation in the form of protein present.

CONTACTIN-ASSOCIATED PROTEIN-LIKE 2 (CNTNAP2)

Contactin-associated protein-like 2 is a member of the immunoglobulin superfamily. The CNTNAP2 gene shows variation in individuals with intellectual disability, but also with seizures, autistic features, and language impairment. Shifts in connectivity in the frontal lobe have also been associated with CNTNAP-2 genetic variants.

MITOCHONDRIAL DYSFUNCTION AND INTELLECTUAL DISABILITY

The role of mitochondrial dysfunction in intellectual disability is evident due to its appearance within numerous conditions associated with low ID, including Down syndrome, Fragile X, Rett syndrome, and autism (Valenti et al., 2014).

EXECUTIVE FUNCTIONS

Executive functions (EFs) include scheduling ability, planning ability, sustained attention, cognitive flexibility, inhibitory control, learning categories, and central coherence (i.e., local processing). Each of these abilities is measured by a number of instruments, but few genetic studies have been conducted to identify genes contributing specifically to variation in these abilities. It is known that individuals with executive function difficulties experience a worsening from childhood to adolescence. Mercado et al. (2015) found high variation among autistics in the area of learning categories.

It is also known that genetic factors for EF variation in ASD may be unrelated to the variation that contributes to ASD risk. McLean et al. (2014) found that parent-reported EF deficits were related to profound decreases in adaptive functioning, regardless of age, IQ, and severity of ASD symptoms. However, they also found that first-degree unaffected relatives of autistics did not demonstrate EF difficulties.

Understanding the dynamic nature of EF during the development lifespan of patients, and the fact that much of the research in autism has occurred during a period in which something is causing a major increase in its incidence, EF worsening may be due to the same factors that contribute to increasing incidence. It may be difficult to derive from studies conducted over the past fifteen years to discern causality for any factor due to a massive cohort effect. Therefore, direct age-matched analyses may be most useful for identifying genetic variation that contributes to EF disparities in autism, and for studying ASD trait variation in general.

References : see envgencauses.com

Chapter 7.

REPETITIVE MOTOR BEHAVIORS AND SEIZURE PHENOTYPES

There are between two and six independent phenotypic subtypes of repetitive motions (Bishop, 2013). Two phenotypes that are well supported are repetitive sensory motor and insistence-on-sameness behaviors. Repetitive sensory motor behaviors include stereotypic motor behaviors, sensory-seeking behaviors, and repetitive manipulation of objects. Insistence on sameness preferences are typified by compulsions, rituals, and difficulties with changes in routine. Insistence on sameness appears to be independent of IQ. The other subtypes include self-injury, rocking, unusual fears, and circumscribed interests. Some of these are correlated with each other and some with IQ (e.g., circumscribed interests; Bishop, 2013). That means that multiple levels of discovery exist. Studies seeking a genetic basis therefore should be conducted as phased studies (pilot, discovery, evaluation, validation) to understand the biological basis and independence of the various potential subtypes.

The main patterns in the autistic brain of simplified synapses and widespread excitatory/inhibitory synapse ratio (with a dearth of inhibitory synapses) make understanding the cellular basis of repetitive movements, stuttering, tics, hyperactivity, and perhaps seizures easy to comprehend. The absence of inhibitory synapses prevents the feedback signals required to shut down motor signals. It also makes the sensory overload experience easy to understand. Our senses become satiated with repetitive input, and the lack of inhibitory synapses may make the satiation process ineffective.

GENETIC VARIATION ASSOCIATED WITH REPETITIVE MOTION

One study found an association between specific genetic variations and repetitive behaviors. Silverman et al. (2008) studied more than 350 individuals with autism spectrum disorder (ASD) and found that those with reduced repetitive motion tended have a mutated SLC25A12 gene, the nuclear-encoded mitochondrial aspartate-glutamate carrier.

IMITATION BEHAVIORS

ASD patients have been found to exhibit increased imitation of hand actions compared with neurotypical controls (Spengler et al., 2010). This increase was associated with lowered brain activation in areas involved in mental state attribution (the medial prefrontal cortex and temporoparietal junction). Differences in theory of mind are suggested.

Diagnosis of autism and ASD usually involves behavioral analysis. Motor movements such as uncontrollable hand flapping, tics, motor imitation, and gaze variations (e.g., aversion) are all useful indicators of autism. Underlying these behaviors are aberrant motor neuron and motor inhibition neurological circuits. It seems highly likely that the impetus for language processing, including input and cognitive processing of language and self-generated language processes (output) may inappropriately trigger motor circuits. Signal-routing errors are accompanied by a trade-off of language and communication activity. Misactivation of primary visual areas and motor brain areas by language stimuli, for example, are supported by the findings of Lambardo et al. (2015).

Stereotypical movements are typical of the severe autistic disorder (AD) experience. According to first-hand descriptions, autistics' sensory world is filled with information that appears to come to them incessantly and unfiltered, and can be overwhelming. Many with ASD exhibit perseveration behaviors, including repeating a behavior, word, thought, or activity long after the stimulus or rationale for the action has discontinued. Exercising a preference for a seemingly restricted number of interests to reduce stress is likely caused by a lack of autonomous feedback inhibition of input signals (see Markram and Markram, 2010). Sometimes the world of autistics can be one of sensory overload. Hypersensitivity to sound was reported in patients with variants in the contactin genes CNTN5 and CNTN6 (Mercati et al., 2016). Kashevarova et al. (2014) described a microdeletion involving CNTN6 and two other genes in a set of twins with atypical autism. The other two genes did not appear to contribute to the AD or intellectual disability (ID) phenotypes. Our firsthand experience should prevent acceptance of these behavioral variations as necessarily pathological, in a clinical sense, as opposed to conscious preferences of a mind attempting to cope with stress. Who would not want to find a way to control overwhelming inputs?

Molecular endophenotypes involved can be understood at the cellular and molecular level; indeed, perseveration can result from physical (e.g., blunt trauma) types of brain injury as well. A lack of ability to prioritize sensory inputs is likely due to profound differences in circuitry among brain regions—not merely multiple instances of first-order filtering. The information from many senses courses through the brain unchecked, activating uncontrolled motor and behavioral phenotypes.

It is important to note that anxiety appears to be independent of ASD and should be handled and diagnosed separately (Gotham et al., 2013).

GENETIC VARIATION ASSOCIATED WITH ASD BEHAVIORAL PHENOTYPES

A variety of genes contribute to the behavioral domain as well. Brune et al. (2006) found an association between a 5HTTLPR long-long genotype in the serotonin transporter gene (SLC6A4) and repetitive sensory-motor behaviors. Mice lacking the gene for the chemokine receptor Cx3cr1 showed depressed microglial activity and lowered synaptic pruning. They also showed increased repetitive movements, as well as reduced social behavior (Zhan et al., 2014). Variation in the GABRB3 locus (with gamma-aminobutyric acid-receptor subunit gene) is associated with insistence-on-sameness factor score in families (Shao et al., 2003). An excellent review for genes that appear to contribute to repetitive motor behaviors is Lewis and Kim (2009).

MOTOR SKILL STUDIES SUPPORT CORE STATUS

Motor skills studied were highly correlated with autism severity and IQ (Hilton et al., 2012). Hilton et al. found that 83 percent of ASD scored at least a full standard deviation below age-matched unaffected controls, whereas only 6 percent of ASD siblings scored that low. Green et al. (2009) found 79 percent of autistics with motor impairment (specific types), and that everyday adaptive behavior was no different once IQ was used to adjust. The coordinations of interpersonal in-phase and out-of-phase rhythmic motor movement (drumming) was found to be impaired in young autistics (Isenhower et al., 2012). Metanalysis supports substantial motor coordination deficits in ASD (Fournier et al., 2010).

Variants in a number of genes—MeCP2, SHANK3, Neurexin 1 (NRXN1) deletion, and AUTS2—have been associated with hypotonia, stereotypes, and/or motor delay. Variants in the RNA-binding protein FOX1 (RBFOX1) have been associated with motor asymmetry (abnormalities restricted to or more pronounced in a specific limb or to limbs on one side of the body).

SEIZURES IN AUTISM SPECTRUM DISORDER

The measles, mumps, and rubella (MMR) vaccine can produce febrile seizures in children with genetic variations in the genes IFI44L and CD46. A direct, simple causal link is apparent: CD46 is a known as a binding site for the measles virus—and it is also lost from apoptotic cells and stimulates phagocytosis by microglial cells (Griffiths et al., 2009). In the same study, variation in the genes ANO3, SCN1A, SCN2A, and TMEM16 were found to be associated with increased risk of febrile seizures in children in which the MMR vaccine plays no immediate role.

Thalamocortical seizures are common in both epilepsy and autism. Using functional magnetic resonance imaging (fMRI), Nair et al. (2013) found both anatomical and functional thalamocortical underconnectivity in both ASD and thalamocortical epilepsy. They also found evidence of microstructural compromise in tracts between thalamus and motor cortex, indicating a role in other motor phenotypes in ASD.

Other genes with variation found in ASD with seizures include the ubiquitin-protein ligase E3A gene UBE3A (Nurmi et al., 2001), TSC1 and TSC2 genes (Duyu Nie et al., 2010), SYN1 (Fassio et al., 2011), and the SHANK genes (Díaz-Anzaldúa et al., 2015). The specificity of any of these genes and their role in seizures is, at yet, unclear. TSC2 is involved in neuronal pathfinding (axon guidance).

Nevertheless, at least with environmentally induced excitotoxicity, it is possible that microglial activation may be involved as a causal factor in seizures (Zattoni et al., 2011). We have seen how microglial activation disrupts serotonin production and prevents the growth of inhibitory synapses. Now we see a possible link between the excitotoxicity and some of the most distressing—and socially isolating—symptoms in autism, as predicted by Chugani et al. (2004).

A NOTE ON SEIZURES

Triggers of seizures in epilepsy are difficult enough to nail down; given severe autistic disorder, nearly impossible. However, parents and caregivers of autistic individuals may do well to use diaries to chronicle events that occurred in the hours or days leading up to a seizure and then, after a few weeks, or months, look for trends. This approach may help identify dietary and sensory inputs that could lead to seizures (e.g., monosodium glutamate and other sources).

The potential clinical indications of this for individuals with autism in terms of biofeedback are immense. If language input, including self-input, is shown to trigger somatomotor areas, biofeedback could help individuals learn to better control their responses, perhaps by visualizing a new channeling of the information into language processing centers of the brain.

SOLUTE CARRIER FAMILY GENES, AUTISM, AND SEIZURES

(This section is dedicated to Brandon G. and his family.)

The Solute Carrier (SLC) family includes more than 300 genes that provide instructions for making solute carrier proteins, which transport various molecules and solutes across cell and organelle membranes. Defects in many of the solute carrier genes are implicated in numerous diseases. Transport of solutes is essential for cellular and intercellular functioning, both for cellular function and for excretion. Without proper function, solutes may further accumulate to toxic levels within and outside of cells.

Solute carrier family genes are implicated in a variety of ways in autism, including risk genes, specific phenotypes (notably seizures), and environmental susceptibility. This reflects the varied roles of SLC genes, which transport glucose, metal ions, neurotransmitters, and creatine. The nature of the contribution of each gene to autism depends on the specific role of the gene. SLC6A4, a serotonin transporter, is discussed in detail with other serotonin transporters in chapter 5. Mutations in SLC9A6 have been associated with X-linked ID (Gilfillan et al., 2008), Angelman-like phenotypes (Gilfillan et al., 2008), and autism (Garbern et al., 2010). Variation in the SLC9A9 gene has been associated with autism (Morrow et al., 2008), ADHD (de Silva et al., 2003), and the age of onset of ADHD (Lasky-Su et al., 2008). SLC1A2 is a solute carrier family 1 (a glial high affinity glutamate transporter member). It is a membrane-bound protein and the primary transporter that uptakes the excitatory neurotransmitter glutamate from extracellular spaces near synapses. If glutamate clearance is inefficient, synaptic formation and reinforcement activation does not occur, and neuronal damage can result from excessive activation of glutamate receptors and microglial excitotoxic activation. SLC1A2 mutations have been found in higher frequency with individuals with autism in WAGR syndrome (Xu et al., 2008).

There is some indication that mutations in the SLC2A1 (solute carrier family 2 member 1) may be involved in autism, but this awaits confirmation. The SLC2A1 regulates the glucose transporter protein type 1 (GLUT1), which mediates glucose entry into glial cells.

Mitochondrial dysfunctions have also been related to seizures in general, independent of ASD (Zsurka et al., 2015).

SEIZURES AND MICROGLIA

Brain inflammation via innate immunity involving microglial is widespread in epilepsy. Dambach et al. (2014) found that valproic acid did not reduce the ill effects of microglial activation in cell culture, whereas treatment with carbamazepine did. Their research supports another positive effect of treatments that return microglia to their ramified state and points to carbamazepine as a likely ameliorative treatment of the seizure phenotype in diseases with persistent brain inflammation, such as autism.

References : see envgencauses.com

Chapter 8.

SENSORY PHENOTYPES AND SENSORY PROCESSING DISORDER

Some of the behavior of autistic children involves reactions to certain sounds, lights, and other stimuli, to which a given individual has a seemingly unwarranted aversion. The stimulus can be a type of clothing, temperature, or a specific texture. These environmental sensitivities are no doubt related to sensory input filtering issues with a biological basis. The answer of whether environment can influence the degree or type of sensitivities is clearly yes. Therapy may involve a controlled environment or a sensory diet. In this chapter, key examples of sensory phenotypes with evidence of genetic basis are presented and discussed. Sensory perception and integration show greater amounts of variation, but not necessarily deficits, in autistics compared to neurotypicals.

Sensory integration differences lay at the core of many autistic phenotypes. These differences suggest the following question: Is the sensory overload phenotypes that are commonly observed in autistics in addition to the morphological and functional differences already considered, or is there a specific set of genes and/or environmental influences that influences the degree to which sensory overload occurs? This is an open research question for some. There are also indications that sensory overload can occur without autism.

In a study of differences between ASD and sensory processing disorder (SPD) patients, Schoen et al. (2009) found that autistics had greater taste and smell and taste-smell sensitivity but lower sensory responsivity compared to individuals with sensory modulation disorder (SMD), whereas the SMD group had more atypical sensory seeking behavior. Their study was focused on two questions. High-functioning ASD males could detect odors at a greater distance than age-matched neurotypicals (Ashwin et al., 2014). Using the Alcohol Sniff Test, the ASD group could detect the odor on average at a distance of 24.1 cm, compared to 14.4 cm for the control group. This ability was also correlated with autistic traits in the ASD group. Autistics have been found to detect motion twice as fast as neurotypicals (Foss-Feig et al., 2013).

The first question addressed by Foss-Feig et al. (2013) was whether children with ASD have different sensory-related behaviors compared to children with SPD. They used measurements of electrodermal activity during sensory challenges compared to children with SPD. They found that skin conductance levels were significantly lower in the ASD group than the SPD group and the neurotypical group. This meant lower arousal-to-stimulus level in ASD. The SPD group did not differ from the neurotypical group in the electrodermal activity measures.

Another study had shown the same difference in SPD patients, as well as slower rates of habituation in SPD patients compared to typically developing control children (McIntosh et al., 1999).

These differences in SPD are primarily due to sensory gating differences. Owen et al. observed that males with SPD have white matter connectivity and that the white matter microstructural differences were correlated with sensory behavior differences. They postulated that the pattern difference could be useful in differential diagnosis with autism and ADHD, although their study was limited to neurotypical controls.

The second question addressed by Foss-Feig et al. (2013) was whether ASD patients have differences in reactivity (sympathetic nervous system) compared with sensory modulation disorder patients; for this, they used the Short Sensory Profile. Reactivity, measured by three different measures, followed the quantitative trend sensory modulation disorder > neurotypical > ASD.

A closer look by the same team (Chang et al., 2014) found similarities in the SPD and ASD sensory integration pathways compared to neurotypicals, but different variations in SPD and ASD in connectivities in social-emotional pathways. Across all groups, they found microstructural white matter variation in connectivity related to auditory processing, working memory, social skills, and inattention defined by specific neural microcircuits.

Teasing these conditions apart may prove difficult, however. Van Campen et al. (2015) found that for patients with childhood epilepsy, comorbidity of autism and attention deficit hyperactivity disorder (ADHD) indicators could predict which patients had more severe sensory processing difficulties. And SPDs are prevalent in otherwise undiagnosed individuals as well, with preterm birth being a strong predictor (Adam, 2015). Individuals with a sibling with ASD have more ADHD traits than individuals whose sibling did not have ASD (van der Plas et al., 2016). Whether this important trait correlation reveals shared genetic risk of ADHD and ASD or shared environmental susceptibility among siblings is unknown.

When asked to inhibit a response or to react in a flexible way to auditory information, individuals with ASD were slower than age-matched controls (Mostert-Kerckhoffs et al., 2015).

It may be useful to study specific variation related to sensory integration issues across the population rather than within a specific diagnosed group. White matter microstructural differences in a specific region have been found to be responsible for inattentiveness (Pryweller et al., 2014), for example, and differences in myelination in other regions have been found to be associated with listening difficulties in children suspected of having auditory processing disorders. Overall, auditory processing appears to be similar between neurotypicals and ASD, but ASD shows measurable delay in response (Roberts et al., 2013). Age-related changes in hearing were also more or less similar between ASD and neurotypicals.

Therefore, the potential clinical utility of white matter microstructural differences for differential diagnosis is intriguing. Lange et al. (2010) found fine-resolution and gross differences in autistics compared to neurotypicals, with high sensitivity and specificity in the use of those measurements as biomarkers, both in the training and independent test set. However, more research is needed given that their study did not test for specificity against other conditions. fMRI biomarkers for high-functioning AD showed weak signal, but performance evaluation measures were not high enough for clinical use, showing 76 percent accuracy compared to 95 percent accuracy of behavioral measures (Plitt et al., 2014).

In some conditions, white matter microstructural differences are clearly caused by genetics. The hemideletions in Williams syndrome is a good example (Marenco et al., 2007). Common behavioral patterns across otherwise diverse neurological and psychological conditions appear to involve the same brain regions and microcircuits (see review by Paul, 2011). Generally speaking, variation in white matter microstructure is under strong genetic control (Kochunov et al., 2010). Variation in white matter structures in a healthy cohort of 467 subjects was traced to marker D15S816 at chromosome 15q25 and marker D3S1754 at chromosome 3q27. Both markers had been previously shown to be associated with psychiatric conditions that show white matter microstructural differences. Variants near D15S816 have also been shown to be associated with early onset depression, bipolar disorder, and inflammatory bowel disease (McAuley et al., 2009). One gene in this region, MCTP2, has variants associated with schizophrenia (Djuorvic et al., 2009) and kidney disease (Sandholm et al., 2012; Schoen et al., 2009). Another nearby gene encodes repulsive guidance molecule for retinal axons (Monnier et al., 2002).

Genes do not always function as light switches. Biological pathways in general are complex circuits, with multiple inputs, feedback loops, nonlinearities, interactions, and redundancies. The structural, electrochemical, and hormonal aspects of brain function are similarly complex and utilize underlying biological pathways. Highly penetrant pathologies in cellular function lead to larger-scale developmental differences. Thus, while it is tempting to say that we understand sensory modalities in autism and other conditions, due to the evidence of some genetic control, microstructural differences are also a source of input and factor for overall brain function. They are both manifested as and interpreted in the setting of the overall genomic and proteomic functions of the brain.

Wherever the structural differences are found both in the brain and on the diagnostic landscape, they often lead to decreased rates of learning and present barriers to social integration. With SPD inside or outside autism and ADHD, it is difficult to process and respond to information received through the senses. This can create challenges in executing many everyday tasks and can result in motor clumsiness, behavioral problems, anxiety, depression, and impediments to learning.

Then again, there is musicality. The ability to identify specific musical notes with extreme accuracy and precision (absolute pitch) in some musicians may be due to local hyperconnectivity in the bilateral superior temporal lobe structures (Loui et al., 2011); it is a trait that shows family aggregation. Absolute pitch is not a static trait, and nongenetic shared family influences play a strong role. Early music training is a major factor in the expression of the trait. The heritable components of accuracy (pitch) and precision (relative pitch) may be fractionable; pitch in chord processing is locally processed, whereas the identification of relations among tones in chords involves global processing (Ziv and Radin, 2014).

Musicians with absolute pitch tend to show a larger number of autistic traits (Dohn et al., 2012). These traits are not social skill-related, and a great deal of the variation in absolute pitch is related to non-autistic variation. This is perhaps not surprising, given that absolute pitch traits are related to those used in language processing (Oechslin et al., 2010), and processing of tones in language and music involve similar circuits. The traits in absolute pitch appear to map to chromosome 8q24.21, a region in which deletions and CNVs have been observed related to autism (Kaminky et al., 2011). A study in the Finnish population traced a major locus for absolute pitch to a locus on 4q22, which has three regions within which numerous studies have found sporadic mutations in genes in cases of autism (SFARI database, 2016, see especially https://gene.sfari.org/autdb/CNVSecDis.do?l=4q22.1 and https://gene.sfari.org/autdb/CNVSecDis.do?l=4q22.3).

References : see envgencauses.com

Chapter 9.

IMMUNOLOGICAL FACTORS IN AUTISM AND ASD

Alteration in immune function caused by early life programming of the immune system can dramatically alter neural function and associated behaviors for the life of the individual. (Schwarz and Bilbo, 2015)

With great compassion for autistic individuals and their families, the study of cognitive science has progressed in part due to our attempts to understand the ways in which autistic brain phenotypes become manifest. Variations are referred to as abnormalities, aberrations, differences, and variance. In cellular and molecular pathology and molecular neurobiology, the use of these terms is never meant to be pejorative; medical professionals and researchers must communicate using such terms to work effectively. The medical significance of the variation is of greatest interest, and these terms are used here in a value-neutral manner.

From a molecular standpoint, autism is clearly immunological, and is therefore a medical disorder. Immunological factors play a role in autism on at least three levels: induced autoimmunity in autistics, maternal immune activation (MIA), and innate immune overactivation from repeated exposure to activating neurotoxins (excitotoxicity). Seeing autism as an immune disorder has been stymied by views on the blood-brain barrier. However, the immune system accesses the brain compartment during early development and during injury and infection (e.g., meningitis, encephalitis), by recruiting peripheral circulating cells to the site of injury or infection. Severe meningitis and encephalitis are systemic and very dangerous.

Vaccines have been observed to alter psychological processes. O'Connor et al. (2014) found that the meningococcal conjugate vaccine can induce depressive symptoms in early adolescence. They found that enhanced vaccine response was associated with depressive and anxious symptoms. They followed 126 eleven-year-olds from prevaccination, four weeks, three months, and six months. Mood symptoms were associated with elevated and persistently higher antibody responses. The associations remained after controlling for numerous possible confounders, such as social class, body mass index (BMI), sleep, psychosocial risk, and pubertal status.

MATERNAL IMMUNE ACTIVATION: IN UTERO ADAPTIVE IMMUNITY AND EXCITOTOXICITY

Early in development, the fetus relies on maternal immunity via immunoglobulins that cross the placenta into the fetal circulation. The types of immunoglobulins present reflect the past and current environmental exposures of the mother, and passive immunity is retained until the child is capable of mounting an autonomous adaptive immune response. Immunoglobulins that react with self-antigens cross the placenta and attack the CNS prior to blood-brain barrier formation and interfere with neural crest development, as well as interregional specialization. Isolated case studies have reported potential roles for a number of infectious agents, including congenital rubella (German measles). Perinatal cytomegalovirus infection has also been associated with aberrant white matter patterns and with autism.

Fever reveals an activated immune system. While healthy in the case of infection, to clear infectious diseases, the immune system can also be fooled into being activated by proteins normally present in the body, including fetal brain proteins. While it may seem logical therefore for women to receive vaccines, especially the influenza vaccine, while pregnant, the most common side effect of vaccines is fever and immune activation. A large percentage of the influenza vaccine recommended for pregnant women in the United States contains thimerosal.

These mechanisms may explain a number of cases of natal autism; however, the genetic determinants of maternal immunological attack are not well studied. The autonomous adaptive immune system of a newborn may play either a primary or a secondary role to prior maternal immunological response. If no maternal response has occurred, a newborn's immune system is still capable of learning to mount a response to brain proteins in the case of natal infection. This may also contribute to the correlation between the use of antibiotics and autism, with the fever being the culprit, not the treatment. Strong antibiotics may exacerbate inflammation and innate immune activation, inducing widespread cytokine release.

Knowledge of the role of fever, especially from viral infection, in natal autism is widespread. Mouse MIA studies have found dysregulation of genes during brain development, including those involved in neural differentiation and migration, axonal pathfinding and synapse formation, maintenance and function, and neurotransmitter synthesis (Parker-Athill and Tana, 2010). The proinflammatory cytokine interleukin (IL)-6 is upregulated as well (Madsen-Bouterse et al., 20 percent), leading to microglial activation. Choi et al. (2016) found that interleukin 17a (IL-17a) activation is involved in producing an abnormal cortical phenotype during maternal immune activation. IL-17a signaling induces microglial activation leading to cognitive deficits (Sun et al., 2015).

Animal models demonstrate that MIA that produces autism phenotypes in mice can be induced with or without involvement of the innate immune system (microglial activation; Smolders et al., 2015; Giovanoli et al., 2015). The generation of antibodies involves the adaptive immune systems. Mothers of autistics, as well as their autistic children, can have antibrain protein antibodies (Rossi et al., 2013), a potential signature of MIA (Braunschweig et al., 2012).

Sequeira et al. (2013) discussed the clinical utility of the use of folate receptor autoantibodies for assessing risk of autism, and Shapira et al. (2015) found that autoantibodies to the folate receptor protein was related to neural tube defects and autism.

POSTNATAL AUTOIMMUNITY PARTLY RULED OUT

Libbey et al. (2008) found lower anti-myelin-basic protein in late-onset, regressive autistics compared to classic autistics and Tourette syndrome patients, but not compared to controls, indicating a lack of signature of autoimmunity in regressive autism. Thus, the results of the Libbey et al. study imply that the adaptive immune system is not particularly involved in the destruction of brain functions during regression.

POSTNATAL NEUROEXCITOTOXICITY

Evidence for a key role for the innate immune system is widespread. After birth, the molecular mechanisms and the genetic and environmental risk factors are better studied than during pregnancy. Microglial activation and neuroinflammation have been observed in autism for some time (Pardo et al., 2005).

Overall, individuals with ASD tend to show the following characteristics:

1. Neuroinflammation (Mead et al., 2015).
2. Increased circulating immunoglobulin autoantibodies that react with components of the central nervous system (Enstrom et al., 2009; Wills et al., 2009; Goines et al., 2011).

3. Glutathione imbalance and oxidative stress in peripheral immune cells (Rose et al., 2012).
4. Decreased levels of T helper-1 (T(H)1)-like cytokines (e.g., interferon gamma) and T(H)2-like cytokines (i.e. IL-4, IL-10) indicated depressed immune cell activity (Abdallah et al., 2012).

Furthermore, individuals with ASD *may* show some of the following characteristics:

1. Increased T-cell activation, with increased proinflammatory or T(H)1 cytokines (Ashwood et al., 2010, 2011; Goins and Van de Water, 2010; Mead et al., 2015).
2. Increased IL-17 when comorbid with asthma (Akintunde et al., 2015).
3. Increased incidence of allergies and autoimmune disorders (Careaga et al., 2010).
4. Enhanced innate natural killer (NK) cell and monocyte immune responses (Mead et al., 2015).
5. Increased glial populations and glial cell size in the brain (Morgan et al., 2014).
6. Inactivation of microglial chemokine CX3C motif receptor 1 (CX3CR1), leading to absence of microglial guidance for proper nerve cell connections and resulting in neuron and synaptic development damage by microglia (Zhan et al., 2014). The authors found that mice lacking the CX3CR1 gene underwent a transient reduction of microglia during the early postnatal period, followed by a deficit in synaptic pruning. They found weak synaptic transmission, decreased functional brain connectivity, deficits in social interaction, and increased repetitive-behavior phenotypes.

Some of the conditions listed above are also found in Rett syndrome (Schwarz and Bilbo, 2015).

Autopsies of autism patients reveal ongoing, active inflammation in the brain (Careaga et al., 2010), including excess activated microglia. Postmortem studies of AD patients reveal aberrations in the fine structure of axons below prefrontal cortices (Zikopoulos and Barbas, 2013); thus, overpruning by microglia may be a permanent facet of neurobiological processes during the life of autistic individuals.

PARACETAMOL (ACETAMINOPHEN)

Paracetamol, also known as acetaminophen, is a common analgesic used to treat pain and fever. The use of acetaminophen after vaccination with measles, mumps, and rubells (MMR) was found by Schultz et al. (2008) to increase the risk of autism. A study by Bauer et al. (2013) similarly found that increased paracetamol use was accompanied by increased autism spectrum disorder (ASD) rates and tied the gender bias to use of paracetamol to the 4:1 gender bias in the diagnosis of autism. Metabolic processing of acetaminophen involves a process called sulphation, required for DNA methylation, which is compromised in autistics (Hartzwell et al., 2012). Its alternative metabolism in autistics induces oxidative stress and immune dysregulation, ultimately leading to microglial activation and lipid peroxidation via glutathione depletion. Paracetamol depletes glutathione, which is also disastrous in a setting of metal toxicity. As a result of this toxicity, normal cellular detoxification of metals involves conjugation with glutathione S-transferase, uptake by vacuoles, and transport and secretion via endoplasmic reticulum pathways. Depletion of glutathione aborts this process, which is essential for normal cellular detoxification.

An excellent description of the disruption of the process in astrocytes in response to aluminum toxicity is given by Prahash et al. (2013):

> *Aluminum (Al) is an environmental neurotoxin that affects cerebral functions and causes health complications. However, the role of Al in arbitrating glia homeostasis and pathophysiology remains obscure. Astrocyte, microglia activation (reactive gliosis) and associated inflammatory events play a decisive role in neurodegeneration and may represent a target for treating neurodegenerative disorders. In this study, we have analyzed the role of aluminum chloride (AlCl3) in causing reactive gliosis in the brain of mice and the ability of fisetin, a flavonoid to attenuate reactive gliosis and neuronal inflammation. Reports suggest that fisetin exerts antioxidant and anti-inflammatory actions. Fisetin at a dose of 15 mg/kg body weight was orally administered, daily (pre-treated for 4 weeks before AlCl3 induction and co-treated until experimental period of 8 weeks) to mice induced with AlCl3 (200 mg/kg b.wt./day/8 weeks, orally). Administration of AlCl3 developed behavioral deficits, triggered lipid peroxidation (LPO), compromised acetylcholine esterase (AChE) activity and reduced the levels of superoxide dismutase (SOD), catalase (CAT), glutathione-S-transferase (GST) and reduced glutathione (GSH) and caused histologic aberrations. These effects were accompanied by increased expressions of Glial fibrillary acidic protein and ionized calcium-binding adapter molecule 1. Pro-inflammatory cytokines, such as tumor necrosis factor alpha, interleukin-1β, inducible nitric oxide synthase, were increased upon AlCl3 administration. AlCl3-induced alterations in the activities of SOD, CAT, GST, AChE and levels of GSH, LPO, activity of AChE, behavioral deficits, histologic aberrations, reactive gliosis and inflammatory niche were attenuated on treatment with fisetin. Collectively,*

> *our results indicate that fisetin exerts neuroprotection against AlCl3-induced brain pathology.*

The level of disruption within astroglial cells dramatically reduces their ability to uptake glutamate. Glutamate buildup in the brain signals microglial activation. Fisetin is found in low levels in apples, blueberries, cucumbers, grapes, kiwis, mangos, onions, persimmons, and strawberries.

A polymorphism (–173G/C) in the promoter of the gene macrophage migratory inhibitory factor (MIF) gene is associated with hereditary periodic fever, asthma, and autism (Becker et al., 2010). In addition to depleting glutathione, paracetamol has an inhibitory effect on the macrophage migratory inhibitory factor gene (Senter et al., 2002). This effect would make microglial cell deactivation more difficult.

PRKCB1

The expression of the gene PRKCB1 is downregulated in some autistics, and the decreased expression is associated with certain isoforms due to mutations that may impact alternative splicing (Lintas et al., 2009). PRKCB1 appears to play the role of dampening a runaway immunological process, but the process may be hampered in some autistics owing to the mutations leading to alternative splice formation (Lintas et al., 2009). Association of haplotypes of PRKCB1 with ASD has been reported (Philippi et al., 2005).

A variety of brain regions are targeted by immunoglobulin, including thalamus, hypothalamus, caudate nucleus, cerebral cortex, and putamen, but most consistently the cerebellum (Piras et al., 2014). There is a reduction in the oligodendrocytes in the amygdala of people with ASD older than twenty years of age compared to controls (Morgan et al., 2014).

EVIDENCE OF VACCINE-INDUCED IMMUNOLOGICAL VARIATIONS IN AUTISM

Singh et al. (2002, 2003) found elevated levels of measles antibodies in autistics, but not in age-matched controls, indicating a hyperactivated immune response to the measles virus proteins. Exposure to the measles virus in these children was via MMR immunization, not measles infection. Greater than 90 percent of MMR antibody-positive autistic sera were also positive for myelin basic protein autoantibodies, indicative of CNS autoimmunity (Singh et al., 2002; Singh, 2009).

Measles-induced seizures in autism are associated with mutations in the gene CD46 (Jabara et al., 2011). CD46 activates phagocytosis by microglial cells (Griffiths et al., 2009) and also CD40 expression, which is required for the activation of microglia (Ponomarev et al., Tan et al., 1999). Thus, live measles virus may be among the many factors that contribute to excitotoxicity leading to autism. Microglial overactivation plays a central role as a lifelong condition that leads to and maintains autism. Note that the expression of both CD47 and CD200 are upregulated during apoptosis, normally shutting down microglia activation into its less active state (Griffiths et al., 2009). Downregulation of CD200 allows increased microglial activation and impaired synaptic plasticity, and disrupts long-term potentiation (LTP; Downer et al., 2010; Lyons et al., 2007). Brain slices from $CD200^{-/-}$ mice show impaired LTP compared with wild-type mice (Costello et al., 2011).

IMMUNOLOGICAL ENVIRONMENTS

When considering immunological factors in natal autism, the intrauterine environment is important, because the interaction between the immune systems of the fetus and the mother may play a role. Two children, one with autism and another with severe language impairment, were born to the same mother, whose serum contained antibodies that were shown to bind to the cerebellar cells of developing fetal mice (Dalton et al., 2003). Piras et al. (2014) found that children with more severe autism had larger amounts of circulating anti-brain protein antibodies. They also noted that immunoglobulins that recognize self-antigens can also cross the placenta and reach the CNS before blood-brain barrier formation. Cabanlit et al. (2007) found increased brain-specific autoantibodies in plasma from AD patients compared to age-matched non-AD controls. As many as 23 percent of mothers of autistics have fetal brain autoantibodies, compared to 1 percent of mothers of neurotypical children, and mothers of autistics also tend to have developed type 1 diabetes (Krakowiak et al., 2016). Interestingly, twins that do not share a chorion may have different immunologic environments (Bohm and Stewart, 2009). This appears to apply to specific phenotypes, with indications of possible effects for personality, cognitive ability, and brain structures. Children born later in a family are at a higher risk of developing autism; this could indicate a sensitization of the mother's immune system and its effect on the developing CNS of her later-born children in some families.

One of the most fascinating aspects of the human mind is the process of adaptive-reinforcement learning. When we are faced with learning something new, a complex process is involved. Axons and dendrons are not static in our minds—they are constantly forming connections, making new growths (extensions), almost feeling each other out with their branch-like extended arms. When we take information in, it is routed through a local circuit—let us call it a microcircuit (as neurologists have for years)—with chemoelectric activity and connections ready to receive that information. If the information is very important—and there are fascinating ways in which our brains tell themselves it is important—the circuit is made stronger and the connections (synapses) between the cells become more reinforced. Administration of adrenaline to rats in tubs of water causes the rats to learn the location of a lifesaving platform more quickly and to retain those memories longer (Hatfield et al., 1999; McIntyre and Roozendaal, 2007).

These local circuits, which manifest in various areas of the brain, depending on the type of memory, are thought to be reinforced while we sleep—and those that remain become our long-term memories. Those that are lost are perhaps still resident in other local circuits, more weakly, only by association, and a thought or memory may be recalled via reactivation of a weak and existing circuit.

GENETIC VARIATIONS INFLUENCE IMMUNOLOGICAL RESPONSE TO VIRAL PATHOGENS

A number of studies report that genetic variations in some genes, especially the toll-like receptor family of molecules, mediate innate immune responses. Variations in these genes have been found that alter (weaken) a person's response to the measles and rubella viruses (see review by Buonaguro and Pulendran, 2011). Such variation likely contributes to variation in response to pathogens in vaccines as well. Whether such mutations confer protection against CMA remains to be determined.

ALUMINUM-MEDIATED MICROGLIAL OVERACTIVATION CAUSES PERVASIVE NEUROLOGICAL DAMAGE

Dr. Russell Blaylock is well known for being an early medical scientist to stress that chronic microglial cell hyperactivation is a likely process involved in neurological damage. He has published his ideas widely, and his work has provided one critical key element of causality to the vaccine/autism link: biological plausibility. He considered chronic microglial activation a "hallmark" of ASD (Blaylock, 2009).

Subsequent independent research has overwhelmingly supported Blaylock's hypotheses. Researchers at the Johns Hopkins University in the Neuroimmunopathology Lab studied autistics aged 5 to 44 and found that their brains had widespread microglial hyperactivation and sensitivity to astrocytes, reflecting interleukin (IL)-6 cytokine-mediated inflammation (Vargas et al., 2005). Chronic inflammatory conditions were most pronounced in the cerebellum, anterior cingulate, and medial frontal gyrus. Critical cells regulating rhythmic nerve transmissions (Purkunje cells) were missing, as were granule cells from the cerebellum. The fact that the hyperactivated state persisted for decades is a critical observation from this study.

Aluminum doses from all sources are cumulative. Oral routes yield minimal absorption, but the common retort to concern with aluminum in vaccines that "we get more from diet, it is everywhere" hides the fact that aluminum from vaccines is above and beyond the baselines. Toxicologists are well aware that dose means everything when it comes to toxicitiy.

Ingested aluminum and vaccine adjuvant aluminum have very different kinetics. Ingested aluminum is ionic and may be excreted by the kidneys. Injected adjuvant in the form of aluminum nanoparticles is too large to be filtered out by the kidneys; instead, these particles may be engulfed by macrophages and carried throughout the body, where they can contribute to chronic inflammation.

Aluminum can cross the blood-brain barrier and accumulate in glial and neural cells (Golub et al., 1999). Large doses of aluminum during vaccination can easily lead to accumulation in the neonatal brain and interfere with postnatal brain development.

The critical key linking preservatives and adjuvants in vaccines to immunoneuroexcitotoxicity has been studied, with numerous studies demonstrating unequivocally that both aluminum and mercury cause microglial hyperactivation. Mercury causes both cell death (apoptosis) and endoplasmic digestion of cellular components (autophagy). Because mercury exposure is additive, exposure to all forms should be avoided. Geier et al. (2009) found that babies born to women with mercury dental amalgams had a 3.2-fold increase in the risk of autism (Geier et al., 2009).

Once in the brain, the effects of aluminum on the brain are manifold—none of them good. Aluminum causes oxidative stress across the brain (Yuan et al., 2012), and oxidative stress leads to microglial activation. Aluminum also induces autophagy and apoptosis in astrocytes. The mechanism is overactivation of the class III PI3K/Beclin 1-dependent autophagy signal (Zeng et al., 2012). These cell deaths in the brain release cytokines, invoking microglial activation.

Shaw and Petrik (2009) found that aluminum caused increased apoptosis of motor neurons, as well as increases in both reactive astrocytes and microglial proliferation in the spinal cord and cortex. Aluminum, including a small portion from the diet and a much larger proportion delivered via injection, has been shown to be picked up by macrophages and deposited in organs, especially the brain (Gherardi et al., 2015). There, it is toxic to astrocytes, reducing their capacity to uptake glutamate. The microglial cells become hyperactivated (neuroexcitotoxic), leading to excessive pruning. The science on aluminum immunoneuroexcitotoxicity is so thorough and complete, it provides an excellent model for how other toxins in the environment may be studied as causes of neurological damage leading to toxin-induced autoimmune disorders.

WHAT ARE MICROGLIA?

Microglial cells scavenge the brain for aberrant proteins and foreign proteins on the surfaces of bacteria and viruses, of which there is an apparent never-ending onslaught, even in healthy brains (Branton et al., 2013). In the healthy brain, microglial cells usually exhibit small central bodies and long processes. This has been referred to as a "surveying" phenotype. As they scan their surrounding environment, they react quickly by converging on the damage attracted and driven by molecular chemotactic signals, such as adenosine triphosphate (ATP) or adenosine diphosphate (ADP) (Davalos et al., 2005). These phagocytes both move existing processing and send new ones to the site of concern. This response is dependent on stimulation of the purine receptor P2Y12 (P2Y12R) expressed by microglia (Davalos et al., 2005).

The proinflammatory substances released by activated microglial cells lead to neuronal cell death. In progressive, age-related neurodegenerative diseases, such as Parkinson's disease and Alzheimer's disease, hyperactivation of microglial cells is known to play a functional role in the causation of learning and memory deficits. Experimental treatments such as Thioflavin T show reversibility of the microglial activated state followed by prevention of beta amyloid plaque formation (Sarkar et al., 2015), further indicating causality. Microglial failure to activate against β-amyloid is reversed by alginate-derived oligosaccharide (Zhou et al., 2015). The duality of the role of microglial cells in Alzheimer's disease, first as a clearance mechanism and then also a toxic mechanism, is well known (e.g., Gold et al., 2015), and research of the use of amyloid signatures as blood biomarkers for ASD seems promising (Ray et al., 2016).

In the absence of infection or cellular damage signals, microglial cells are also responsible for monitoring and negotiating nerve connections, actively interacting with axons and dendrites, taking up the role of constant pruners of the axonal buds and branches and extensions of neurites, fine-tuning circuit and synaptic architectures.

This process was once thought to only involve removal of "excess" branches and extensions. The dynamic role of microglial cells is now much better understood: They foster and maintain synapses, the connections between axons of one nerve cell and dendrites of another. They are constantly busy, remodeling and sculpting connections, whittling away at weak connections (primarily dendrites) that release cytokines during autophagy, but also reinforcing connections as they become reinforced. This activity is required for both canonical brain development (Paolicelli et al., 2011) and learning.

A fundamental role of the brain's innate immune system in memory was not imagined until studies demonstrated that microglial cells are essential for proper memory formation. Mice depleted of microglia show deficits in learning tasks, including a significant reduction in motor-learning-dependent synapse formation, fear conditioning, and novel object recognition. Twenty-one of the 61 proteins found in microglia-depleted mice had functions involving synapses. Similar effects are seen when microglia are activated in BDNF–mice (Parkhurst et al., 2013). The injection of lipopolysaccharide (LPS) into the hippocampus of rats moves microglia into crisis mode and was seen to cause a decrease in glutamatergic transmission and aberrant microglial activity, leading to learning and memory deficits (Tanaka et al., 2009). Memory formation deficits are evident in rats that experience early-life intracranial infections (Williamson et al., 2011). Remarkably, the deficits are seen again in later life when infection is produced in a limb, not directly involving the brain. Microglial-mediated emergency response is seen after the second infection. This important study has obvious implications for environmentally induced encephalopathies in autism, including encephalitic reactions following booster shots.

Learning involves reinforcement of specific connections synapses between and among groups of neurons, with the formation of more connections. Each connection involves a dendrite (a branching arm) from one cell reaching to and connecting with a bud (axon) on another cell.

All replication processes are imperfect, and our perception is also hardly ever perfect. This may explain why we do not remember things precisely and exactly. Some people with photographic memories may have endogenous circuit building/reinforcement/duplication driven by a process that is greatly simplified and involves less chance—perhaps reinforcement only occurs in local circuits that are already identical to those formed by initial perception, and thus their memories are not only more solid but can also be instantaneous and seemingly more permanent.

In autism, the ability to form memories—essential for learning language and motor skills and perceiving others as typically developing people do—may be greatly diminished via a two-step process. First, early brain development may involve rapid growth of many neurites and too many connections. This may reflect the initial cellular toxicity of environmental factors on microglia. Numerous studies support initial hyperconnectivity. This by itself may yield altered learning capacity, which is not necessarily negative. The process may contribute to macrocephaly in approximately 20 percent of patients. Thus, the capacity for learning may originally be enhanced. If a pair or so of genetic mutations, or modulation in gene expression, exist or are activated by one or more environmental insults that activate microglial cells against synaptic proteins, the ability to prune synaptic structures in a meaningful and useful way may be abrogated, or compromised, as the microglial cells may overact in their immune system capacity. Excessive microglial brutality on endogenous, native, normal dendritic extensions can be systemic and devastating.

Perinatal exposure to air pollution has been shown to be associated with ASD (Roberts et al., 2013). Air pollution also causes microglial cell activation (Allen et al., 2014), a clear indication of brain injury or infection (Allen et al., 2014). The effects of third-trimester exposure of mice to air pollutants include reductions in size of the corpus callosum, hypomyelination, aberrant white matter development, structural integrity with ventriculomegaly (VM), elevated glutamate and excitatory/inhibitory imbalance, increased amygdala astrocytic activation, and repetitive and impulsive behaviors (Allen et al., 2016). It is extremely well known in disease epidemiology that risk due to exposure is cumulative. Thus, individuals in areas of high air pollution may be already "primed" and experience a higher load of immunoneuroexcitotoxicity from other sources. Environmental toxins and endogenous proteins that are expressed in response to injury, infection, and toxins can cause microglia to enter an overactivated state and release reactive oxygen species (ROS) that cause a positive feedback loop—these endogenous ROS cause further cellular damage and apoptosis, eliciting the activated state. Microglial cells change shape under these conditions and enter a state that has been described as a fully activated, amoeboid, microglial phenotype. They can produce high quantities of the self-excitatory neurotransmitter glutamate. The destructive effects of microglia on surrounding cells cause the release of cytokines, which is a signal for continued activation. Both glutamate and the released cytokines sustain microglial activation, thereby establishing one part of a vicious circle in which neurodegeneration and neuroinflammation sustain each other. Microglial cells in this state are referred to as *excitotoxic.*

Normal activation in microglia can occur via a number of routes. One important route involves Toll-like receptor (TLR) molecules on the surface of the cell. These molecules, of which there is a variety, are specialized to uptake different signals around the cell called cytokines, which tell the microglia what is going on around them and what they should be doing. Microglial roles change depending on the neurochemical signals in which they are bathed. For instance, the cytokine CD154 and toll-like receptor ligands cause extensive microglia to promote excess cholinergic neuron differentiation (Ni et al., 2007).

In the activated state, microglia cells change shape. They pull in their arms, become more rounded, and become macrophagic (amoeboid), capable of moving and engulfing molecules and parts of cells around them. Microglial cells uptake extracellular glutamine, which is metabolized to glutamate via glutaminase. Glutamate is then released by microglia via the connexin hemichannels of gap junctions that are formed in response to brain injury and inflammatory mediators (Dantzer and Walker, 2014). The result is neuroinflammation and, if it involves sufficient tissue (locally or diffuse), attendant encephalitis.

This process can, but not necessarily, also involve peripheral (adaptive) immune cells (T or B lymphocytes) that can traffic to the brain parenchyma. The presence of T or B lymphocytes in the brain is rare; indeed, any sign of adaptive immunity in the brain is unusual, unless there are serious injuries or ongoing infections. Numerous routes for the adaptive immune system to pass the blood-brain barrier are now recognized. The typical innate immune response of the brain—a weak response—involves the routine harmless scavenging by activated microglial cells. Prolonged activation causes microglia to send an "SOS" signal to the adaptive immune system, recruiting the T cells, and thus the body learns what is present and how to mount a response. Chronic activation can cause microglia to release cytokines that induce microglial activation, establishing a permanent state of innate-immune system hyperactivation and a type of semi-inflammation that may or may not involve adaptive immune cells.

The lifelong hyperactivation of microglial cells observed in ASD reported by Vargas (2005) has been confirmed by other follow-up studies. Experts have expressed doubt of the pathological indication of astroglial cells, as they have a less clear-cut role in the innate immunity of the brain. Some even doubt the utility of the presence of cytokines (classical immune red-alert signals), given that they have also appear to have multitude of roles in the brain for neurological homeostasis. However, a great deal of experimental evidence exists on the cytokine signaling among microglia themselves, and from microglia to and from other cells of the CDS, including astrocytes.

A study of immunological markers in the blood and cerebral spinal fluid of autistic patients revealed no immunological anomalies (Pardo et al., 2014); however, microglial status itself was not assessed, and given the results of animal studies, the more relevant measures would be done during a secondary infection or environmental exposure of the first type.

Fever and encephalitis induced by vaccines is a commonly reported precursor adverse event prior to regressive autism. Acetaminophen depletes glutathione, adding oxidative stress to astrocytes and microglia; this encumbers their ability to perform their duties and leads to excitotoxicity. These individual occurrences of regressive autism are not only observations consistent with the hypothesis of a pathological role of excitotoxic microglial cells: they have provided test after test of the hypothesis that vaccines followed by acetaminophen can cause autism in some people. Further, treatments aimed at modulating microglial activation are being developed. If such studies also ameliorate the effects of autism, it will provide absolute confirmation of a persistent role for microglial cells in autism. The available evidence, however, is sufficiently strong.

Cunningham et al. (2013) showed that microglia also control neural precursor cells during cortical development. Importantly, they showed that microglia selectively colonize the cortical proliferative zones, where they phagocytose (engulf and destroy) neural precursor near the end of neurogenesis. When they deactivated microglia in utero with tetracyclines, or eliminated microglia with liposomal clodronate treatment, they found a significant increase in the number of neural precursor cells. When they activated microglia in utero through maternal immune activation, they found a significant decrease in the number of neural precursor cells.

The implications of this research for autism are profound: microglial cells regulate the size of the precursor cell pool in the developing cerebral cortex. The authors concluded that "any factor that alters the number or activation state of microglia in utero can profoundly affect neural development and affect behavioral outcomes."

MICROGLIAL ACTIVATION IMPLICATED IN LOW CONNECTIVITY

Microglial hyperactivation is brain-wide and self-sustaining in autism/ASD. Rodriguez and Kern (2011) provide a major review of the evidence of microglial activation in autism and evidence showing that it causes underconnectivity. Tang et al. (2014) found underpruning of axons in autistics. Accompanied by overpruning of dendrites, there is an imbalance in the target of microglia.

LACK OF MICROGLIA IMPLICATED IN CONNECTIVITY VARIATION IN ASD

Mice lacking CX3CR1 are born with impaired social interaction due to nerve cell damage by microglia (Zhan et al., 2014). A normal phenomenon called synaptic multiplicity follows normal trimming of unused connections; the links reinforced by learning then become physically reinforced with many connections. In some models of autism, a different architecture is seen. Mice without the gene CX3CR1 have fewer microglia and show reduced functional brain connectivity. They also avoid social interactions and engage in repetitive behavior. Examination of the cells in the neocortex showed primarily one-to-one synaptic architectures, as opposed to the canonical many-to-many synapses, as though the additional synapses reinforced through learning could not be made. Their functional magnetic resonance imaging (fMRI) studies also showed that long-range and global functional connectivities were weakened due to the absence of microglia.

Long-range connectivity variation involved in social function is seen in both high-functioning autism and schizophrenia as variation in white matter, whereas variation in gray matter associated with complex reasoning is unique in the two conditions. Specifically, autistics demonstrated bilateral prefrontal and anterior cingulate increases in gray matter, whereas schizophrenics exhibited prefrontal and left temporal reductions in grey matter (Katz et al., 2016).

ASD-ASSOCIATED MUTATIONS FOUND IN MICROGLIAL STATE REGULATING GENES

PTEN gene mutations, associated with higher risk of ASD, compromise normal mTOR signaling (autophagy) and consequent microglial proliferation and activation (Theoharides et al., 2013). The direct mTOR signaling based microglial activation is now well characterized (Dello Russo et al., 2009; Xie et al., 2014) and its roles in autism established.

MICROGLIA USE INDISCRIMINATE CHEMICAL WARFARE ON NEARBY CELLS

In their activated state, especially when aroused by mitochondrial dysfunction, microglia release a burst of chemicals in a process leading to lipid peroxidation (Barget et al., 2007). These chemicals include inducible nitrous oxide synthase (iNOS), which induces cell death. This can occur at some distance.

EFFECTS OF ENVIRONMENTAL TOXINS ON MICROGLIAL BIOLOGY

Long-term subclinical methylmercury (MeHg) exposure leads to increased microglial cells and decreased astrocytes (Charleston et al., 1996). While the activation state of the glial cells was not determined in that study, an overall increase in microglial density is consistent with an innate immune response. The same study concluded that MeHg was also deposited in microglial cells in the highest concentration compared to other cells. The injection of aluminum into mice, at levels bioequivalent to those encountered by infants and children on the Centers for Disease Control and Prevention (CDC) pediatric schedule, was found to result in increased reactive astrocytes and microglial proliferation in the spinal cord and cortex, as well as increased apoptosis of motor neurons accompanied by loss of learning and memory function, as well as hyperphosphorylated tau protein (Shaw and Petrik, 2009).

Prenatal exposure to terbutaline, an inhaled treatment for asthma, was found to affect brain development, showed high levels of microglial activation and an increased innate immune response (Zerrate et al., 2007). Earlier studies had established an increased risk of ASD diagnosis following terbutaline exposure (Connors et al., 2005; Coren et al., 2011). Connors et al. (2005) found that overstimulation of adrenergic receptors caused by terbutaline had the same effect as a genetic polymorphism of the adrenergic receptors that caused a desensitization of those receptors. Both effects resulted in ASD anomalies in the fetal brain. Croen et al. (2011) found that exposure to terbutaline for more than two days during the third trimester resulted in a fourfold increased risk of ASD diagnosis.

In an editorial comment, which included revelation of a conflict of interest by two authors due to their service as expert witnesses in litigation that involves the use of terbutaline during pregnancy, Rodier et al. (2011) attempted to dismantle the published evidence for a causal link between late-term terbutaline exposure and autism. However, none of their concerns relieve terbutaline as a putative cause when used long-term during pregnancy (as for management of asthma). Most of their concerns with inferences based on studies of late-term exposure were hypothetical. For example, in criticizing a study that found a correlation of ASD in dizygotic twins and in males with late-term exposure to terbutaline, they wrote, "It is unclear why such a subgroup (males) would ever be selected for study a priori. If it was selected a posteriori, then the results should be considered 'hypothesis-generating' at best." Why they would suspect a specific post-hoc comparison and yet cite the negative results of the other subgroup analyses is unclear. This type of cherry-picking of results and "speculative targeting" of results showing evidence of association with a toxin is profoundly unscientific. It has been, unfortunately, pervasive among those writing or speaking in defense of specific neurotoxins.The findings are consistent with increased risk due to shared haploinsufficiency in dizgotic twins and consistent with additive or multiplicative interactive risk of gender × terbutaline interaction. One would not impeach birth order × terbutaline interaction, for example, as they are independent factors.

They criticized the Zerrate et al. (2007) study as using behavioral outcome measures not related to autism; however, the study measured hyperreactivity to both novelty and to aversive stimuli when assessed in a novel open field, which are both easily seen as reflecting the degree of preference for sameness. Insistence on sameness is a common phenotype in AD and elsewhere within ASDs.

After their review, Slotkin et al. (2013) studied the mechanisms of damage of terbutaline and confirmed that it operates through trophic interactions with β2-adrenoceptors, affecting both the brain and systemic norepinephrine, and concluded that autonomic dysfunction seen in autistic children born to women who were exposed to terbutaline is also likely causally related.

Terbutaline had been used as a subcutaneous injection to stem preterm labor; the Food and Drug Administration (FDA) changed the label for terbutaline in 2011, and it now that warns against using the medication for preterm labor citing a lack of evidence of safety for preterm use. The presence of microglia in the activated state found by Zerrate et al. (2007) is indicative of a resident pathological condition, whereas the surveillance state is normal homeostatic state. In this state, they provide routine cleanup services of cellular debris, awaiting signals to kick into the activated state and rapidly clean up damaged or weakened nerve endings and nerve cells.

Although the presence of microglial cells alone is not sufficient to indicate excitotoxicity, the findings of significantly higher activated microglial cells (Zerrate et al., 2007 and others) strongly indicates a causal role of excitotoxicity in autism. Findings of microglia in persistent activated states are similarly strong indicators of ongoing molecular and cellular immunologic pathology in numerous other neurodegenerative conditions and cannot be attributed to homeostasis if those conditions are found to be more prominent in autism cases than in typically developing individuals. The more recent studies showing that overexcitation of microglia in rodents leads to disrupted memory functions (Parkhurst et al., 2013; Tanaka et al., 2009) serve as key indicators of a causal, not merely correlative, relationship.

Activated microglial cells are also found in the dorsolateral prefrontal cortex (dlPFC) of autism patients (Morgan, 2010). Specifically, the visualization of microglial cells showed marked activation in 5 of 13 autism patients studied and marginal (but significant) activation in an additional 4 patients. Measured changes included stockier cellular bodies, a higher density, and elongated projections (Morgan, 2010), clearly indicating the activated microglial populations. While the study was small, the patterns are impressive in light of the bulk of the evidence pointing to activated microglial cells as contributing causal factors of autism.

DO MATCHING AUTOLOGOUS AND FOREIGN ANTIGEN PEPTIDE SEQUENCES CONTRIBUTE TO VACCINE-INDUCED ACUTE DISSEMINATED ENCEPHALOMYELITIS (ADEM)?

There are two recent case studies of individuals undergoing complete demyelination within a day of receiving the influenza vaccine.

Case 1: Influenza Vaccine-Induced CNS Demyelination in a Fifty-Year-Old Male

> *A fifty-year-old Caucasian male with a course of progressive, focal, neurologic deficits within 24 h after receiving the influenza vaccine. Subsequent workup revealed the possibility of an acute central nervous system (CNS) demyelinating episode secondary to the influenza vaccine, best described as either CIS or ADEM. . . . Case reports of CNS demyelination following vaccinations have been previously noted, most often occurring in the context of recent influenza vaccination. This report . . . document(s) a case of CNS demyelination occurring 24 h after influenza vaccination in a middle-aged patient and will describe some salient features regarding the differential diagnosis of CIS and ADEM*" (Sacheli and Bauer, 2014).

Case 2: Influenza Vaccine-Induced Acute Disseminated Encephalomyelitis in a Seventy-Five-Year-Old Woman

> *A 75-year-old woman developed acute disseminated encephalomyelitis within 3 weeks of receiving the seasonal influenza vaccine. The patient subsequently passed away, despite treatment with methylprednisolone and plasma exchange therapy.* (Shoamanesh and Traboulsee, 2011).

Clearly, the idea that vaccines have caused aphasia, paralysis, and nerve damage is not overruled from an immunological standpoint. Additional case studies include ADEM after H1N1 vaccination in a two-year-old boy (Fuji et al., 2012); ADEM in an eighty-three-year-old woman, who recovered after plasma exchange (Machicado et al., 2013); and two reports of ADEM following influenza vaccination in a sixty-two-year-old man and in a sixty-year-old man (Nakamura et al., 2003).

Vaccines, like the pathogens they are designed to protect us against, induce an immune response. It is possible that any given pathogen, and therefore its vaccine, has within it antigens that have a high match to an individual's myelin sheath protein sequences—an unfortunate coincidence of the genetics of the individual and the pathogen. Sequence-based match typing might be possible in the future to check for homology between a person's proteins and each and every vaccine. Such matching should be based computationally on 3-D protein shapes, not merely the protein sequence, because proteins with divergent sequences can share the same shape, and antigen/antibody matching is based on shape, not sequence alone. This idea has been called *molecular mimicry* (Menge et al., 2007); it is a case of potential convergent evolution. Given the size of our genome and the millions of strains of pathogens, it seems likely that this type of convergent evolution has occurred.

It may also be possible that a small percentage of people have part of a pathogen's genome embedded in their own genome—inherited from their parents, eliciting an attack on their own tissues. This has been observed in the high mortality of Borna virus infection that causes a serious neurological disorder in horses. In this disease, a previously normal-acting horse may bang its head on the ground after infection until death; mortality is estimated between 80 and 100 percent. These two possibilities can be readily explored by validated high-throughput sequencing, even years after suspected vaccine-induced injuries. If enough autoimmune disorders are shown to be due to shared sequence similarity/identity, a sequenced-based screening protocol may be worth exploring, to exclude individuals at high risk of adverse events including central nervous system (CNS) demyelination and resulting ADEM. The role of aluminum as an immune system activating agent may be important for inducing such autoimmune disorders.

OTHER CAUSES OF MICROGLIAL ACTIVATION

Long-term exposure to the psychostimulant methylphenidate reduces dopamine and activates microglial cells in the basal ganglia (Sadasivan et al., 2012). This is a cause for concern for children diagnosed with both ASD and ADHD, and some clinicians question the utility of additional diagnosis of ADHD given ASD. I review the grave dangers of overtreatment of false positive ADHD cases in *Cures vs. Profits: Successes in Translational Research* (World Scientific, 2016). Psychostimulant use is associated with numerous motor behavior anomalies, among these agitation, tremor, hyperkinetic and stereotypical movements, cognitive impairment, and hyperthermia and cardiovascular dysfunction (Asser and Taba, 2015).

Other factors could play a role in activating the innate immune system during pregnancy, leading to neuroexcitotoxicity (microglial overactivation).

A high-fat diet during pregnancy induces a systemic, low-grade proinflammatory condition. High-fat diets fed to pregnant mice induced microglial activation (Kang et al., 2014). This is likely especially true with polyunsaturated fats, whereas other fats may well be protective. Add obesity-induced interleukin (IL)-6 to the equation and neurological abnormalities are seen, especially in the growth of neurites (Sanders, 2014). Fetal responses to maternal obesity is evidently gender specific (Edlow et al., 2016).

Five human studies have found association between high body mass index (BMI) or high gestational weight gain during pregnancy and elevated risk/severity of autism spectrum disorder (ASD; Dodds et al., 2011; Krakowiak et al., 2012; Bilder et al., 2013; Reynolds et al., 2014; Moss and Chugani, 2014). Weight gain often involves low micronutrient absorption, or cortisol imbalance associated with systemic inflammation. Gestational diabetes also increases the risk of autism (Xiang et al., 2015), as does exposure to abuse from an intimate partner within two years prior to the birth year (Roberts et al., 2016).

Neurological pathways may also be determined in part by maternal dietary fat consumption in the perinatal period (Sullivan et al., 2014).

These risks, however, may be correlative, not causal. A careful analysis by Gardner et al. (2015) showed that although maternal BMI appears associated with ASD at the population level, analysis of sibling and paternal BMI strongly suggests that maternal BMI is likely a proxy marker for other familial risk factors. It appears that the same genetic or environmental factors shared among family members that predispose mothers to high BMI may also predispose offspring to ASD. This kind of analysis is essential for ruling out cause and correlation, and is only really possible in studies at the family level. Population association studies are only important as a first-pass discovery tool, and their utility in the case of rare, heterogeneous diseases is limited to positive results. Just as genetic association studies at the population level do not warrant conclusions about cause, association studies of environmental factors also should not be used to draw final conclusions about cause. This is especially so because negative results of environmental association do not prove no effect: the effect, as we have learned in autism, may be limited to unknown genetic susceptibility subgroups.

The same pattern of significance at the population level, but loss of significance at the family-level analysis was found by Roberts et al. (2016) for the effect of intimate partner abuse. Both Gardner et al. (2015) and Roberts et al. (2016) are to be commended for studying these risk factors in a "genetic effects in autism are clustered within families" aware approach. The use of population-wide association studies that ignore genetic clustering of effect results in poverty of knowledge, whether the finding is a positive or negative association. The age of genetic-agnostic association studies should come to a close.

Postmortem studies routinely show chronic microglial activation in autism. Chronic microglial activation is seen in autistic brains from age five years to age forty-four years (Vargas et al., 2005), and more recent studies show how microglia control serotonin (MacFarlane et al., 2015). Imaging studies show microglial activation in autism as well (e.g., Suzuki et al., 2013), and the signature of microglial activation in autism is obvious at the transcriptome (gene expression) level, which corresponds to anticorrelated signatures of neuronal activity (Gupta et al., 2014).

Microglial cells are dynamic cells with multiple roles in the brain: they perform routine surveillance and cleanup of cellular debris, viruses, and bacteria. They also monitor and maintain a balance between the number of dendrites and axons. Upon infection or serious brain damage, however, they become activated, change shape, and go on the attack as macrophages. They can damage dendrites and destroy neural precursor cells. The neurotoxic effects of aluminum salts are also apparent: they increase levels of glial activation, inflammatory cytokines, and amyloid precursor protein within the brain (Bondy, 2010). Amyloid precursor protein is one of the main suspected causes, or end product of processes, that lead to Alzheimer's disease.

We now have a more complete picture of how vaccines induce immunoneuroexcitotoxicity, as Dr. Russell Blaycock theorized so many years ago.

ADAPTIVE IMMUNITY AND EXCITOTOXIC MITOCHONDRIAL DYSFUNCTION

All of the above is sufficient reason to conclude that vaccine adjuvants can cause autism in some people via an immunological route. Skeptics sometimes point to the absence of evidence of involvement of the adaptive immune system, which rarely (but sometimes) crosses the blood-brain barrier. Recruitment of T cells from the periphery constitutes a major problem for the mammalian brain due to extensive damage that can occur during encephalitis (brain swelling). Studies have shown how peripheral viral infection can lead to the trafficking of CD8+ T cells, encephalitis, and death in mammals (Matullo et al., 2011). Half of all mice given a dual viral infection died of seizures, CD8-dependent edema, and brain herniation. The VAERS includes many cases of people who died of seizure after vaccination.

The evidence for the role of autoimmunity in autism is mounting (Cabanlit et al., 2007; Croen et al., 2008; Croen et al., 2008; Braunschweig et al., 2008; Rossi et al., 2013). Chronic microglial activation is a form of chronic (lifelong) autoimmune-induced brain injury, with microglia devouring nascent brain tissue and failing in their function to negotiate, foster, and, via intercell signaling, help sculpt the creation of synapses. So many roads in the molecular studies of autism ultimately have led to microglial activation, to the extent that focus on treatment of autism should begin with attempts to minimize exposure to toxins that elicit microglial activation, and treatment with compounds that coax microglia into their less aggressive, ramified state.

In addition to the general glutameric trauma induced by macrophagic delivery of aluminum into the brain leading to CMA, aluminum also may have a specific interaction with the pesticide glyphosate, inducing hypoxia and dysfunction in the pineal gland and disruption of gut biota, leading to excessive overgrowth of *Clostridium difficile* (Seneff et al., 2015). This could explain some of the sleep disorders observed in numerous neurological conditions, including ASD (Seneff et al., 2015). This hypothesis also brings a biologically plausible introduction of hypoxia into the cell, which could elicit glutamate-induced or excitotoxic mitochondrial dysfunction. Glyphosate alone was found to depress mitochondrial respiration by 40 percent due to partial inhibition of Complexes II and III, but not IV (Peixoto, 2005).

FUTURE STUDIES

Antigens used in vaccines in any form should be scanned for incidental homology (sequence similarity) to human proteins to avoid induced autoimmunity. This should be a standard feature of safety screens for vaccines. Full depictions of signaling between axons, neurons, and microglia during microglial balancing of dendrite:axon ratios, excitatory/inhibitory synapse ratios, and effects on dopamergeric/GABA transmission are needed.

SUMMARY

Cautions urged in interpreting microglial overexcitation as neurotoxic and causally linked to autism are no longer warranted. A direct causal link from aluminum accumulation to autism has been established. Regardless of the cause, chronic microglial overactivation clearly causes damage to neurites and may dispense with the homeostatic maintenance role, instead inducing apoptosis of healthy neurites, blocking the formation and reinforcement of local memory patterns. Immunoneuroexcitotoxicity is especially dangerous, and a straightforward, clear path has now been established demonstrating how neurotoxins, including mercury and aluminum, can induce a chronic, lifelong autoimmunity that targets neurites and neural precursor cells. Treatments designed to depress the excitotoxic state of macrophagic microglial cells, or to shut down IL-6 and mechanistic target of rapamycin (mTOR)-mediated proinflammatory responses, may show promise in the amelioration of deficits in learning and memory associated with autism. Autistic children carry signatures of their environmentally induced immunological exposures in their blood (antibodies against self-antigen); these markers should be studied in individual cases to identify likely causes and compared to age-matched typically developing children.

Autism may be a form of innate autoimmunity. An excellent review on *adaptive* immunological factors in autism is by Goines and Van de Water (2010). The best available review on innate immunological factors in autism is by Rodriguez and Kern (2011).

References : see envgencauses.com

Chapter 10.

GASTROINTESTINAL AND RENAL PHENOTYPES IN ASD

The gut is by far the largest interface the human body has with our environment. The autism gastrointestinal (GI) phenotype is often characterized by extremely poor GI functioning, with serious attendant health and development consequences. A very common clinical course involves ear infections (otitis media), potentially caused by mycoplasma infection (Armstrong et al., 2010; Welsh, 2015). This is most frequently followed by treatment with antibiotics and is accompanied by acid reflux, manifestation of loose bowels, and watery diarrhea. This can develop into daily explosive diarrhea during the course of a year.

Clinical examination may find pervasive lesions; ulcers and inflammation sporadically or throughout the gut, indicating a resident pathological process. Because initial signs of GI issues often appear after strong antibiotics, it is sometimes the gut microflora—viruses, bacteria, and yeast—that are the cause of the GI inflammation. Parents may find clinical diagnosis and treatment stressful and filled with dead ends.

While the history of GI issues in autism has a controversial past, a growing body of scientific findings confirms both GI and renal disorders are common in autistic disorder (AD). In this chapter, the degree to which these issues are genetic or environmental (behavioral or dietary) is examined. Also, the molecular basis is explored.

Most of the consideration of autism as a condition has focused on the central nervous system (CNS) and the brain in particular. However, autism is recognized as a multiorgan systemic condition, with dysfunction in the gut and with urinary dysfunctions, among others. Autistics often experience severe abdominal pain, accompanied by head banging and other *stimming* (i.e., repetitious, self-stimulating, sometimes injurious) behaviors. The chronic diarrhea, constipation, vomiting, gastroesophageal reflux, and intestinal infections add significant discomfort and distress to the patients and their families.

Initially, an hypothesis of a "leaky" gut was proposed, which would have helped explain much of the increased exposure to CNS measles infection and to neurotoxins from the environment (Wakefield et al., 1998). Subsequent studies failed to replicate the results of the Wakefield study, especially the presence of latent (aka persistent) measles infection that exists past the normal period of clearance. Hornig et al. (2008) studied 24 autistics and found persistent measles infection in one patient. Although the persistent infection does not seem to be universal, studies like that of Hornig et al. (2008) validate the plausibility association of GI issues with regressive autism.

There are major design issues with pasthuman vaccine studies, which focused on measles, mumps, and rubella (MMR) versus no MMR vaccine. These studies suffer from a number of possible biases, including that "no-MMR" equates to low overall vaccination rate and MMR equates to a higher vaccination rate. That is, differences between the two groups, when found, cannot be attributed to MMR alone. All studies that focus on MMR versus no MMR and do not consider other vaccines are confounded. Thus, future discussions on vaccine safety need to move well beyond MMR and the Wakefield controversy.

For a time, discussions of a leaky gut were considered nearly taboo, tantamount to scientific fraud. Studies now show that a large percentage of cases of food allergies in ASD have lesions throughout the intestine; one study reported intestinal permeability (thus, *leaky gut*) of 25.6 percent for children with ASD compared to 2.3 percent of healthy children (de Magistris et al., 2013). Children can be checked for antibodies against substances in food, including casein from milk and gluten from wheat. However, whether food allergies are due to immunological sensitivity, permeability of the gut, or both is unknown (de Magistris et al., 2013).

Approximately 30 percent of individuals in the general population have common genetic variants in either the HLA-DQA1 or HLA-DQB1 genes that predispose them to inflammatory-induced damage to tissues and organs when their immune system is confronted with a protein in wheat gluten (gliadin). Removal of the antigen from the diet dramatically improves the health of people with gluten sensitivities.

Although studies that have followed up on the initial report of Wakefield et al. (1998) have not isolated measles virus from the gut of ASD patients, Wakefield et al. may have been onto other factors that involve viruses on the CNS. The Wakefield study ostensibly examined "MMR vaccinated" individuals; however, the MMR vaccinated patients also likely had other vaccines, and models of persistent vaccine-borne virus-mediated gut inflammation (and autism) now seems plausible without requiring latent viral infection in the gut.

Two cases illustrate how infections can lead to autism. Consider the case of a girl who at age fourteen developed every symptom of autism due to herpes simplex encephalitis (Gillberg, 1986). A similar case involved a thirty-one-year-old man (Gillberg, 1991):

> *The author describes a previously healthy man who contracted herpes encephalitis at the age of 31 years and over the following months developed all the symptoms considered diagnostic of autism. This case report casts doubt on the notion of autism as an exclusively developmental disorder. It is suggested that temporal lobe damage may cause autism in some cases.*

Damage to the developing brain can occur due to infections by organisms, including the flu virus (*Haemophilus influenzae*) and cytomegalovirus. This damage can lead to autism when they significantly damage the developing, immature brain.

A study by Deykin and MacMahon (1979) found that a clinical history of common viral illnesses in the first 18 months of life, including mumps, chickenpox, fever of unknown origin, and ear infections were all significantly associated with increased risk of ASD. Congenital and perinatal rubella infection are accepted risk factors for autism. Viral infections activate the immune system, and, for some people, this can lead to autoimmunity and to hyperactivation of the innate immune system. MMR vaccines, as with all vaccines, are designed to activate the immune system. These findings allow us to ask if vaccine-induced immune system activation—by the presence of antigen, or by adjuvant (other vaccines), or both—may have been behind Dr. Wakefield's results after all.

Recent studies have demonstrated a strong correlation between a diagnosis of autism and maternal-reported incidence of GI problems. Gut issues appear early in ASD. In a large prospective birth cohort study, autistics were found to have significantly increased odds of constipation and food allergy and intolerance (Bresnahan et al., 2015), confirming past results. McElhanon et al. (2014) performed a meta-analysis that revealed that autistic children have four times higher incidences of constipation and diarrhea, twice as much abdominal pain, and are more than five times as likely to have general GI symptoms than children in the general population. Chaidez et al. (2014) showed that GI problems are higher in autistics and developmental delay patients compared to neurotypicals. Also, Welch et al. (2005) reported that areas of the brain associated with autism show signs of inflammation in a rat inflammatory bowel disease (IBD) model. And in keeping with approximately 20 percent of cases of autism involving either genetic or environmentally induced mitochondrial dysfunction, Gorrindo et al. (2013) found that plasma levels of F2t-isopostanes were elevated in autistics with gastrointestinal disorder, relative to autistics without GI disorders and to neurotypicals.

A robust and biologically sound hypothesis that could explain the high frequency of GI issues in the ASD population is the high frequency of immune-imbalance-related otitis media (ear infection). This state may also reflect an altered immune system and leads to treatment with strong antibiotics. This altered immune system in turn can lead to a dramatic change in the microflora of the gut (e.g., as reported for patients after coronary bypass surgery by Poeran et al., 2015). *Clostridium difficile* can overtake the gut, leading to chronic diarrhea. The severity of ASD and GI symptoms are strongly correlated. Fecal matter transplants can be used with great success to reintroduce the lost flora (Lyons-Weiler, 2016). Success has been reported within autism (see major review by Frye et al., 2015, who also outline GI in ASD research priorities).

MICROBIOMICS

It is becoming increasingly evident that signals—both neurological and molecular—from the gut can influence brain function. Pathogenic toxins and peptides can cross the blood-brain barrier, for example, eliciting a host of changes in the cellular activity of various types of brain cells. Disease-related variation in the gut microbes, *dysbiosis,* can affect anyone, especially after a course of strong antibiotics. A course of probiotics may be prescribed.

However, in autistics, there appears to be a manifold increase in the severity of GI issues. Some of these issues are no doubt due to the reduced ability for self-care. Walker et al. (2001) found that

> *ASDGI children have a gastrointestinal mucosal molecular profile that overlaps significantly with known inflammatory bowel disease (IBD), yet has distinctive features that further supports the presence of an ASD-associated IBD variant, or, alternatively, a prodromal phase of typical inflammatory bowel disease.*

Medically, however, and at the molecular level, researchers often see a drastic and desperate GI tract, including multiple lesions, ulcers, and dystonia, when they focus on a diagnosis of the tract itself.

VANCOMYCIN MAY HELP WITH GI ISSUES BUT HAS RISKS

A promising case report of a young autistic boy whose overall ASD symptoms appeared to improve after treatment with vancomycin is described by Rodakis et al. (2015). A very moving story of the boy's improvement includes increased eye contact, improvement in energy, and how the boy used his tricycle without prompting for the first time after months of seemingly unproductive training.

This case study was presaged by a study by Sander et al. (2000), who found nonpersistent overall ASD benefit (severity reduction) from treatment of 11 children with regressive autism in an intervential trial. Follow-up revealed loss of benefit; however, the authors noted the importance of understanding the mechanism of activity of vancomycin and its effects on ASD phenotypes.

ENTERIC MICROGLIA EXCITOTOXICITY?

There are numerous links between the immune system, gut-brain connections, and autism. Enteric reflexes are required for proper intestinal functioning. These reflexes trigger a complex array of signaling via the enteric nervous system. The GI tract contains such a large number of nerve cells and such a diversity of subtypes of nerve cells that it has been called "the second brain" (Grubišić and Parpura, 2015).

The intestinal mucosa contains various types of macrophages. It is now known that cytokine signaling from enteric neurons keep microglia-like macrophages in their ramified (nonactivated) state. Verheijden et al. (2015) presented an excellent review of the topic. The following passage from this review is particularly germane:

> *Intestinal macrophages are strategically located in different layers of the intestine, including the mucosa, submucosa and muscularis externa, where they perform complex tasks to maintain intestinal homeostasis. As the gastrointestinal tract is continuously challenged by foreign antigens, macrophage activation should be tightly controlled to prevent chronic inflammation and tissue damage. Unraveling the precise cellular and molecular mechanisms underlying the tissue-specific control of macrophage activation is crucial to get more insight into intestinal immune regulation. Two recent reports provide unanticipated evidence that the enteric nervous system (ENS) acts as a critical regulator of macrophage function in the myenteric plexus. Both studies clearly illustrate that enteric neurons reciprocally interact with intestinal macrophages and are actively involved in shaping their phenotype. This concept has striking parallels with the central nervous system (CNS), where neuronal signals maintain microglia, the resident macrophages of the CNS, in a quiescent, anti-inflammatory state. This inevitably evokes the perception that the ENS and CNS share mechanisms of neuroimmune interaction. In line, intestinal macrophages, both in the muscularis externa and (sub)mucosa, express high levels*

of CX3CR1, a feature that was once believed to be unique for microglia. CX3CR1 is the sole receptor of fractalkine (CX3CL1), a factor mainly produced by neurons in the CNS to facilitate neuron-microglia communication. The striking parallels between resident macrophages of the brain and intestine might provide a promising new line of thought to get more insight into cellular and molecular mechanisms controlling macrophage activation in the gut.

CX3CR1 is a chemokine receptor expressed by microglia in the brain. In mice that lack the gene, microglial cell numbers decreased and synaptic pruning was delayed (Paolicelli et al., 2011).

Because a person only has one genome, mutations that effect microglial activation signaling will impact their function in the gut as much as in the brain.

All of the mutations associated with autism that influence CNS function are therefore also candidates for enteric nervous system malfunction. Just as in the brain, enteric microglial cells provide guidance and neuroprotection by releasing antioxidants (Abdo et al., 2010, 2012) and trophic (growth) factors (Boyen et al., 2006). Enteric glial cells work against excitotoxic neuron death by regulating extracellular potassium (Hanani et al., 2000; Costagliola et al., 2009). Also, as in the brain, excesses of glutamate and/or nitric oxide cause excitotoxicity and neuronal death (Kirchgessner et al., 1997). The same study found that glutamate causes enteric neurites to express kainate (GluR5/6/7) receptor subunits. Recall that mutations in these receptors are known in ASD (Uzunova et al., 2014); therefore, in individual ASD cases, GI dysfunction could be wholly genetic, wholly environmental, or a mix of both factors.

The brain-gut link may also include serotonin involvement. The 5-HT2A receptor is underexpressed in the GI tract of autistics compared to controls, indicating altered serotonin signaling (Kazek et al., 2010). Increases in blood levels of serotonin in autistics appear to reflect a gene dosage pattern.

In addition to being a neurotransmitter, serotonin functions as a regulator of smooth muscle function and platelet aggregation, managing permeability of the intestine and inflammation of the intestinal tract (nonspecific enterocolitis; Kazek et al., 2010). A serotonin receptor in the brain acts as a switch for fear-induced defecation (Ohmura et al., 2015). Therefore, at least some of the gut-mind link is serotonin mediated.

Mutations in serotonin, serotonin transporters, and serotonin receptors and their involvement in ASD are reviewed in Chapter 5.

Considering the autistic phenotypes related to the serotonin pathways, the GI issues do not appear to be a core symptom of autism, but the view looks very different from the perspective of altered molecular signals that activate both enteric and brain microglia. The early appearance of symptoms found by

Bresnahan et al. (2015) provides a clue that something may be amiss in the gut of some children prior to the appearance of other symptoms. In their study, developmentally disabled children also show significantly more GI issues than those without AD or developmental disorder (DD) diagnosis, but the effect is larger in ASD.

A review of GI issues in autism is provided by Samsam et al. (2014). They reviewed studies that are inconclusive on whether the incidence of GI issues is higher in the ASD population than in neurotypicals. This inconclusion is the expected result if there is high genetic heterogeneity linked to the incidence of enteric dysfunctions. General studies for possible gene × vaccine interaction should be conducted (including individuals with mutations in the genes of interest for GI issues). Focused studies, which ask whether individuals with mutations in specific genes in ASD are more likely to have GI issues, could be informative not only on risk but on etiology.

Gastrointestinal issues can also have a syndromic cause resulting directly from genetic duplications (e.g., 15q duplication syndrome; Shaaya et al., 2015).

RENAL PEPTIDURIA

Renal function problems exist in a subset of autistics, and for these individuals it is a serious condition. These problems often lead to complications such as high blood pressure, heart disease, and neurodevelopmental problems.

In a study of patients from seven countries, Reichelt et al. (1997) found increased peptides in the urine profiles of autistics to be reversible by dietary modulation. Patients who stayed on a gluten- and milk-free diet did not progress, while those who did not stay on the diet did progress.

In a massive genome sequencing study of more than twenty thousand children, 7.4 percent of patients with chronic kidney disease were found to have copy number variations (CNVs), most frequently in the HNF1B gene (Verbitsky et al., 2015). They noted that many of the CNVs associated with chronic kidney disease were also associated with developmental delays, intellectual disabilities, and seizures. Notable among these was the 16p11.2 deletion, which was identified as a highly penetrant risk factor for autism (Weiss et al., 2008). Language deficits and intellectual impairments in autism due to 16p11.2 deletion appear as separate endophenotypes; specifically, left-hemisphere arcuate fasciculus mean and radial diffusivities were found to be negatively correlated with clinical language ability but not nonverbal cognitive ability (Berman et al., 2015). Some people with 16p11.2 deletions do not show signs of autism or any other condition, suggesting autosomal recessive mode with one or more environmental modifiers.

Vaccines given in the past typically contained thimerosal. A study of postmortem autistics by Palmieri et al. (2010) found that excessive calcium (Ca^{2+}) levels were responsible for boosting aspartate-glutamate carrier activity, mitochondrial metabolism, and, to some extent, oxidative stress in autistic brains. The excessive Ca^{2+} levels produced an unbalanced Ca^{2+} homeostasis in genetically vulnerable individuals. Palmieri et al. (2010) ruled out mitochondrial dysfunction, as no mutations were identified. Renal function is strongly influenced by Ca^{2+}-mediated efflux.

Palmieri et al. (2010) also pointed to whole-body effects of thimerosal as follows:

> *Thimerosal is a Ca2+-mobilizing agent, capable of releasing Ca2+ from intracellular stores and increasing Ca2+ entry. . . . Despite its short half-life compared to inorganic mercury, it undergoes preferential accumulation in the CNS, affecting the microglia and producing strain-dependent neurotoxic effects in rodents.*

Intestinal and renal glial excitotoxicity could be due to chronic exposures. The herbicide glyphosate (Roundup®), for example, causes glutamate-induced excitotoxicity (Cattani et al., 2014). Exposures that in general do not lead to intestinal and renal issues may be toxic to individuals with mutations that also confer risk to autism.

Given a genetic predisposition to excitotoxicity, otherwise non-toxic amounts of aluminum from any source could pose problems for the gut in ASD, especially via diet. Care should be taken to help children reduce their lifetime exposure to aluminum, mercury, glutamate, and other causes of chronic microglial activation to reduce risk of neurological and GI issues.

Similarly, keeping in mind that repeated episodes of chronic exposures are at least additive in their lifetime effects, it is interesting to note that renal impairment and nephrotoxicity induced by aluminum in pregnant rats involve inflammation marked by increased CD68 (a microglial marker), and the symptoms are alleviated by vitamin E and selenium (Abdel-Hamid et al., 2013).

Available research supports that chronic microglial activation is not merely an important process in the autism spectrum disorder (ASD) brain, but it seems to be a central factor in overall ASD phenotypes.

References : see envgencauses.com

Chapter 11.

NEUROTOXIN-INDUCED AUTOIMMUNE-MEDIATED NEUROLOGICAL DAMAGE IN AUTISM

Hundreds of scientists and doctors have come forward to emphasize that autism is an environmental disorder (Project TENDR, 2016). Preliminary estimates from the Project TENDR experts suggest that if exposure to top neurotoxic chemicals could be reduced by 20 percent, rates of autism, attention deficit hyperactivity disorder (ADHD), and/or learning disabilities could be reduced by 15 to 40 percent. This is reflected in the scientific literature as well. A major review found evidence that autism was associated with pesticides, phthalates, polychlorinated biphenyls, solvents, toxic waste sites, air pollutants, and heavy metals, with the "strongest evidence found for air pollutants and pesticides" (Rossignol et al., 2014). The Rossignol et al. review excluded studies concerning potential toxicant exposures related to medications (e.g., mercury or aluminum in medicinal preparations, including vaccines and dental amalgams), food additives, cocaine, alcohol, smoking, allergens, maternal stressors, and infectious agents (e.g., viruses, yeast, and bacteria). The review also excluded vaccines. A group of 140 research scientists, many from the National Institutes of Health (NIH), published a letter stating that autism is caused by environmental factors, including mercury (Project TENDR, 2016).

A systematic study of temporal trends of autism prevalence and environmental factors (Nevison, 2014) found that the increase in autism rates could not be explained by changes in diagnostic criteria and identified three environmental factors (out of all those studied) that had increasing trends that make them serious candidates for causal factors. The environmental candidates include polybrominated diphenyl esters, the herbicide glyphosate, and aluminum adjuvants in vaccines. Polybrominated diphenyl esters are commonly used flame retardants incorporated into textiles, motor vehicle parts, building materials, furniture, and electronics. Glyphosate appears as brand names Roundup™, Rodeo™, and Pondmaster™. Thimerosal was likely the cause of the first cases of autism diagnosed by Kanner in the 1930s. Some excellent sleuthing by Dan Olmsted and colleagues revealed that the first case Kanner described was born in 1931, just as diphtheria vaccines with thimerosal were introduced. Even more compelling was the identification made by Kanner of the occupation of another patient, who worked with thimerosal as a lumber preservative in his occupation as a plant pathologist.

Nevison's study did not start with the assumption of a correlation for any of the environmental factors; these factors showed themselves. Thus, the observed correlations can be thought of as a hypothesis that can be tested by cell tissue and animal and human studies.

Maternal ingestion or injection of valproic acid at the time of neural closure (Arndt et al., 2005) induces gamma-aminobutyric acid (GABA) signaling in the brain and has been used to treat epilepsy. Use of valproic acid (VPA) during pregnancy (gestational exposure) is known to cause autism. Kumamaru et al. (2014) found that VPA selectively prevents the formation of inhibitory synapses, the same mechanism of action of other activators of microglia. VPA also disrupts serotonin-2A receptor signaling (Sullivan et al., 2004).

Snow et al. (2008) found complex morphology in apical dendrites of pyramidal cells, indicating an initial lack of pruning (consistent with early brain overgrowth and initial hyperconnectivity). The arborization was more complex in VPA-exposed animals than controls.

Although no particular mutation appears to be necessary for VPA to induce autism, its activity highlights an important parallel role for some mutations. VPA induces the expression of Homeobox 1A gene (Hox1A; Rodier, 2003), and a common polymorphism in HOX1A doubles the risk of autism (Ingram et al., 2000). Mutations in Hox1A are correlated with macrocephaly in children with autism (Conciatori et al., 2004). Another effect of VPA is aberrant serotonergic neurons (Miyazaki et al., 2005).

Rodier et al. (1996) found that thalidomide caused a reduction in the number of neurons in facial nucleus, absence of superior olive (important for hearing), and shortening of the brain stem. Motor neurons in the brain stem are unlikely to develop normally. Hindbrain abnormality is highly correlated with Hox gene expression; specifically, pattern formation of the hindbrain is disrupted during neurulation (Rodier et al., 1996).

The fact that so many obviously high-potential molecular bases of core autism features can be caused by these compounds highlights the futility of *either/or* thinking in terms of genetics versus environment origin for autism. It also shatters two important logic flaws sometimes used in assigning causality, and a serious logic flaw concerning diagnosis. The first logic flaw commonly made is that for a factor to be a cause of autism, it must always cause autism. Some environmental factors will not cause autism in the absence of a given genetic factor. The second logic flaw is that for a factor to be a cause, it must be specific: that is, it and only it must cause autism.

The serious logic flaw in diagnosis is that a given case cannot be autism if a molecular etiology is known. For this logic to be solvent, no genetic influence is allowed in autism—clearly a nonviable position. It is nonviable because it is overly simplistic: multifactorial causality may or may not apply, and a factor can still be causal. (For this logic to apply, only one stage of a multistage rocket can be allowed to cause it to achieve escape velocity.) Clearly, some genetic variation will predispose some to being more sensitive to toxins in the environment than others. If combinations of genetic or environmental factors conspire to disrupt neuronal development or function in a manner than yields core autism and autism spectrum disorder (ASD) symptoms, diagnoses should be made according to phenotype, not genotype, because not every person with an ASD risk genotype will develop ASD. Treatment may be refined by molecular profile.

LOW DOSES OF MERCURY HAVE LARGE EFFECTS

Even small amounts of thimerosal induce major gene expression changes in the cerebellum. Minami et al. (2010) concluded: "The present study helps to support the possible biological plausibility for how low-dose exposure to mercury from thimerosal-containing vaccines may be associated with autism."

Animal studies have long confirmed that ethylmercury at vaccination schedule doses or lower causes neurological damage (Burbacher et al., 2005; Magos et al., 1985; Olczak et al., 2009; Qvarnstro et al., 2003; Rodriques et al., 2010). Yet the Centers for Disease Control and Prevention (CDC) has recommended thimerosal-containing influenza vaccines for pregnant women. They have never been asked by Congress to explain this policy recommendation. They seem to exhibit a *willful ignorance* of vaccine toxicity. They are not the only ones.

ALUMINUM: PAGING DR. OFFIT

Dr. Paul Offit earned millions of dollars from the sale of his jointly owned patent for a rotavirus vaccine, after he voted toward having rotavirus included in the pediatric vaccine schedule. He also appears unfamiliar with the body of peer-reviewed literature that demonstrates that aluminum is a serious neurotoxin, with well-characterized mechanisms of neurological damage.

In his book *Deadly Choices: How the Anti-Vaccine Movement Threatens Us All* (Basic Books, 2010), Offit is irresponsibly and recklessly dismissive of aluminum as a serious threat to the health of nearly all people by falsely reporting that ". . . aluminum has been found to be harmful in only two groups of people: severely premature infants who receive large quantities of aluminum in intravenous fluids and people on chronic dialysis (for kidney failure) who receive large quantities of aluminum in antacids."

Adults usually consume between 1 and 10 mg of aluminum per day (Greger et al., 1992); however, adults absorb only a tiny proportion of dietary aluminum. Babies, toddlers, and adults absorb 100 percent of the aluminum injected via vaccines. Offit claims, incorrectly, and without citation, that aluminum is very quickly cleared from the body. He cites "researchers" (without citations) who studied aluminum concentrations in blood before and after receipt of aluminum-containing vaccines and reported "No difference."

Offit's book was published in 2010. Unfortunately, it is evident that Offit did not bother to conduct a search of Pubmed Central® (http://www.ncbi.nlm.nih.gov/pmc/), a wonderful public scientific research literature database at the United States National Library of Medicine at the National Institutes of Health. Pubmed Central, which is the standard resource for the latest on research topics in medicine, biology, psychiatry, and many other disciplines. A Pubmed Central search reveals more than 200 studies or papers on aluminum neurotoxicity *before* 2011. As of January 2015, there were 399 studies or papers returned by search on *aluminum neurotoxicity*.

Some of these studies include direct discussions on the risk of aluminum in adjuvants in vaccines and provide data that demonstrate aluminum's mechanisms of neurotoxicity. Other studies discuss ways to alleviate neurotoxicity of aluminum. Yet other studies describe aluminum as a well-known neurotoxin responsible as a causal agent for neurodegenerative diseases.

Surely, Offit—an expert who served on on Advisory Committee on Immunization Practices, the body in the Department of Health and Human Services responsible for making decisions on changes to the pediatric vaccine schedule—would have checked the literature prior to 2011 while writing his book, in order to form his own opinion based on the current state of knowledge. If he had, he would have found studies with some compelling titles. The papers are condemning evidence against the use of aluminum in vaccines.

A large number of important studies completed prior to 2010 indicated aluminum adjuvants may induce self-sustaining and therefore chronic exitoneurotoxicity in microglial cells, motor neuron death, and behavior and cognitive deficits. Yet Dr. Offit omitted reference to these studies.

PRE-2011 KNOWLEDGE ON ALUMINUM NEUROTOXICITY

Nine of eleven available studies reviewed by Flaten et al. (2001) concluded that Alzheimer's disease incidence was greatest in regions with highest concentrations of aluminum in residential drinking water. Measures of inflammation, particularly in the brain, also correlated with increased levels of aluminum in for drinking water samples (Campbell et al., 2004); importantly, microglial cell activation was also increased. Piyasirisilp et al. (2002) lists autism among a variety of neurological adverse events reported after vaccination, including macrophagic myofasciitis attributed to aluminum. Polizzi et al. (2002) found that inhalation of aluminum dust in preclinical mild cognitive disorder might prelude Alzheimer's disease or Alzheimer's disease-like neurological deterioration, and suggested that monitoring blood levels of aluminum might be important to mitigate neurological deterioration observed in aluminum foundry workers. Savory et al. (2006) found neurofibrillary tangles in rabbits due to exposure to aluminum, which are precursors in the etiology to Alzheimer's disease. Aluminum adjuvants bioequivalent to the vaccine schedule for Gulf War military personnel led to motor neuron death and to behavioral and learning deficits in mice (Petrik et al., 2007). In mice, subcutaneous aluminum injections resulted in significantly increased death of motor neurons and increases in reactive astrocytes and microglial proliferation within the spinal cord and cortex. Reduced spatial memory capacity and impairment of motor function was observed after six doses (Shaw et al., 2009). Aluminum also influences cells other than microglia; aluminum alters mitochondrial metabolism, globular astrocyte shape, and astrocyte function (Lemire et al., 2009).

Vaccine-derived aluminum hydroxide responsible for macrophagic myofasciitis not only results in pain, fatigue, and depression, but also in cognitive deficits (Couette et al., 2009). The Couette et al. study is a peer-reviewed study and should not be ignored, especially by those who deny the existence of aluminum-induced neuroexitotoxity, who claim to base public health policy on peer-reviewed research but ignore this (and many other) studies. A critical passage in the Couette et al.(2009) paper:

> *Macrophagic myofasciitis (MMF) is an emerging condition, characterized by specific muscle lesions assessing long-term persistence of aluminum hydroxide within macrophages at the site of previous immunization. Affected patients mainly com-*

> *plain of arthromyalgias, chronic fatigue and cognitive difficulties. We designed a comprehensive battery of neuropsychological tests to prospectively delineate MMF-associated cognitive dysfunction (MACD). Compared to control patients with arthritis and chronic pain, MMF patients had pronounced and specific cognitive impairment. MACD mainly affected (i) both visual and verbal memory; (ii) executive functions, including attention, working memory and planning; and (iii) left ear extinction at dichotic listening test. Cognitive deficits did not correlate with pain, fatigue, depression, or disease duration. . . . In conclusion, long-term persistence of vaccine-derived aluminum hydroxide within the body assessed by MMF is associated with cognitive dysfunction, not solely due to chronic pain, fatigue and depression.*

Studies conducted since the publication of Dr. Offit's book have confirmed aluminum-induced neuroexitotoxity. Injection of aluminum silicate into the cisterna magna of ferrets resulted in an increase in reactive microglial in white matter, cortex, and hippocampus (Di Curzio et al., 2013). Akinrinade et al. (2015) demonstrated that oxidative stress impacts the activation of astrocytes (glial fibrillary acid protein [GFAP]) and mediates proinflammatory responses (microglia and B-cells: CD68 and CD20, respectively). Aluminum toxicity caused increased microglial activation and learning and behavioral deficits in Wistar rats (Stevanović et al., 2011). Aluminum nanoparticles also activate microglia (Li et al., 2009).

VACCINE ALUMINUM DOSAGE EXCEEDS FDA ALUMINUM LIMITS

Aluminum neurotoxicity has been known for decades. A study of perinatal exposure to intravenous aluminum (Bishop et al., 1997) found negative effects of aluminum on the neurologic development of infants born prematurely. Babies given standard IV solution were more likely to have a Mental Development Index of less than 85, and increasing aluminum exposure was associated with a reduction in the Mental Development Index. The authors noted that the decrease in Mental Development put these babies at risk of "subsequent educational problems." Furthermore, Bishop et al. wrote: "For all 157 infants without neuromotor impairment, increasing aluminum exposure was associated with a reduction in the Mental Development Index ($P = 0.03$), with an adjusted loss of one point per day of intravenous feeding for infants receiving the standard solutions."

Aluminum in breast milk impairs long-term memory in Wistar rats, with neuronal and synaptic ultrastructure exhibited pathological changes (Zhang et al., 2014), with disrupted cyclic adenosine monophosphate (cAMP)–protein kinase A (PKA)–cAMP response element-binding protein (CREB) activity. PKA is one of the mediators of microglial activation (Kyong-Jin et al., 2004).

Intraperitoneal injection of aluminum-containing vaccines into mice caused an increase in brain tissue aluminum levels two to three days after injection (Redhead et al., 1992). Aluminum was also shown to reduce glutamate-induced activation of nitric oxide (NO) synthase and NO-induced activation of the cyclic guanosine monophosphate (cGMP)-generating enzyme, guanylate cyclase in rats (Canales et al., 2001). They found strongly impaired glutamate-NO-cGMP pathway in cerebellum of rats chronically treated with aluminum. These authors wrote:

> *Aluminium is a neurotoxicant and appears as a possible etiological factor in Alzheimer's disease and other neurological disorders. . . . These findings suggest that the impairment of the Glu-NO-cGMP pathway in the brain may be responsible for some of the neurological alterations induced by (aluminum).*

Nayak et al. (2001) found that glutamate levels were increased in the cerebrum, thalamic area, midbrain-hippocampal region, and cerebellum in response to aluminium exposure in rats. They presaged: "The aluminium-induced differential regional accumulation of glutamate or other alterations in enzymes of the glutamate-GABA system may be one of the causes of aluminium-induced neurotoxicity."

Nayak et al. (2002) later found that protein malnutrition may influence the specific manifestation of aluminum-induced neurotoxicity.

El-Rahman (2003) also found increased glutamate and glutamine levels and decreased GABA level in rats chronically exposed to aluminum.

The hepatitis B vaccine, given the day of birth, is unsafe by Food and Drug Administration (FDA) standards for a typical (8-pound) baby with nearly 250 μg. By two months, babies have typically received more than 1200 μg more aluminum than is considered safe for their typical (12-pound) body weight. The FDA policy at the time of vaccine approval, for safe daily exposure to aluminum for full-grown adults (all sources), was 50 μg. Dosage per body weight considerations, important in pediatric drug dose toxicity (Lu and Rosenbaum), seem all but ignored in pediatric vaccinations—an afterthought that is discovered only after grave harm has been done to the population. This was also seen in the foot-dragging by the CDC to remove thimerosal from pediatric vaccines.

The risk of neurological damage from aluminum is more than autism. Aluminum can be deadly to a fetus. A study of mortality of neonates in Israel (Karakis et al., 2014) found that more than 25 percent of the mothers of the deceased has tested positive for aluminum, while 31 percent tested positive for semimetals. Cell proliferation rates were also at elevated levels, indicating oxidative stress.

Increased microglial activation results from elevated aluminum levels and can be attenuated by some chelators (Yokel et al., 1998). Some parents have attempted to reduce the risk of autism due to vaccines by administering Tylenol®; however, it is thought that the mechanism of action of acetaminophen depletes glutathione, inhibiting the natural antioxidant and detoxification pathways in the brain. Some doctors prescribe "buffers" prior to vaccination; however, no prospective randomized clinical trial has been conducted that demonstrates reduced autoimmunological reactions using such approaches. The reason that no clinical trial of such "buffers" has been undertaken is clear: repeated findings of positive associations of vaccines and autism have been hidden from public view (Thompson, personal communication to Brian Hooker; see Barr, 2015; Thompson, 2015).

IS VACCINE-INDUCED MACROPHAGIC MYOFASCIITIS ADULT-ONSET AUTISM?

A full decade before publication of Offit's book, Authier et al. (2001) reported central nervous system ailments eerily similar to those found in autism in patients. The patients were diagnosed with macrophagic myofasciitis (MMF) and displayed symptomatic demyelinating CNS disorder, hemisensory or sensorimotor symptoms, bilateral pyramidal signs, cerebellar signs, visual loss, cognitive and behavioural disorders, bladder dysfunction, supratentorial white matter hyperintense signals, and corpus callosum atrophy.

Clinical features of MMF as described by Rigolet et al. (2014) are also strongly reminiscent of autism, such as marked cognitive deficits (not related to pain, fatigue, or depression), dysexecutive syndrome, and visual memory impairment. Some cognitive deficits in MMF can be unusually severe. Cognitive dysfunction was found to be stable with time. Rigolet et al. also report that "classical therapeutic approaches are usually unsatisfactory making patient care difficult." Autism also involves cognitive deficits, executive function issues, memory impairment, low-level vision deficits, and can involve severe cognitive deficits that are recalcitrant to treatment.

Mice that have been injected with aluminum adjuvant doses equivalent to those given to US military service personnel undergo both neuroinflammation and cell loss in the spinal cord and motor cortex, with consequent memory deficits (Petrik et al., 2007).

The cause of MMF has been identified as aluminum hydroxide from vaccine lesions (Authier et al., 2006; Gherardi et al., 2001, 2012; Rigolet et al., 2014). Patients with MMF have an unusually long reaction at the site of injection of aluminum-containing vaccines in their muscles, and biospies show infiltration of muscle tissue by macrophages.

Authier et al. (2001) reviewed seven cases of MMF, accompanied by demyelinating CNS symptoms. All seven patients had received an aluminum-containing vaccine 3 to 78 months before the presentation of symptoms. Gheradi et al. (2001) reviewed immunizations for 50 patients presenting with macrophagic myofaciitis. Similar to the Authier results, all 50 individuals in the Gheradi et al. study had received aluminum hydroxide-containing vaccines 3 to 96 months before biopsy.

The World Health Organization Vaccine Safety Advisory Committee, long before 2011, had reported a subset of predisposed individuals who may be sensitive to aluminum-containing adjuvant (Authier et al., 2001).

ALUMINUM-INDUCED CHRONIC MICROGLIAL ACTIVATION

Gherardi et al. (2015) presented a chilling description of the effect of aluminum when used as an adjuvant:

> *. . . poorly biodegradable aluminum-coated particles injected into muscle are promptly phagocytosed in muscle and the draining lymph nodes and can disseminate within phagocytic cells throughout the body and slowly accumulate in brain.*

This description by Gherardi et al. (2015) is important because it clearly shows that activated microglial cells are macrophages with dual roles in the brain. These cells perform routine surveillance and cleanup of cellular debris, viruses, and bacteria. Upon infection or serious brain damage, however, the macrophages become activated, change shape, and begin to attack dendrites and neural precursor cells. Microglial overactivation is a leading candidate for increased apoptosis and neurological damage associated with autism.

The neurotoxic effects of aluminum salts are also apparent: they increase levels of glial activation, inflammatory cytokines, and amyloid precursor protein within the brain (Bondy, 2010). Amyloid precursor protein is one of the main culprits for Alzheimer's disease. An increasing cline in aluminum concentration has been seen in vasculature in proximity to the cerebrum, leading Bhattacharjee et al. (2013) to conclude that the epithelium of the vasculature leading to the brain has a high affinity for aluminum. Prolonged exposure to aluminum induced conformational changes in beta-amyloid protein and enhanced its aggregation in vitro (Kawahara et al., 2001).

Aluminum-induced encephalopathy and dementia have occurred due to environmental exposures (e.g., Meiri et al., 1991). A study of scalp hair samples from 397 people with neurological disorders showed that aluminum and manganese occurred in greater concentrations in afflicted people than 201 age-matched controls with no known disorder (Arain et al., 2015). In a similar study, patients with multiple sclerosis showed elevated levels of aluminum and rubidium compared to healthy controls (Tamburo et al., 2015).

Aluminum has been shown to be remarkably biopersistent, with variation in delay of peak concentrations by organ and by site of injection (Crépeaux et al., 2015). Lower doses in mice showed brain transport (being detected 45 days after injection in the brain), but greater doses showed no transport (likely due to toxic effects of aluminum on transporting macrophages). The authors concluded that "long-term biopersistence of alum in lymphoid organs is clearly undesirable and may cast doubts on the exact level of long-term safety of alum-adjuvanted vaccines."

Most dietary aluminum does not pass from the gut into the bloodstream. We absorb 0.1 to 0.3 percent of aluminum present in food and water, leading to approximately 0.05 to 0.4 μg/kg per day (Yokel, 2012). The pH of the gut makes dietary aluminum largely biologically inert.

In contrast, 100 percent of aluminum from vaccines estimated at 125 to 300 μg per dose is absorbed, leading to approximately 0.07 micrograms/kg/day (Yokel, 2012). Aluminum derived from vaccines has not been bathed in acidic and alkaline digestive juices.

Studies of the biopersistence of aluminum from dietary sources are reviewed by Yokel (2012), and the data indicate that while most aluminum is cleared within weeks, some remains in the body for *decades*. Aluminum accumulates in the brain as humans age (Roider et al., 1999).

IS ALUMINUM EVEN USEFUL AS AN ADJUVANT?

The medical community and the public should indeed revisit the issue of whether aluminum is a necessary adjuvant for vaccines. Use of virus-like particles with sufficient antigen loading requires no adjuvant. Such vaccines should be, but rarely are (if ever), screened for unsafe peptides with high homology to human proteins. Further, recent controlled trials found that the immunologic response to certain vaccines with aluminum adjuvants was no greater, and in some cases less, than that after identical vaccination without aluminum adjuvants (Willhite et al., 2014).

HOW ALUMINUM ENTERS THE BRAIN

Aluminum is far from biologically inert. It reacts to form complexes with oxygen-atom donor sites, including carboxylate and phosphate groups in biological systems (Kreski et al., 2007).

The form of aluminum and the environment in which it is found (gut, plasma, brain interstitial fluid, membrane-bound, etc.) are important. Willhite et al. (2014) provided a major review of the forms of aluminum (oxides, hydroxides, oxyhydroxides, and salts, and the soluability of particles) and wrote:

> *The toxicity of soluble Al forms depends upon the delivered dose of Al+ 3 to target tissues. Trivalent Al reacts with water to produce bidentate superoxide coordination spheres [Al(O2)(H2O4) + 2 and Al(H2O)6 + 3] that after complexation with O2•–, generate Al superoxides [Al(O2•)](H2O5)] + 2. Semireduced AlO2• radicals deplete mitochondrial Fe and promote generation of H2O2, O2 – and OH•.*

Thus, the mechanism for aluminum-mediated mitochondrial dysfunction in ASD is clear as well: "Thus, it is the Al^{+3}-induced formation of oxygen radicals that accounts for the oxidative damage that leads to intrinsic apoptosis."

The basis of the use of $Al(OH)_3$ and $AlPO_4$ as vaccine adjuvants is their affinity for antigens. A variety of cellular environments influence the degree of reactivity with biological systems, including properties of the biological surfaces to which these constituents bind (Gupta, 1998). Lesions at the site of injection of vaccines into cynomolgus monkeys included mostly macrophages three months after injection (Verdier et al., 2005).

EFFECTS OF VACCINE-DELIVERED ALUMINUM

Adenosine triphosphate synthesis is reduced by aluminum exposure, resulting in neurological and liver disorders by transforming astrocytes into globular "fat producing machines" (Han et al., 2013). Female mice given aluminum adjuvant gain weight, and males show signs of autism.

After the compulsory vaccination of sheep against bluetongue in Spain in 2008, a devastating incidence of autoimmune or autoinflammatory syndrome induced by adjuvants (abbreviated ASIA syndrome) was observed. These effects were reproduced by inoculation of adjuvant alone (Luján et al., 2013). Symptoms of ASIA include acute neurological episodes, with low response to external stimuli, acute meningoencephalitis, weakness, extreme cachexia, tetraplegia, and death. ASIA has been proposed to include vaccine-induced adverse events, including Gulf War Syndrome and MMF (Shoenfeld et al., 2011), and has been reported in a sudden onset of "pseudo-neurological" disorder following human papillomavirus (HPV) vaccination (Poddighe et al., 2014).

Shaw et al. (2013) gave mice vaccine-level doses of aluminum and saw weight gain, especially in male mice. The mice showed changes in behavior;

female and male mice showed a reduction in novelty-seeking behavior (males by a whopping 80 percent at 22 weeks after exposure). Considering available evidence, they also concluded that the correlation between ASD rate and aluminum adjuvant amounts shows dose-dependence and satisfies eight of nine Hill's criteria for causality, after also finding that aluminum caused weight gain in female CD-1 mice and CNS disturbance in male CD-1 mice.

In a study of the fate of two types of aluminum in rabbits, Flarend et al. (1997) found that a only 6 percent of aluminum hydroxide and only 22 percent of aluminum phosphate were eliminated 28 days after exposure: most was distributed to organs throughout the body, including the brain.

Bondy (2014) found parallels between the neurological insults of prolonged exposure to low levels of aluminum and premature aging of the brain. He reviewed further a significant body of literature showing that aluminum exposure leads to higher levels of inflammatory activity within the brain, even at low levels of exposure (Bondy et al., 2015). Further evidence is revealed by a case study of a man who died from Alzheimer's disease that reported elevated aluminum in his brain (Exley et al., 2014).

The most important facts about aluminum neurotoxicity:

- Risk due to exposure is cumulative and can be due to multiple exposures. Discussions of single dose amounts of aluminum are not useful.
- Although most aluminum is cleared during the short term, some persists, even for *decades.*
- Lifetime risk of neurodegenerative disease due to aluminum is cumulative.
- Childhood vaccination schedules surpass FDA limits per body weight.
- Aluminum activates the innate immune system and can cause gliosis.
- Aluminum has multiple routes into the brain.

ANIMAL CLEARANCE STUDIES ARE NOT FOR EVERYONE

Clearance studies of aluminum in animals should never merely look at serum concentrations, due to its higher affinity for organ tissues. Only a total recapture of all dosed aluminum from all body fluids and tissues can provide reliable measurements of the fates of the dose—something that is rarely done. Further, given a genetic risk predisposing some to aluminum retention, clearance studies in wild-type animals may be misleading, as they do not represent the population of individuals with genetic risk of ASD.

It is also not known if mutations in proteins in the gut make aluminum transfer more likely in ASD, or if mutations in protein in blood vessels and membranes might exist that predispose ASD patients to aluminum neurotoxicity. Mutations in proteins in astroglial cells could exist that would make uptake of aluminum more likely; alternatively, mutation in waste removal (detoxification pathways) could cause greater aluminum retention in the brains of some autistics. They include the genes that encode proteins in the endoplasmic reticulum for cellular waste removal and genes that regulate them.

Interactions among metals in situ have not been adequately studied for synergistic or ameliorative effects (Pohl et al., 2011). However, aluminum is known to form toxic complexes with other elements, such as fluorine, to interact negatively with mercury, lead, and glyphosate. Each complex can have a unique biological effect (Shaw et al., 2014).

The net implications of the studies discussed in the previous paragraphs are that aluminum toxicity by loading is very likely to be occurring during the CDC pediatric schedule.

MICROGLIAL ACTIVATION BY MERCURY

Mercury is used as a preservative in some vaccines. Many vaccines that were part of the pediatric schedules used thimerosal, which contains ethylmercury (EtHg). The evidence for biological plausibility for EtHg was outlined extensively by Kennedy et al. (2015). The evidence of microglial activation by mercury was reviewed by Kern et al. (2012).

The evidence of microglial activation by mercury is overwhelming and includes the following:

- Eskes et al. (2002) found that cultured microglial cells could be activated by noncytotoxic methylmercury chloride (MeHgCl). Activated microglia interactions with astrocytes increased interleukin (IL)-6 release, whereas microglia under normal conditions serve to further neuroprotection.
- Microglial cell counts were increase by exposure of mice to methylmercury (MeHg) in drinking water (Fujimora et al., 2009). Fujimora et al. also observed reduced numbers of neurons and evidence of necrosis and apoptosis in the cerebral cortex. They also reported a decrease in the number of neurons and an increase in migratory astrocytes.
- Prairie dogs exposed to mercury in their water showed increased expression of the proinflammatory cytokine, tumor necrosis factor (TNF)-α in a gender-specific manner (Thomas Curtis et al., 2011), with males showing more inflammation.

- Long-term exposure of rats to mercury led to microglial activation (Monnet-Schudi et al., 1996).

The doses used in many of these studies were low, and yet discovery of microglial activation has been repeatedly validated:

- One dose of $HgCl_2$ in rats resulted in an increase in microglial cell counts and deposits of mercury in nerve and glial cells (Gajkowska et al., 1992).
- Perinatal exposure of MeHg in drinking water in rats resulted in microglial activation, among other changes indicative of microglial hyperactivity (Roda et al., 2008).
- Neurotoxicity in rats was accompanied by glial involvement (Vicente et al. 2004).
- Long-term subclinical exposure of monkeys (*Macaca fascicularis*) to methylmercury resulted in an increase in microglial activation in the thalamus (Charleston et al., 1995).
- All of the neurons examined by Charleston et al. (1995) in monkeys exposed to long-term subclinical exposure to methylmercury and mercuric chloride had small deposits of IHg, whereas astrocytes and microglia had larger deposits.
- Microglia were found to be more responsive to methylmercury (Ni et al., 2011).
- MeHg stimulates the microglial secretion of lysosomal proteases, which cause lysis of nearby cells and lead to neuronal toxicity in vivo (Sakamoto et al., 2008).

Although the methyl form of mercury is not the same as that used in vaccines, the evidence of microglial activation is compelling. The fact that these are animal studies may be off-putting to some; however, the basic mammalian neurobiology is consistent across wide ranges of the mammalian order. Both inorganic mercury and an excess of glial cells were found in human patients with acute Minamata disease, with accompanying loss of neurons (Eto et al., 1999).

Past controversies concerning the role of mercury in vaccines as a cause of autism should be reexamined in light of the evidence showing microglial activation via neurotoxins. Similarly, aluminum is unsafe for use in vaccines. As increasing numbers of vaccines are added to the pediatric schedule, awareness of the neurotoxicity is also increasing, with repeated calls for action. Immunotherapy is the latest biomedical discipline to discovery aluminum neurotoxicity (Exley, 2014a; 2014b; Jensen-Jarolim, 2015). Exley et al. (2014) are among the latest to sound the alarm and call for reform in response to adverse outcomes resulting from aluminum neurotoxicity during subcutaneous allergy immunotherapy. They have also called out "industry propaganda" and "political interference" as futile against the truth of the causal role of aluminum exposure in neurodegenerative diseases. Jensen-Jarolim (2015) agreed with the expression of concern.

Other vaccine injuries involve autoimmunological pathologies as well. The increase in incidence of multiple sclerosis after the introduction of hepatitis B vaccine in France was explored by Le Houézec et al. (2014), who found seven of nine of Hill's criteria for causality to apply, with a maximum correlation at two years following vaccination.

A CALL FOR REFORM

It is critical that aluminum be removed from vaccines immediately! Furthermore, we need to understand how activating the immune systems (innate and adaptive) so as to induce fever 60–70 times effects children, even without an adjuvant. Chronic microglial activation occurs due to neurotoxins, that much is known. It is also certain that this is the primary route for postnatal autism. Maybe postnatal autism can also be induced via antigens alone. The scientific research needed to answer that question has not been undertaken. Perhaps neurological damage requires the interaction of neurotoxins × antigen (unlikely given that valproate and thalidomide induce CMA and autism in mice). Injection into muscle bypasses the subdermal dendritic cell reaction, and microdermal abrasion or similar techniques may confer more lasting immunity. The answer to these questions are critical to a fuller understanding of the link between vaccines and autism.

We need to remove thimerosal from *all* vaccines, especially from the CDC-recommended flu vaccine for pregnant women. It is unconscionable to continue to expose developing fetuses to mercury in any form, even in trace amounts.

In the meantime, genetic testing can potentially identify patients—and families—who are susceptible to developing autism both as a result of vaccinations (as currently formulated) and as a result of their genetic predispositions alone and exposure to background toxins. The ethical considerations concerning genetic testing in autism and mental disorders are explored by Gershon and Alliey-Rodriguez (2013). People with even a single gene indicating risk should avoid aluminum-containing vaccines.

Numerous additional environmental exposures increase the risk of autism. Risk is at least additive, and all sources contributing to chronic microglial activation (CMA) are harmful. For example, aluminum from roadside dust increases the risk of autism. And it is not just autism. It is Alzheimer's disease, schizophrenia, and Parkinson's disease. The research discussed in this and previous chapters supports medical exemptions based on the parents' desire *to reduce the cumulative lifetime risk of neurodegenerative diseases in their child by reducing exposure to known neurotoxins.* Parents may also wish to express their desire *to reduce the risk of autoimmune disorder development in their child.* These are both medical concerns that parents are entitled to express, and they are not addressed by sweeping generalizations about vaccine safety.

In rare instances, some families with two or three hits are likely to have children that develop autism without vaccines, especially if there is an inherited risk and a de novo mutation is present. Such occurences are exceedingly rare. I expect the combination inherited loss of function (LoF) + inherited CNV is extremely rare. I expect a slight increase in autism risk due to genetics. The human genome is at least two hundred thousand years old. Many common variants have existed for a long time—long enough to time our departures from Africa and trace our migratory routes around the world. Vaccines are approximately one hundred years old and the massive vaccination schedule only a scant 35 years old.

In this arrangement of factors, what then is necessarily the cause of autism? Instead of merely "genetics," the combination of increased rates of de novo mutations combined with an ever-increasing toxic environment matching toxins to variants seems more likely. The causes must be environmental factors such as vaccines and other industrial and agriculture exposures. Genetic variation does not condemn us to a fate of autism or other disease. We can mitigate the risk by our choices of environmental exposures to which we subject ourselves. The history of how society handled the link between smoking and cancer, and other lifestyle choices and cancer, supports this understanding of genes as secondary causal factors. Mutations that predispose individuals to cancer do not alleviate carcinogens of their role as a primary cause.

De novo mutations are more frequent in autistics, and they show variation in methylation. This implies that their environment is mutagenic—or that their parents' was, or both. Either way, the liability again easily falls to environmental factors as causes of de novo mutations and CNVs.

Clearly common variants are absolved from genetic liability as a primary cause because generations of individuals with those mutations do not have autism. Happenstance, rare de novo mutations, may contribute directly to cause autism. To understand or measure primary genetic liability, the immediate pressing challenge is to differentiate between de novo mutations caused by exposure to toxins concentrated in space and time by human endeavors from mutations that could have arisen without those exposures, and to separate the contribution of environmental toxins on some common variants. Unraveling these factors would be difficult.

It will not help to be dogmatic about the question of genetics or to pose the question as either/or. It will be more useful to ask what percentage of cases might be attributed to environment alone, to environment + vaccines, environment + vaccines + one-, two-, and three-mutation risk. Of course, the study would have to be retrospective, because it would be highly unethical to vaccinate any child who has known predisposing risk factors.

Each day that passes with aluminum in vaccines sees more cases of autism. Each person born has a natural right to express their genotypes without fear of being burdened by disease or disorder due to the artificial introduction of chemicals in their environment. At the same time, we have natural, constitutionally, and internationally recognized rights to informed consent, free from coercion and manipulation. Clearly, the imposition of vaccinations on a population in which a minority of people are much more susceptible to perverse outcomes than others does more than reveal the neurotoxins in vaccines as a primary cause. It reveals who we are as a culture and as a people. It defines the very moral fabric of our society.

The reasons presented above are enough to encourage prompt reform. But, as in Ebola, perhaps we need a selfish reason to care. The sum of the research studies strongly lead to the conclusion that given a large enough dose of neurotoxic insults leading to neuroexcitoxicity, *everyone* would develop autism. It is simply a matter of dose tolerance. The warning bells have been sounded. Now it is time to enact the changes needed to make vaccines safe, to protect the inherent rights of patients to refuse medical treatments, and to provide fully informed consent for those who choose to vaccinate.

References : see envgencauses.com

Chapter 12.

VACCINE-AUTISM STUDIES IGNORED BY THE CDC

On February 10, 2015, Rear Admiral Anne Schuchat, Principle Deputy Director of the Centers for Disease Control and Prevention, testified before Congress that vaccines were "highly effective and safe" and, specifically, that vaccines do not cause autism. By that date, the majority of the studies published in this book had been published; in 2012, the Institute of Medicine had rejected 17 of 22 studies conducted by the CDC as flawed, and the incidence of autism and ASD had risen to 1 in 68. In some states, the rate is now over 2 percent.

Massachusetts Senator Elizabeth Warren asked Dr. Schuchat a few softball, leading questions, and in each response, Schuchat reassured her that vaccines were highly safe and effective and that "dozens of studies" had been conducted that showed no association between autism and vaccines.

> Warren: "*Is there any scientific evidence that vaccines cause profound mental disorders?*"
>
> Dr. Schuchat: "*No.*"

Near the end of her testimony, the following interchange occurred:

> Warren: "*Parents should know that* all of the credible scientific evidence *suggests that modern vaccines are safe, modern vaccines are effective and modern vaccines are our best chance of protecting our children from diseases that can kill them, is that right?*"
>
> Schuchat: "*That's right.*"

The emphasis on *all of the credible scientific evidence* is mine, but the words are Warren's, agreed to by Schuchat, and they are critically important.

Schuchat dismissed most of the evidence cited to this point in this book, which is a very large number of peer-reviewed, credible scientific studies. As she agreed with Warren's statement, it follows that Schuchat testified that *all* of the evidence that contradicted her own was not credible. Her testimony, and the CDC's positions on vaccines and autism, are not credible.

Rear Admiral Schuchat's conclusion is inconceivable. All of those studies, paid for by the American people and government, were treated as if they never occurred and were never published. As if the National Institutes of Health, who funded those studies, did not exist. As if none of the rounds of peer-reviewed effort for grants and publications mattered. As if the hundreds of thousands of research hours were not spent. As if all the human effort and toil never occurred.

None of the intellectual effort from the US medical research institutions and universities mattered to Shuchat. None of it, according to Shuchat, was worth considering. She found *none* of it credible. That includes most of the science reviewed in this book.

A relevant question is whether she believed her testimony, or whether she intentionally misled Congress with her testimony.

Regardless of what her motives were, in my opinion *she was misleading the American public.* The rest of the science, reviewed in this book, debunks her testimony.

Further, many of the CDC studies on vaccine safety are retrospective epidemiological studies, which are fraught with risk due to the lack of proper experimental control. The interpretation of such studies hinge on the researchers' and/or the communities' agreement to consider unmeasured, uncontrolled, potentially confounding variables using underpowered studies. In retrospective studies, groups being studied are not random samples from the same population, and thus biases may exist that can impeach any findings of association. The same concerns can impeach findings of no association. Double-blind, randomized, prospective trials provide better control than retrospective studies. This is the FDA gold standard for approval of pharmaceutical and other treatments in medicine because they prevent unwarranted knowledge claims. The use of before-and-after measurements in clinical trials is rarely considered valid or important due to possible unseen confounders.

There are methods to accommodate the inherent biases of retrospective studies, such as matching, balancing, and alternative randomization schemes. In retrospective vaccine studies, statistical control is sometimes used, but the selection of "control variable" is subjective, and the history of the CDC research has been one of performing many rounds of analysis, until an initially detected association of autism with vaccines disappears. This topics is reviewed in greater detail in my book *Cures vs. Profits: Successes in Translational Research* (World

Scientific, 2016) and in Kevin Barry's book *CDC Whistleblower: Exposing Autism Research Fraud at the CDC* (Skyhorse Publishing, 2015).

Thus, much of the scientific research that Shuchat described as "credible" was, in fact, "highly suspect." And for good reason. Not only are retrospective studies notoriously susceptible to biases and confounding, but the outcome of the analysis can be manipulated to a particular desired—or expected—result. More important, vaccines have long been suspected of inducing (in some people) lifelong autoimmunological conditions. Peanut oil used in vaccines (Hobson, 1973) has been considered a possible cause of the rise of peanut allergies, but no studies have been conducted that demonstrate an increase or decrease in people exposed to peanut oil in vaccines. Autoimmune diseases induced by vaccine via epitope redundancy—the sequence or structural similarity of peptides in humans and pathogens—have been called the *elephant in the room* (Moise et al., 2015). The evidence for increases in vaccine-induced autoimmune disorders after vaccination is reviewed very clearly by Orbach (2010).

A more recent example of research on vaccine-induced autoimmune disease is the finding that the onset of central nervous system demyelinating syndromes was found to be associated with "vaccines of any types" within 30 days after vaccination in a case-control study in individuals younger than 50 years (Langer-Gould, 2014).

It does not take a stretch of the imagination to see how the immune system may learn to respond to self-antigens that resemble those in pathogens, when adjuvants like aluminum so effectively activate the adaptive immune response. This topic has been extensively studied by Yehudah and colleagues (e.g., Agmon et al., 2009; Rinaldi et al., 2014).

But then one does not need a stretch of the imagination when we have the bulk of scientific research that so clearly indicates that as more vaccines have been added to the pediatric schedule, we have been putting more and more immunostimulants into the bodies of our youth, inducing increasing numbers of autoimmune reactions to an increasing diversity of antigenic peptides, and stronger *innate autoimmunity*, especially immunoneuroexcitotoxicity, in human studies.

HUMAN STUDIES THAT SUPPORT A VACCINE-AUTISM LINK

Below is a list and brief description of peer-reviewed publications of studies that stand, in addition to those cited in previous chapters, in direct contradiction to Schuchat's testimony to Congress.

Gallagher and Goodman (2010): A cross-sectional study of the National Health Interview Survey from 1997 to 2002 found that the odds of a diagnosis of autism is threefold greater in neonates who received hepatitis B vaccination than those who did not, and that minorities had an even greater risk of autism attributable to vaccination status. They reported a ninefold increase in the rate of developmental disabilities associated with vaccination overall for boys. The others concluded: "U.S. male neonates vaccinated with the hepatitis B vaccine prior to 1999 (from vaccination record) had a threefold higher risk for parental report of autism diagnosis compared to boys not vaccinated as neonates during that same time period. Nonwhite boys bore a greater risk."

Delong (2011): This study found, after correcting for family income and ethnicity, that a 1 percent increase in vaccination rates resulted in 680 children with autism or specific language impairment (SLI). The author concluded: "The results suggest that although mercury has been removed from many vaccines, other culprits may link vaccines to autism."

Sharpe et al. (2013): This study showed increased thimerosal hypersensitivity in B cells grown from autism spectrum disorder (ASD) individuals from four families, compared to controls. Cellular proliferation and mitochondrial function measures were taken. The authors concluded that "certain individuals with a mild mitochondrial defect may be highly susceptible to mitochondrial specific toxins like the vaccine preservative Thimerosal."

Tomljenovic and Shaw (2011): In looking for a triggering effect, this study examined a given year's total aluminum dose and the rates of autism diagnosis. Autism spectrum disorder incidence in each year (1991–2008) increased overall with increasing aluminum content, consistent with an epidemiological model of more and more children surpassing their individual dose tolerance. In addition, they found that a sufficient number of causality criteria applied to support causality of the observed correlation.

Geier and Geier (2007): The authors describe details of nine patients whose ASD symptoms and mercury exposure could only be attributed to thimerosal-containing vaccines. "Eight of nine patients (one patient was found to have an ASD due to Rett's syndrome) (a) had regressive ASDs; (b) had elevated levels of androgens; (c) excreted significant amounts of mercury post chelation challenge; (d) had biochemical evidence of decreased function in their glutathione pathways; (e) had no known significant mercury exposure except from Thimerosal-containing vaccines/Rho(D)-immune globulin preparations; and (f) had alternate causes for their regressive ASDs ruled out."

Young et al. (2008): These researchers examined the available data in the Vaccine Adverse Events Reporting System and found an association of exposure to thimerosal-containing vaccines with "[c]onsistent significantly increased rate ratios were observed for autism, autism spectrum disorders, tics, attention deficit disorder and emotional disturbances with Hg exposure from TCVs."

Nataf et al. (2006): These authors studied urinary porphyrin levels in ASD, Asperger syndrome, and internal and external control groups. Coproporphyrin, a measure of exposure to environmental toxicity, was found to be elevated in children with autistic disorder relative to control groups, but not Asperger syndrome. The authors concluded : "These data implicate environmental toxicity in childhood autistic disorder."

Yasuda and Tsutsui (2013); Yasuda et al. (2013): Scalp trace element scans were studied for scalp hair concentrations for 1,967 autistic children. "In the 1,967 subjects, 584 (29.7 percent) and 347 (17.6 percent) were found deficient in zinc and magnesium, respectively and the incidence rate of zinc deficiency was estimated at 43.5 percent in male and 52.5 percent in female infantile subjects aged 0–3 years old. In contrast, 339 (17.2 percent), 168 (8.5 percent) and 94 (4.8 percent) individuals were found to suffer from high burdens of aluminum, cadmium and lead, respectively and 2.8 percent or less from mercury and arsenic. High toxic metal burdens were more frequently observed in the infants aged 0-3 years-old, whose incidence rates were 20.6 percent, 12.1 percent, 7.5 percent, 3.2 percent and 2.3 percent for aluminum, cadmium, lead, arsenic and mercury, respectively."

Blaurock-Busch et al. (2012): This study compared hair metal concentrations of autistic and nonautistic children and found that "elevated hair concentrations were noted for aluminum, arsenic, cadmium, mercury, antimony, nickel, lead and vanadium. . . . There was a significant positive correlation between lead & verbal communication . . . and general impression." The authors concluded that "heavy metals play a role in the development of ASD."

Molina and Shoenfeld (2005): In considering the link between vaccine and pediatric autoimmune neuropsychiatric disorders, this analysis (not a new study) concluded that "Vaccines, in several reports were found to be temporally followed by a new onset of autoimmune diseases."

Bradstreet, et al. (2003): This study examined urinary mercury levels in vaccinated versus unvaccinated children after a three-day treatment with meso-2,3-dimercaptosuccinic acid (DMSA), an oral chelating agent. They found that mercury concentrations were significantly higher in children with autistic spectrum disorders compared to neurotypical controls and that vaccinated (treated) cases showed a significantly higher urinary mercury concentration than did vaccinated (untreated) controls. The authors concluded: "The observed urinary concentrations of mercury could plausibly have resulted from Thimerosal in childhood vaccines, although other environmental sources and Thimerosal in Rh (D) immune globulin administered to mothers may be contributory. Regardless of the mechanism by which children with autistic spectrum disorders have high urinary mercury concentrations, the DMSA treatment described in this study might be useful to diagnose their present burden of mercury." Notably, a later comparison of autistic and nonautistic urine mercury levels—without treatment—reported to show no difference in removable mercury, but their analysis was not standard, leading DeSoto (2008) to comment, "your data shows autistic children have higher levels of heavy metals."

McDonald K et al. (2008): In a study 11,531 children, those who delayed vaccination had a much lower risk of asthma (McDonald et al., 2008). According to the authors, "Early childhood immunizations have been viewed as promoters of asthma development by stimulating a T(H)2-type immune response or decreasing microbial pressure, which shifts the balance between T(H)1 and T(H)2 immunity." Reversibility of effect is key in determination of causation, and while this study does not demonstrate reversibility, it demonstrates dose effect. The authors concluded: "We found a negative association between delay in administration of the first dose of whole-cell DPT immunization in childhood and the development of asthma; the association was greater with delays in all of the first 3 doses. The mechanism for this phenomenon requires further research."

Singh et al. (1998): Using standard measurements of presence of antibodies, Singh et al. found that ASD children had elevated measles antibodies and increased brain autoantibodies relative to age-matched controls. Dr. Paul Offit claimed in his book *Autism's False Prophets* (Columbia University Press, 2008) that this study did not measure antibodies; indeed, the study used standard enzyme-linked immunosorbent assay (ELISA). Offit would have to impeach hundreds of thousands of studies that used ELISA to warrant his patently false claim and untold numbers of official findings by the CDC, including, for example, Atkins (2002). His claim also potentially defames the authors of the Atkins study with libel. The authors concluded: "This study is the first to report an association between virus serology and brain autoantibody in autism; it supports the hypothesis that a virus-induced autoimmune response may play a causal role in autism." Note that Dr. Rosalyn Yalow, co-inventor of ELISA, won the Nobel Prize for medicine for her work with the then-deceased Solomon Berson in 1977 in the development of ELISA.

Holmes et al. (2003): This study looked at the mercury content from infants' first haircuts: "First baby haircut samples were obtained from 94 children diagnosed with autism. . . and 45 age- and gender-matched controls. . . . Hair mercury levels in the autistic group were 0.47 ppm versus 3.63 ppm in controls, a significant difference. The mothers in the autistic group had significantly higher levels of mercury exposure through Rho D immunoglobulin injections and amalgam fillings than control mothers."

Li X et al. (2009): This study compared cytokine levels, measures of immune activities, in the brain tissue of ASD patients and matched normal subjects and found a clear signature of autoimmunity. They found proinflammatory cytokines with an immunological Th1/Th2 ratio swayed toward Th1 overrepresentation. The authors concluded: "ASD patients displayed an increased innate and adaptive immune response through the Th1 pathway, suggesting that localized brain inflammation and autoimmune disorder may be involved in the pathogenesis of ASD."

Vargas et al. (2005): This study showed that microglial activation, a sure sign of excitotoxicity and neuroinflammation, are both found in autistics. The vaccine link to microglial activation has been established by other studies. The authors concluded that "innate neuroimmune reactions play a pathogenic role in an undefined proportion of autistic patients."

Seneff et al. (2012): This study examined the trends in the reported occurrence of autism in Vaccine Adverse Event Reporting System (VAERS), noting an increase in reports that may be attributed to the increased burden of aluminum in vaccines as mercury was being phased out. They found that adverse events in individuals who had received aluminum-containing adjuvant attributable specifically to aluminum decreased after 2003. The data showed a marked decline, as would be expected due to the removal of thimerosal from vaccines if a thimerosal × aluminum interaction was present. From the authors:

> *While we have not shown that aluminum is directly causative in autism, the compelling evidence available from the literature on the toxicity of aluminum, combined with the evidence we present for severe adverse reactions occurring much more frequently following administration of aluminum-containing vaccines as compared to non-aluminum-containing vaccines, suggests that neuronal damage due to aluminum penetration into the nervous system may be a significant factor in autism.*

Seneff et al. also noted a strong correlation between autism and the MMR, which contains neither aluminum nor mercury, but which they thought might be explained as an increased sensitivity to acetaminophen administered to control fever. It is now known that acetaminophen depletes glutathione levels in the brain.

Poling et al. (2006): Many people think that Hannah Poling was never diagnosed with autism. In fact, her claim of vaccine-induced autism was conceded by medical experts from the Department of Health and Human Services. The Special Master court has repeatedly found in favor of vaccine-induced injury of encephalopathy with "autism-like features."

I will let the case description speak for itself and let the reader decide. This is the opinion of Hannah's neurologist, Dr. Andrew Zimmerman, who provided a diagnosis of autism and was prepared to testify in her behalf:

> *Within 48 hours after immunizations to diphtheria, tetanus and pertussis; Haemophilus influenzae B; measles, mumps and rubella; polio; and varicella (Varivax), the patient developed a fever to 38.9°C, inconsolable crying, irritability and lethargy and refused to walk. Four days later, the patient was waking up multiple times in the night, having episodes of opisthotonus and could no longer normally climb stairs. Instead, she crawled up and down the stairs. Low-grade intermittent fever was noted for the next 12 days. Ten days following immunization, the patient developed a generalized erythematous macular rash beginning in the abdomen. The patient's pediatrician diagnosed this as due to varicella vaccination. For 3 months, the patient was irritable and increasingly less responsive verbally, after which the patient's family noted clear autistic behaviors, such as spinning, gaze avoidance, disrupted sleep/wake cycle and perseveration on specific television programs. All expressive language was lost by 22 months. The patient continued to have chronic yellow watery diarrhea intermittently for 6 months, which was evaluated with negative testing for Clostridium difficile, ova/parasites and culture. Four months later, an evaluation with the Infant and Toddlers Early Intervention program for possible autism was initiated. Along with the regression, her appetite remained poor for 6 months and her body weight did not increase. This resulted in a decline on a standard growth chart for weight from the 97th to the 75th percentile.*

Dr. Jon Poling, Hannah's father, felt compelled to write a letter to a blogger named Steven Novella because of his representation of the case online. Novella, a neurologist, posted a reply that included his assessment (without full evaluation) of Hannah's condition as not likely autism because, in his view, "Hannah Poling's history has many features that are not typical of autism—like a history of otitis media with frequent fevers, seizures and what sounds like a rare encephalitis that probably did result from vaccines. Even if we put her mitochondrial mutation aside—this is not a typical case of autism."

At the time of Novella's reply (July 2008), Rosenhall et al. (1999) had already reported that at least 25 percent of cases of ASD had otitis media, and a more recent study (Deavenport-Saman, 2015) has found that otitis media is one of the top three reasons for autistics to appear in emergency rooms. And, of course, seizures are often reported as comorbid with autism (approximately 25 percent). Frequent fevers is consistent with autoimmunity and chronic microglial activation, both part of the immunological inducement of AD and ASD. It is important to pay attention to evidence in medicine in support of positions that might influence public health policy.

Palmer et al. (2006): These authors found a 43 percent increase in the rate of special education services and a 61 percent increase in the rate of autism for every one thousand pounds of environmentally released mercury.

Mohamed et al. (2015): Concentrations of mercury, lead, and aluminum were measured in hair samples from one hundred autistic children and one hundred controls. All three metals were found to be higher in autistic children compared to controls. The authors concluded that "environmental exposure to these toxic heavy metals, at key times in development, may play a causal role in autism."

Each one of these studies described above provides peer-reviewed results that stand in direct contradiction to Schuchat's testimony to Congress, as well as other testimony from other CDC scientists, including Dr. Coleen Boyle, who attempted in 2012 to convey a message of no link between vaccines and autism but, when asked by Rep. Bill Posey whether a "vaccinated versus unvaccinated" study had been done, finally relented that no such study had been conducted. The evidence in the book stands in stark contrast to the current stagnant CDC policy on vaccine safety research. What if the CDC also knew there could be an association with neurological disorders but never brought it forward as a publication? See, for example, the following unpublished report.

Verstraeten et al. (2000) (unpublished CDC internal report) found a positive association for all ASD and ADHD and vaccination exposure. This result was never included in a published study, but some of the text of the report, obtained via a FOIA by Safeminds, is interesting:

> *As for the exposure evaluation at 1 month of age, which is basically an evaluation of the neonatal hepatitis B dose, we have found a significant relationship to the outcome only for* misery and unhappiness disorder *(ICD9 code 313.1). We were not able to produce a graph for the RRs at 3 months of this condition as no or few cases occur in the two lower categories. The relative risk for this condition was significantly increased (2.04, 95% CI:1.09–3.82) when comparing those with a cumulative exposure above 62.5 ug at three months compared to those with cumulative exposure equal to or less than 62.5 ug.*
>
> *There is a nearly significant increased risk for the category exceeding 12.5 ug at 1 month for attention deficit disorder. This group includes children that received 2 doses of HepB or the first dose of Hib or DTP in the first month of life. At three months, this positive relationship is no longer significant for any category.*
>
> *As for the exposure evaluated at 3 months of age, we found increasing risks of neurological developmental disorders with increasing cumulative exposure to*

Thimerosal. Within the group of developmental disorders, similar though not statistically significant increases were seen for the subgroup called specific delays (ICD9 code 315) and within this sub-group for the specific disorder developmental speech disorder (dysalia, ICD9 code 315.39) and for autism (ICD9 code 314.0) and attention deficit disorder (ICD9 code 314.0). This increase, when comparing each category of exposure to the lowest exposure group was significant only for the entire category of developmental disorders. For specific delays and speech disorder this increase occurs only about 25 ug.

Later in the same report:

7. Comparison to the number of vaccines, aluminum

The purpose of these analyses would be to differentiate between the effect of Thimerosal and the vaccines themselves. Unfortunately (nearly) all vaccines in our analysis were either Thimerosal containing (DTP, DTaP, HepB and Hib) or Thimerosal free (polio). Any analysis of the number of vaccines or aluminum as an exposure variable would show a correlation to the Thimerosal analysis and not be helpful in this distinction. I ran analyses with the number of Hib, DTO, HepB and polio vaccines as exposure and found a relationship of the risk [of ADHD] *to the number of DTP and Hib vaccines received at three months, which was to be expected. I also found a relationship to the age at which the first Hib vaccine was given (the later the vaccine given, the less chance of neurological developmental delay), which was also to be expected. Surprisingly, I did not find this for DTP.*

These are the findings of the CDC. They never appeared in any peer-reviewed publication, and were released only after a Freedom of Information Act request.

These passages cited above show a huge lapse in logic on the part of the analyst. If they cannot comment on aluminum because it is confounded with the dosage of thimerosal, the reverse is equally true (such is the nature of confounding). They seem to be oblivious to this rather obvious fact. And yet, the analyst was willing to apply the knowledge from the thimerosal analysis leading to the expectation of results—in which they even showed surprise to not find an association for DTP!

None of this text reads remotely like any of the association studies from the CDC on vaccines. Anywhere one looks for CDC statements, they state unequivocally that "Vaccines Do Not Cause Autism" and "Vaccine Additives Do Not Cause Autism." Officials at the CDC have testified under oath before Congress to the same effect. These officials have offered neither qualifiers nor caveats, just absolute knowledge on vaccine safety, with no exceptions.

The congressional testimony of CDC officials reveals that they are not dealing in science. Knowledge in science is asymptotic. There are almost always exceptions to the rule. Their position is so unqualified that even a single case of autism resulting from vaccination would make their statements absolutely false.

If there had been only one or two studies, Schuchat might be excused for dismissing the evidence of a vaccine-autism link. However, a huge number of studies that point to immunoneuroexcitotoxicity were available at the time of her testimony, and more are available now. There is no excuse for her testimony, but her behavior was consistent with other examples of grossly misleading information from CDC officials.

The literature is filled with studies that the CDC ignores. Most of the studies to date in this book have been either animal studies (completely ignored by CDC), or correlation studies (weak science), and studies that show microglial activation in the brain involving human subjects. But now we turn to both the studies conducted by the CDC and those conducted by others not associated with the CDC.

NEGATIVE RESULTS FROM EPIDEMIOLOGICAL STUDIES OF INDIVIDUAL VACCINES ARE NOT SUFFICIENT "EVIDENCE"

The CDC has relied on negative results from retrospective epidemiological studies for their positive claims of the safety profiles of vaccines and vaccination schedules. Results from these types of studies are not acceptable by the FDA for other medical treatments. They insist on prospective, randomized clinical trials. The problems with the types of studies on which the US national policy on pediatrics is based are numerous:

- Population level association studies can miss important associations when they ignore or are unaware of genetic substructure within the population. This is especially so in autism, in which local clusters of risk exist due to different genes, different alleles within the same gene, or de novo mutations (i.e., private alleles) across families.
- The studies are often not powered sufficiently to detect small but important shifts in frequencies of events. This is important because autism only occurs in 1 to 2 percent of the population currently. Underpowered trials are unethical because they are wasteful of resources, and their negative findings are misleading.

- People who tend to get vaccinated may have more access to health care, creating a healthy-user bias, in which the vaccinated group has fewer poor health outcomes simply because they are more likely to be seen by doctors. This is a type of confounding. Another type of healthy-user bias is that individuals with conditions such as autism tend to be excluded from the studies.

Another type of confounding confuses a signature of an adverse event within a vaccine schedule as due to just one vaccine of interest. This type of confounding has occurred for years in the discussion of the measles, mumps, and rubella (MMR) vaccine apparently without much previous notice. Studies of any individual vaccine that compare rates of autism in groups receiving varying amounts of other vaccines are not informative, because people in both groups also received other vaccines. Yet such studies continue to be published (e.g., Jain et al., 2015; Uno et al., 2015). Groups may not differ because the contribution of a specific vaccine of interest; "vaccinated" versus "vaccinated except MMR" is a fairly weak comparison, especially if only 0.6 to 2 percent of the population is at risk of autism at that level of exposure. Also, "MMR vaccinated versus not" comparisons will not likely be able to attribute any findings to "MMR," because "MMR vaccinated" individuals will also likely have received other vaccines. Much of the discussion on vaccine controversies focuses on MMR vaccines, whereas a more useful study would be "fully vaccinated" versus "never vaccinated."

Similarly, animal studies have been conducted in a rather fruitless manner. In a study of a small number of monkeys given doses of neurotoxins of thimerosal that match (per body weight) the doses received according to the 2003 CDC Pediatric Schedule, not a single animal developed autism-like symptoms. However, it is obvious to anyone who has conducted such studies in the past that, given the low prevalence of ASD, the study was not powered for a relatively rare condition diagnosed in 1 to 2 percent of the individuals. Animal studies in which each animal had a constellation of mutations influencing the pathways known to be disrupted, given the doses and compared genetically with matched animals with no dose of adjuvant or preservative, would be more informative.

In correlational studies, the failure to find an association is not evidence of no association, especially when the studies are underpowered and cannot expect to find an association if one indeed exists, due to these undesirable source of systematic variation (i.e., bias). Power analyses should be published as a matter of routine for studies that influence public health policy, and underpowered studies with negative results should not be published.

POPULATION LEVEL STUDIES MISS FAMILIAL RISK AGGREGATION FOR BOTH GENETIC AND ENVIRONMENTAL RISKS

Genetic studies inform us unequivocally that autism genetic risk is highly heterogeneous. Studies at the population level can therefore miss specific associations that are discernable. Subphenotypes within autism that are missed at the population level are detected with family aggregation studies (e.g., Liu et al., 2011; Yirkud et al., 2009). Studies of association of overall disease with environmental factors that are agnostic to genetics, when there is also a genetic risk, are extremely poorly defined. Studies that ignore population substructure, or that do not account for admixture, may similarly miss important associations. The shortcomings of these types of studies have been known in genetics since Wahlund revealed it in 1928.

Interaction terms are also frequently ignored in vaccine safety studies, and yet they are critically important in genetic and environmental studies. The study of interactions between factors requires even larger sample sizes.

ACCESS TO HEALTH CARE BIAS?

A study of the relationship between autism rates and socioeconomic status in New Jersey found that children in wealthier areas tended to have a higher rate of autism (Thomas et al., 2012). While it was not the intentions of the authors of that study, the fact that they attributed the higher rate of diagnosis of autism to better "access to pediatric and developmental services" is ironic, considering that "access to pediatric and developmental services" could thus be considered a risk factor for autism. Any ecological attribution of improved diagnosis is likewise similarly confounded with higher compliance to vaccine schedule in a direction supportive of the role of vaccines in autism.

References : see envgencauses.com

Chapter 13.

CONCEPTS OF COMORBIDITY IN AUTISM AND AUTISM RESEARCH

Concepts on the co-occurrence of conditions with autism, and autism with other conditions, are sometimes unclear. The use of comorbid conditions to exclude patients from safety trials, for example, may exclude individuals whose second clinical condition (e.g., seizures) may be caused by the same factors that led to a diagnosis of autism. Understanding molecular pathology of disease is best done from a molecular point of view, rather than imposing specific medical assumptions into the design of a study. Some seemingly unrelated conditions may share common causes.

CONDITIONS THAT MAY CO-OCCUR WITH AUTISM AND ASD

Approximately 70 percent of cases of autism occur with intellectual disability and 25 percent with seizures (Tuchman et al., 2002). Many autistics also have gastrointestinal ailments, including bloating, gassiness, and chronic constipation, and many have attention deficit hyperactivity disorder (ADHD). Many of the genes contributing to autism are also not specific to autism risk; thus, any number of additional diagnoses are possible (e.g., co-occurring). Discernment of when co-occurrence of any particular conditions (e.g., seizures) is comorbid, or part of an autistic diagnosis, is more than a semantic distinction. If the mutations or copy number variations (CNVs) that lead to diagnosis of autism also cause seizures, separating the phenotypes clinically and medically for a given patient is not reasonable. If, however, distinct pathways are disrupted for a given phenotype, the patient may in fact have two separate conditions, and separate routes to treatment will likely be successful. Generalizations about whether seizures are part of, or co-occur with, autism are not likely to be meaningful. Only a full spectrum of genotype assays followed by biochemical assays will confirm separate or identical etiologies. An excellent treatment of the various etiologic juxtapositions of autism with schizophrenia is given by Crespi et al. (2010), who found twenty genes that overlap in the etiology of autism and schizophrenia. It is apparent that two or more conditions may be subsumed, separate, diametric, and overlapping all at the same time, depending on the gene or pathway at which one is looking.

COMORBIDITY AS A CONFLATED CONCEPT IN NEUROLOGICAL DISEASES

Just as the classification of autism is complex, the relationship of autism to other conditions is also complex and conceptually challenging. For example, intellectual disability is observed in approximately 70 percent of individuals diagnosed with autism (Bryson et al., 2008; MMWR Surveill Summ, 2014; Yeargin et al., 2003). Is this a symptom, a phenotype, or a comorbid condition? Most would see it as a symptom and a phenotype. It is certainly likely to be useful as a composite diagnostic indicator.

Similarly, seizures and epilepsy are often seen to occur in autistic individuals (Canitano et al., 2007; Nazeer et al., 2012). If taken, within autism, as comorbidity rather than phenotypes, it would seem to simplify the unraveling, especially because the molecular etiologies of some of the other phenotypes of autism are shared with those of seizures. This is true for other neurological diseases and conditions as well. High rates of comorbidity of epilepsy are not limited to autism; up to 50 percent of individuals with epilepsy were reported to also have some psychiatric disorder (LaFrance et al., 2008) and, in an odd reversal of relativistic focus, 28 to 40 percent of individuals with intellectual disability were reported to have other autistic features (Bryson et al., 2008; La Malfa et al., 2004). Damage done to the brain by seizures may also accentuate existing, or introduce autistic, features.

MOLECULAR MARKERS AND MOLECULAR SYNDROMES

As many as 10 percent of autistics have obvious chromosomal aberrations, and approximately 10 percent of children with autism have some other single-gene condition that also has an additional formal diagnosis, such as tuberous sclerosis complex, epilepsy, or Fragile X syndrome. It must be noted that the presence of a molecular marker must not be used to automatically provide a diagnosis (e.g., mutations and even large-scale chromosomal rearrangement are not always specific to a condition). Autism can be found within, or to co-occur with, these conditions.

Fragile X syndrome is a good example of a condition with known molecular etiology. If Fragile X syndrome is considered a separate syndrome, it can be considered to co-occur with autism, or to overlap with autism, or for Fragile X syndrome patients to have autism-like symptoms. However, not all people with Fragile X syndrome are autistic. If they were, one would consider it "autism within Fragile X syndrome." Instead, when autism occurs with Fragile X syndrome, it should be studied as "Fragile X syndrome with autism."

Rett syndrome was nearly removed from the autism spectrum because it has a known molecular cause (Abbeduto et al., 2015). There are reasons to keep Rett syndrome within autism spectrum disorder (ASD), such as the high degree of overlap of mutations found in individuals with Rett syndrome and ASD.

Similar clarification is helpful clinically in Dravet syndrome. Dravet syndrome is an infant-onset epileptic encephalopathy characterized by generalized seizures. The specific types of seizures include clonic, tonic-clonic, or hemiclonic. Patients may also develop other types of seizures, including myoclonic, absence, or partial seizures. The seizures are often unresponsive to conventional antiepileptic drugs. Typically normal development, prior to onset, is followed by decline of cognitive development. Behaviors indicative of autism are also often noted. Behavioral comorbidities include delay or loss of language abilities, hyperactivity, and impaired social behavior, all clear indicators of autism.

Many cases of Dravet syndrome involve mutations in the SCN1A gene. The existence of this mutation is often seen as a distinguishing characteristic *between* autism and Dravet syndrome, and yet autism clearly co-occurs with Dravet syndrome. SCN1A mutations, thought to be specific to Dravet syndrome, have now been repeatedly found to be risk alleles for autism. If seizures are thought to bring on autism, then any environmental cause of a case of Dravet syndrome can also be seen as an ultimate cause of the ensuing case of autism. Decisions on diagnosis should not waiver on this point and merely list "autism-like symptoms." If sufficient symptoms exist for placement on the spectrum, it should be thusly diagnosed. A comprehension of the molecules involved does not relieve any environmental trigger of liability, and it should not cause a clear-cut case of autism to be reclassified. Some studies refer to "autism within Dravet Syndrome"; this arrangement of relationships clarifies admission of autism occurring due to, not merely coincidental with, Dravet syndrome.

Some have questioned whether a subclinical condition called alexithymia, which is the general inability to identify one's own and others' emotions (lack of empathy), should be considered to be part of autism, or something that co-occurs with autism (Bird and Cook, 2013). The authors, interested in raising alexithymia from a subclinical to a clinical condition outside of autism, in part because it may co-occur with autism, concluded that:

> *. . . Crucially, matching autistic and control samples for alexithymia should therefore become as routine as matching for age, gender and IQ. . . . Where the affected networks relate principally to social cognition and cognitive control, a "pure" autism phenotype may emerge.*

Bird and Cook (2013) cited a functional magnetic resonance imaging (fMRI) study (Silani G et al., 2007), which found that within awareness of one having one's feelings, a third order of experience exists in which one is aware that one *exists* and is having emotions, a necessary but not sufficient condition for one identifying *their* emotions. Silani et al. (2007) continued:

> *Lambie and Marcel (2002) have reviewed models of emotional experience and argued for a framework where a distinction is made between the neurophysiological arousal associated with emotions (first-order experience) and the awareness of this arousal, often referred to as interoception (second-order experience). In addition, we need to consider a third level, arising from the requirement to introspect on one's inner experience, an aspect that is particularly relevant for autism. This level involves an awareness of a self who has emotions and can monitor them and is different from a second-order bodily awareness of emotions. If impaired introspection or self-reflection characterizes autism (Kennedy, Redcay, & Courchesne, 2006), then we would expect the self-reflective system to be less active. In individuals with autism who also have a high degree of alexithymia this activity might be reduced still further when they are required to introspect on their emotions.*

The aspect of alexithymia found by Silani et al. (2007) to be predictive of alexthymia, but not autism per se, was evidence (or lack thereof) of the second order of experience. Because any of the three orders of experience could lead to a failure to identify one's feelings, alexithymia is not an interceding condition; its root cause when studied in autistics involves any deficit in knowing one is alive (third order), is having emotions (second order), thus being able to identify those emotions as their own (combination of third and second), and is capable of having that emotion in the first place (first order). Alexithymia would seem to be easily embedded as one of the phenotypes of autism that is not required for, and not specific to, a diagnosis of autism, as is the case of many others. Thus, one would consider "autism with alexithymia," not "alexithymia versus autism."

Alexithymia is known to occur with many other conditions outside of autism; however, when alexithymia is considered to occur with autism, studies that seek to understand causes could lose power-to-detect significant causes, if case and control groups are balanced for percentage of alexithymia. The specific aims of the study would determine balancing; that is, if the goal is to study alexithymia within autism, for example, balancing across groups would negate the comparison. The use of alexithymia as an overall control variable in autism studies seems a terrible idea for general studies in autism, as it would preclude understanding the molecular and environmental causes of a core feature, the social affective disorder phenotype in autism. Control for alexithymia, or any particular phenotype within autism, could be done by nested case-control studies. If balanced overall, or "corrected for" by using a statistical model, such restricted studies would fall into the type of study of "rates of phenotype X in autism independent of phenotype Y," which would be very informative. However, selecting one of the mosaic features of autism and "correcting for" it as a matter of routine would necessarily warp general studies in a manner responsive to that one particular phenotype and could lead to many false negative findings of association between molecular and environmental factors. Given the seemingly haphazard distribution of autism phenotypes, this would seem unsafe from a design-of-analysis perspective.

This thinking is followed up in other studies, including one entitled "Alexithymia, Not Autism, Predicts Poor Recognition of Emotional Facial Expressions" (Cook et al., 2013). This thinking is flawed due to the seeking of prediction or causal inference of one phenotype (alexithymia) to explain another (poor recognition of emotional facial expressions). The dissection of alexithymia based on argumentation is insufficient; a distinct molecular or environmental cause of alexithymia would be needed in each case to pull the alexithymic attributes of social affective phenotype out of autism. If the molecular etiologies or environmental triggers are the same, we have something closer to a syndrome

(Asperger syndrome [AS] with alexithymia), perhaps indicating a different route for therapy for AS with alexithymia than for those with AS without alexithymia. That is to say, Cook et al. (2013) may be correct in attributing poor facial expression interpretation to alexthymia, but it almost certainly then contributes to difficulty studying spoken language, reading social situations, and so on, as phenotypes.

Such practice would remove a significant part of the autism experience deserving of explanation to satisfy a proposed disease classification device (i.e, elevation of alexithymia to a clinical condition). It is better to study phenotypes in their setting and to study the relationships among the phenotypes in terms of their severity and root causes. No one would, for example, propose to balance case and control studies in cancer for the rate of cellular division, although numerous diseases involve hyperplasia. For example, I cannot imagine controlling for hyperplasia in the study of precancerous prostate tissue and prostate cancer: it would remove a fundamental signature of cancer. Studies in autism that have manipulated explanatory covariates as "control variables" should be stricken from the publication record, as they profoundly stifle or corrupt our ability to understand autism.

A better representation is given by Griffin et al. (2015), titled "Alexithymia in Children with and without Autism Spectrum Disorders." They found that alexithymia is elevated in ASD on both self- and parent-report measures. However, they found no evidence of correlation between the two measures and concluded that parents of autistics and their children may be using different sources of information. They found that parent-rated alexithymia was associated with increasing severity of autistic traits.

Like molecular syndromes, I am deeply concerned that anyone who wishes to elevate a specific phenotype of interest to its own syndrome may, in a concerted fashion, end up chipping autism away to nothing—nothing to be explained, or studied, except bits and part of autism with their own esoteric names. Worse, it could leave the appearance of a valid, objective study design but leave no ability to detect key signatures of causes of autism. I am advocating for the retention of a many-to-many relationship framework. The *Diagnostic and Statistical Manual of Mental Disorders, Fifth Edition* (DSM-5) in this capacity scores well for moving clinical decisions forward: autism or ASD can be diagnosed with additional conditions noted. But for research on etiology and cause, the utility of dissected designations remains to be shown.

Conditions other than alexithymia co-occurring with higher frequency in autistics include allergies and autoimmune diseases, including psoriasis (Zerbo et al., 2015), perhaps reflecting a common environmental causal factor.

Neurofibromatosis, an apparently genetic neurological disorder, may be comorbid with autism, but the relationship is not completely understood (Bilder et al., 2016).

ORDERS OF COMORBIDITY CONCEPT

Understanding comorbidity and familial genetics of complex phenotypes requires careful consideration of the attributes being studied. Evidence of heritability of autism is strong; therefore, the phenotypes of autism that are synonymous with core symptoms are the characteristics encoded by genes. The complexities of the patchwork quilt of autism phenotypes manifest in patients on the spectrum disappear when individual phenotypes are studied. Considering proximate and ultimate causes helps to clarify as well, and therefore I propose various levels, or orders of comorbidity as follows:

First-order comorbidity: The co-occurrence of subclinical or clinical conditions, directly traceable to the same molecular and environmental etiologies for the key symptoms, leading to a diagnosis of a condition on the spectrum. These causes share a biological basis, and one phenotype is not the consequence of another.

Second-order comorbidity: The co-occurrence of subclinical or clinical conditions that are not directly derived from the same molecular or environmental causes of autism and instead are attendant *consequences* of autistic phenotypes. Examples are the increase in the occurrence of dental issues due to improper dental maintenance care or frequent illness due to a bland diet or poor self-care. Another example is one biological pathway disrupted by mutation, leading to downregulation of a related biological pathway. In these cases, the genetic cause of phenotype may suggest the molecular cause of another.

Third-order comorbidity: The co-occurrence of subclinical or clinical conditions that are not directly derived from the same molecular or environmental causes of autism and are not attendant consequences of autistic phenotypes. These are truly independent comorbidities, lacking any obvious causal or correlative link, that seem to co-occur with frequencies greater than expected by chance. This category may hold comorbidities for which evidence is merely lacking, for want of study, or due to limitations on the current state of knowledge of genomic and systems biology.

Fourth-order comorbidity: The co-occurrence of subclinical or clinical conditions that are not derived from, but instead have their own independently occurring molecular (usually genetic) cause and are not attendant consequences of, but may amplify the severity of (but not cause), other autistic phenotypes. This can occur due to co-segregation (physical linkage on chromosomes) of loci (genes) that contribute to autism and contribute to other conditions otherwise unrelated to autism.

With these four orders, consideration of the existence and nature of the functional relationships among autistic phenotypes and comorbid conditions can be discussed. Such discussions should include the types and levels of the evidence required for categorization of the types of relationship of autism and comorbid conditions.

However, the genetic, genomic, and comorbid information is likely to be far more important in the consideration of likely effective treatments and therapies than for revisiting diagnoses. Under DSM-5, treatment considerations are given in terms of severity, but not necessarily in terms of the constellation of phenotypes aggregated in a patient's presentation.

SEVERITY OF AUTISM AND FOURTH-ORDER COMORBIDITY

The core phenotypes of autism appear to stem from a myriad of inherited and de novo genetic mutations, and in many cases are due to some (usually unspecified or undiscovered) environmental trigger. The specific biological pathways leading to individual core phenotypes are sometimes known to interact; thus, the impact of one core phenotype may exacerbate or ameliorate another. While diagnosis may be better informed via genetics, potential treatments may be ruled in and ruled out on the basis of research that has been shown to demonstrate specific targeted mechanisms of action.

For example, some individuals with autism and ASD have language delay partially caused by sensory variance. For these patients, it seems likely that oxytocin may increase attention and may enhance the duration of time for social bonding. For parents, these moments of clarity and presence can be very touching, and they may represent windows of opportunity within which learning may be more feasible. Research on the timing of the treatment to help the patient learn more effectively may be fruitful.

It is basically impossible to cleanly tease apart many medical and psychiatric conditions that involve the brain. Different conditions involve disruptions of overlapping pathways. Depending on one's focus or specialization, a primary diagnosis of, for example, epilepsy may be specific *with autism* . . . without a primary diagnosis ever being made or considered. However, in another specialist's consideration, the diagnosis could be *autism with seizures specified.* The consequences to the patient to understanding that both diagnoses need attention and that one may be functionally correlated and not causally linked must be made very clear when it comes to autism. The mutations and environmental injuries that lead to autism can also lead to seizures. It makes little sense from a molecular biology standpoint to say "seizures caused this case of autism" if in a given case the root cause to both conditions is identical. Encephalopathy itself is a generic description of "something wrong" with the brain, not a specific clinical endpoint, and thus cannot cause autism but rather helps describe autism (e.g., "encephalopathic autism" would apply to all cases of autism). By contrast, a serious infection or a cold may exacerbate certain autistic traits, and thus may modify the intensity of certain autistic phenotypes, an example of fourth-order comorbidity.

Sometimes molecular biological mechanisms of conditions prevalent in comorbid with autism are very well worked out, and they can be rather illuminating. Wang et al. (2015) also found pervasive pleiotropy, where one gene influences many phenotypes, among psychiatric conditions and immune disorders. This is not surprising given that the immune system is so clearly involved in the processes that lead to manifestation of autism.

FIRST AND SECOND-ORDER COMORBIDITY

Life with autism is challenging. Physicians are keenly aware that autistic children and adults suffer from less-than-optimal health care in part due to core phenotypes. Communication may be impaired, for example.

However, as more becomes known about autism, all subtypes of autism should not be removed from ASD merely because we better understand the molecular etiology. Breast cancer, for example, is not removed from cancer when a familial mutation is identified. Comorbid conditions should not be used administratively to move cases away from ASD unless the ASD phenotypes are not present. That is, we should address autism wherever it presents itself.

Thus, it is useful to specify and distinguish first- and second-order comorbidity. In first-order comorbidity, the two conditions are completely independent—they are neither causally linked from an etiological standpoint nor correlated. Second-order comorbidities allow that some relationship exists between two conditions. Second-order type 1 is causal, and second-order type 2 would be correlational. Autism shares a second-order relationship to encephalopathy, because the mechanisms of causation of autism outlined thus far are types of encephalopathy. As vaccines are known to bring about the cellular dysfunctions that cause autism, it clearly follows then that vaccines cause autism. Doctors should be careful to diagnose suspected cases of vaccine-induced autism as "vaccine-induced encephalopathy-mediated autism," allowing families to seek financial remedy as well as services.

IS OUR THINKING ON COMORBIDITY DRIVEN BY ACADEMIC SPECIALIZATION?

If comorbidities between physically distant regions of the body can be attributed to the same ultimate etiology (e.g., brain and gut dysfunctions due to maternal immune reactions during development), then perhaps the issue of fine-tuning a diagnosis based on so-called comorbid conditions in physically proximal parts of the body is putting too fine a point on the issue of comorbidity. DSM-5 calls on clinicians to conduct diagnoses and to note comorbid conditions, which, while inclusive and clinically actionable, does not portend to elucidate common or independent (coincidental) co-occurences of, for example, autistic disorder and intellectual disability or seizures. Without knowledge of the etiological relationships among the conditions, the term *comorbid* may prove to be a presumptive misnomer for those relationships in any specific case. The precedent of the core features defines the condition; that is, genetics informs.

We can consider variations of autism, as in the spectrum concept, and we can consider etiologic overlap within ASD and overlap with other conditions. There has been much confusion on this issue, and the clearest example is in the extreme: in a possible future in which the etiology of each and every case of autism is clearly described, each individual will have his or her own molecular syndrome, and autism will cease to exist.

It would be much more useful to develop decision rules and nomograms for clinical diagnosis that are generated via machine-learning optimization of diagnostic rules using a variety of inputs that match phenotype constellations within autism to effective treatments informed by genetics.

A DEVELOPMENTAL VIEW ON COMORBIDITY AND BRAIN DEVELOPMENT

Arm-waving at the time of babbling observed by Iverson and Wozniak (2007) suggests failure of specialized development and confusion of motor operations. The special relationship between somatomotor and language processing indicated by Lambardo et al. (2015) is likely to be a trade-off in real-time abilities, or at least a failure of the dampening of motor operations during language processing. Either way, the link between language processing and motor operations seems to be causal, and thus they may be examples of second-order comorbidity type 1, even though the severity of the trade-off in abilities may vary greatly even within autistic disorder and across the spectrum. Such variation often reveals the funcational relationships among variables population, rather than indicating dichotomies. We see confusion of sensory input with motor impulse throughout autism in part due to inhibition dysfunction and in part due to developmental miswiring.

COMORBIDITY AND STUDY DESIGN

Handling comorbidity in the study of etiologies of autism is clearly a complex maneuver that should not be undertaken lightly. The use of variables in model specification and model definition for multivariate models such as multiple-regression analysis of variance (ANOVA) and analysis of covariance (ANCOVA) must be carefully thought out. Known causal relationships among variables must be clearly spelled out first to avoid model misspecification. Statistically correcting for immunological status, for example, would obviate the study of any effect on medical outcomes that are mediated via immune system differences. Data analysis in this space is not for the weak of heart, especially given that Dr. William Thompson of the CDC has alleged scientific misconduct on the part of the agency in association with studies that use multiple variables (Barr, 2015).

Responsible data analysis plans will conduct and report an a priori causal relationship check among pairs of variables via open discussion—with literature citations—to determine if any a priori reason exists for two or more variables to be causally linked. When they are not independent variables, one can perform model selection with one or the other but often not both, as the inclusion of both (or more) may lead to model overfit due to multicollinearity. Such is the case of the Verstraeten et al. (2003) study.

Thus, before one decides to "correct for" conditions that are clinically considered comorbid, one should be sure that the clinical designation has not missed an important previously known functional relationship among variables, and one must not decide to correct for variables based on mere suspicion. Measures of collinearity should be reported. To do so is to ignore prior knowledge, with potentially disasterous consequences, and is very poor science. There are also formal measures such as Mallow's Cp; however, when actionable knowledge exists to guide model specification, informed models can prevent lost opportunities for discoveries of important causal inference. A finding that "correcting for" birth weight, gestational age, and mother's income "removes" an initial association with an environmental variable, such as vaccination, requires consideration of the interaction term and a conclusion that association exists but is modified by they key variables. Birth weight and gestational age and age of mother and mother's income are functionally related and should not be used as in independent variables.

Because they involve diagnoses, congenital rubella infection and pre- and postnatal infections by *Haemophilus influenzae* and cytomegalovirus are also considered comorbid conditions. While the comorbid category of these infections does not rule them out as causal factors, studies of other factors should not enroll patients whose cause of autism is likely already known unless interaction terms are to be studied. Thus, exclusionary criteria should include patients with causally comorbid, but not attendant nor consequent comorbid, conditions.

WHAT COMORBIDITY MEANS FOR ENVIRONMENTAL RISKS SUCH AS VACCINE STUDIES

Association studies comparing the incidence of autism at varying exposures to vaccines tend to exclude individuals that have comorbid conditions known to confer genetic risk of autism. For example, cerebral palsy is a static motor deficit of brain origin, present from early life, and is found in 2.1 to 2.9 percent of individuals with autism and mental retardation. A vaccine safety study that excluded people with cerebral palsy would be irrelevant for the population of people with cerebral palsy.

Conclusions such as "there is no association between vaccines and autism" are overreaching, as they do not allow for the fact that certain excluded clinical groups may be at increased risk of ASD (or any other adverse event) because they were never studied.

References : see envgencauses.com

Chapter 14.

STUDY DESIGNS FOR MEANINGFUL FUTURE CAUSAL RESEARCH IN AUTISM

Retrospective association studies are correlational, and thus any positive result is criticized for not demonstrating cause and is rejected ex post facto as "merely correlation." These types of studies are also woefully prone to the intrusion of confounding variables, and the results are subject to the whims of the vagaries of data analysis. When the data analysis is repeated over and over until an expected or desired result is found (e.g., "no association"), the exercise falls outside of the realm of science. If the habit of continuing weak, merely correlational studies continues, no assessment of causality will ever be made.

Prospective trials are better suited to allow causal infererence. The definition of clinical population is critical for the success of studies aimed at understanding the causes of disease. In autism, the various categories are not fully fleshed, but they are almost certainly not hierarchical. The removal of Rett syndrome means that individuals with Rett syndrome might then also be found to have other, autism-like features. However, the primary diagnosis of Rett syndrome will likely be the driver for therapies. Opportunities for effective treatments that are discovered for autism should not be overlooked or denied for patients with Rett syndrome. On a case-by-case basis, this problem can be solved via individualized approaches to genome-sequence informed treatments.

However, targeted therapies might not even be discovered if the initial subcategories are not correct. Exclusion of individuals from specific subtypes defined for such studies could limit investigators' abilities to achieve sufficiently large numbers of enrolled patients, robbing the subgroup analysis of sufficient power to detect significant effects of treatments.

The reverse effect may also apply. When a genetic subdivision exists within a population but is undetected, the opportunity to create significant discovery can be hampered. Functional correlations that exist can be missed. This artifact is widely known as the Wahlund effect (Wahlund, 1928).

Autism research therefore has a significant classification paradox. Failure to consider the correct, clinically important molecular subtypes could result in failure to detect positive effects of treatments and therapies. Splitting the spectrum on the basis of incorrect or clinically irrelevant markers may cause a loss of ability to make significant discoveries. Where autism may be most meaningfully split may be at the level of functional groups of genes. Loss of function mutations and deletions in glutamate receptors, for example, more likely define an etiologically and clinically distinct molecular subtype of ASD than those with mitochondrial dysfunction, synaptic gene dysfunction, of direct microglial cell function. Whether a specific mutation is inherited or de novo is not as important as the consequences of that allele for the sake of the individual. A dichotomous classification scheme does not work because any individual could have any combination of these gene classes. A multidimensional tesseract model appears to be most appropriate.

VACCINES BACK ON THE TABLE

There is a mountain of evidence now that a subset of people are highly susceptible to toxic environmental factors that might contribute to autism, and a great deal of the evidence points to vaccines, as currently formulated with aluminum adjuvant, as one of many causes of autism.

Vaccines are produced in a manufacturing environment, and their components change with time. It is rational to be concerned that a particular configuration of vaccine epitopes, adjuvants, and additives will be stumbled upon that in short-term study appears effective, but upon long-term postmarket follow-up is found to have caused massive numbers of injuries and deaths. We are uninformed participants in an uncontrolled, post-market experiment.

The manifestation of specific disease states or conditions results when both necessary and sufficient factors are present. In this sense, the low penetrance and variable expressivity of autistic phenotypes is best understood and difficult to predict with blinded prospective outcome studies that consider both genotype and environmental factors. Sufficient causal inferences about environmental factors, however, are classically examined via studies that focus on the prevalence of disease in populations made of specific genotypes and genotype combinations, in the presence versus absence of environmental challenges. These factors are more or less important to individual cases of autism, thus the challenge. Animal models designed to reflect specific individuals' genotype combinations could be used in treatment and control studies to screen suspected environmental factors as contributing causes. More important, such animal models could also be used to predict the efficacy of specific treatments for individuals or groups of individuals with particular constellations of mutations. Genetic predisposition, including very high predisposition by itself, does not reduce the importance of environmental factors in individual cases.

RECOMMENDED STUDY DESIGNS

As an expert in study design, I am well positioned to point out flaws that can compromise the generalizability of findings from retrospective as well as prospective studies. There are a number of major problems with past studies that have impeached their results. These study design errors must be avoided in the future to ensure that the appropriate types of studies are funded and conducted so we do not waste further time and resources on meaningless research. Important factors in designing studies are discussed in the following pages.

FOCUS ON ASSOCIATION INSTEAD OF PREDICTION

Studies that focus on mere association will rarely be convincing of a causal inference regardless of their result (however, see Shaw et al., 2013). Use of studies that are restricted to association alone miss the opportunity to assess whether the findings can be generalized to new sample sets from the same or similar populations and thus often can be found to show low reproducibility.

Further, prediction models provide clinically actionable utilities (e.g., biomarkers and nomograms).

EVALUATION OF GENERALIZABILITY OF FINDINGS ON INDEPENDENT TEST SAMPLES

These studies can be phased (discovery, evaluation, validation), and machine-learning techniques can identify diagnostic or prognostic markers and decision rules providing clinically actionable algorithms that can incorporate a diversity of types of information, from demographic and clinical risk factors to biomarkers.

Rather than weak association analysis, carefully conducted machine-learning-based prediction modeling will inform not only on which variables are important, but also which variables carry redundant information. Generalizable performance evaluation measures during external clinical class prediction validation will either not change or will suffer when nearly redundant variables are included. Numerous types of models are available (e.g., Lasso, Ridge Regression, Random Forests, etc.). If multiple classes of models are trained on a training set (e.g., cases vs. controls), all of their performance evaluation measures (sensitivity, specificity, accuracy) should be reported, and both the training set values and test set values should be reported. Such studies should occur in phases, with independent validation sets to assess generalizability. Control variables can be used as cofactors in explanatory and prediction models, and thus their contribution and interactions appropriately assessed.

Very large studies with preplanned subgroup analyses in comorbid conditions are needed to assess the safety of the pediatric vaccine schedule and for other vaccines. The minority of people afflicted with other conditions should be placed at risk of additional harm to knowledge and patients due to abject ignorance or malfeasance in the area of model selection.

HEALTHY-USER BIAS

In vaccinated versus unvaccinated studies of causality, autistics, and those at high risk of autism, can end up in the unvaccinated group because families may avoid vaccines. This is a type of allocation bias and leads to an enrichment of autism in the unvaccinated group. Thus, association studies will tend to find no difference in rates of autism between groups.

This problem further invalidates studies that purport to show that vaccines are safe, unless *autism* and *siblings with autism* are used as exclusionary criteria for both groups. That step, however, may remove individuals with risk of autism from the study altogether. On this issue, Fine and Chen (1992) reported: "Confounding of this sort is a general problem for studies of adverse reactions to prophylactic interventions, as they may be withheld from some individuals precisely because they are already at high risk of the adverse event."

CONFUSING MMR VERSUS NO MMR WITH VACCINATED VERSUS UNVACCINATED

Studies that purport to report the effects of individual vaccines based on patients' records of receiving MMR confound *MMR* with *likely to have received vaccines.* Thus, conclusions about any single vaccine in such studies are not warranted.

USING ONLY CATEGORICAL VARIABLES RATHER THAN STUDYING CUMULATIVE LIFETIME DOSE

Lumping patients into "vaccinated" versus "unvaccinated" weakens the power to detect intensity effects. Studies that find association and also find, for example, that the severity of ASD is related to cumulative lifetime dose are in much better position to claim fulfillment of Hill's criteria of causality. For example, the observation of dose effect supports Hill's criterion of Biological Gradient.

CONDUCTING ASSOCIATION STUDIES AT THE POPULATION VERSUS THE FAMILY LEVEL

We know that the risk of autism is clustered in families, not randomly spread across the population due to a large number of genes. The consequences for the validity of population-level genetic association studies are clear: initially, genes were rejected, as they were not "major loci." The assumption that a few genes contribute risk has been shown to be false. This is widely known and appreciated.

What is generally not appreciated is that conducting population-wide association studies that ignore familial clustering will similarly tend to doom those studies to fail in finding an association with environmental factors, in the same way and for the same reason that they fail to find significance at the population level. Familial studies nested within environmental exposures will bear fruit.

None of the studies on which the CDC bases their childhood vaccination schedule were designed to detect events that occur in fewer than 2 percent of the population. And if vaccines are among a myriad of environmental factors that can contribute to vaccine risk, their studies comparing the rates of vaccination among autistic versus nonautistic children, and studies comparing rates of autism in vaccinated versus unvaccinated, are extremely likely to have missed the effects of vaccines as well.

Findings of a significant effect at the population level of association can also be lost when studying familial association. This issue is likely to happen when shared environmental risks, not genetics, are responsible for patterns of inheritance, but then those shared environmental risks are heterogeneous across families. Environmental factors tend to be spatially and temporally autocorrelated. Researchers need to consider environmental variables in the same way they think of genetic cluster effects.

Unless studies are designed for comparisons of specific molecular subtypes, for example, by enriching the entire study with individuals with genetic risk factors, the main effect of the environmental factor will likely be missed. It is very important that future studies incorporate the prior knowledge of familial and genetic risk aggregation. Studies that do not, but that report "no association," are suspect.

ABUSE OF COFACTORS AS "CONTROL VARIABLES" AND IGNORING THE INTERACTION TERM

Studies that statistically "correct for" clinical factors such as birth weight, age of mother, income level, or breastfeeding can miss golden opportunities for understanding. By removing a component of variance with ascribing explanatory power, and then not examining an interaction term, one might conclude, for instance, that once birth weight, age of mother, and so on are "removed" from the data, there was no main effect (e.g., exposure to vaccines). One is required at that time to report the significance of the interaction term, because removal of a covariate as a control factor will commonly cause the main effect to become insignificant, moving its significance to the interaction term. Consider these two hypothetical conclusions, for example:

> *Birth weight and age of mother were used as control variables and were found to be significant. After controlling for birthweight and age of mother, "vaccination" was no longer significant. This result supports the idea that autism is not associated with vaccination.*

Note the absence of a mention of the interaction term in the above passage.

> *Both birth weight and age of mother were found to be significant factors in explaining variation in autism outcome. After inclusion in the model, "vaccination" was no longer significant. However, the "vaccination × birthweight" interaction was significant. This supports the idea that toxicity of vaccines is more pronounced in low birthweight babies and that vaccines are a potential causal factor in autism.*

In retrospective case-control, treatment-control, and cohort studies, variables such as ethnicity, age, income level, body mass index (BMI), and other variables should not be considered to be sources of intruding variation that must be removed before the true, underlying variation remains (in the residuals); these variables should be considered cofactors. Risk prediction modeling and outcomes modeling should take precedence over association.

If covariates are used as control variables, the functional relationship between them and the main effect (e.g., vaccination) should be known, not assumed, to be independent. The specific hypothesis of an environmental variable should be examined in the interaction term when covariates are significant. This is widely understood, and there is no good reason why interaction terms have been ignored.

Researchers on studies that can impact public health policy must always be forthright with their interaction terms, and on power. Blocking, stratified, and enrichment designs are more appropriate especially if they focus on cumulative exposures [see unpublished report of Verstraeten et al. (2000) for a good example of forthright reporting].

DEFINING UNINFORMATIVE SPECIFIC AIMS

The specific aims of a study are the questions being addressed, the hypotheses being tested, and the level of discovery at which knowledge can be generated. Much of the medical focus on autism has been on observed regression at approximately 19 months, and yet studies that use any and all available ASD patients, regardless of age of onset, may be combining clinical heterogeneous populations. Safety studies should always include comparison to true placebo, not to adjuvant, nor to similar vaccine. It is imperative to conduct studies of children who had no previous medical record of ASD, no developmental delays, and so on to identify shared events in their lives—and in their genes—that could be responsible for their sudden regression.

WILD-TYPE ANIMAL STUDIES

Use of wild-type animals to demonstrate the safety of chemicals and elements or of vaccine schedules (e.g., Gadad et al., 2015; Curtis et al., 2015) are fundamentally flawed. We know that autism has a genetic risk; therefore, findings of no autism or autism-like effects in groups of wild-type animals do not demonstrate lack of causation. Animal models that incorporate one, two, or three mutations in the key pathways challenged with aluminum toxicity, true placebo (saline), antigen-only, and adjuvant + antigen are needed to assess a 3 × 3 patterns of risk of autism (three levels of environmental exposure, three levels of genetic exposure). Mouse, rat, or monkey studies that ignore the massive amount of genetic knowledge are of severely limited value. This includes the very promising but fatally flawed studies recapitulating vaccine schedules in small numbers of non-human primates, specifically one study of fifteen rhesus macaque monkeys given the CDC 1993 vaccine schedule during those five years modeled by Gadad et al. (2015) and a similar study of thimerosal in monkeys that showed no effect (Curtis et al., 2015).

Unpublished retrospective power-to-detect analyses revealed that for Gadad et al. to detect adverse events (of any kind) due to the vaccination schedule, the effects would have had to have been present in 38 percent of monkeys (between five or six monkeys; see VaccinePapers.org). Instead, the incidence of autism in humans is at most 2 percent (in the mostly vaccinated population, which is not the true null incidence).

All studies in autism should publish power-to-detect analyses that are informed by prevalence or risk, and they should examine interactions. Human studies should be done at the family level and consider the effects of stratification on power (Sebro et al., 2010).

It is imperative that studies be conducted testing the effects of specific mutations and combinations of mutations with dose sensitivity of suspected environmental factors. The Gadad et al. (2015) and Curties et al. (2015) studies could also be replicated to test the interaction effects of vaccines and acetaminophen.

ABSENCE OF RANDOMIZED, DOUBLE-BLINDED, PLACEBO-CONTROLLED CLINICAL TRIALS

The FDA gold standard study design for approval of drugs is the randomized, prospective clinical trial design, in which patients are randomly allocated to a treatment and control group. Vaccine-autism human studies have, for the most part, been retrospective case-control or cohort studies, which are notorious for being susceptible to bias and can easily be manipulated.

The CDC has cited expense as a reason why retrospective, ecological studies are used instead of prospective trials. This is not an acceptable reason for using the weakest type of study design for factors that influence billions of lives around the world, and untold expense. No further retrospective studies should be accepted as evidence of a positive claim of safety. It is time that we allow the National Institutes of Health to oversee extramural vaccine clinical trials and to require the same longitudinal safety studies required of any other drug, treatment, or procedure. In plain terms, the CDC has failed.

The NAS/IOM report from 2012 (National Academy of Sciences, 2012) found sufficient flaws in 17 of 22 studies cited by the CDC as demonstrating no link between vaccines and autism, leaving a scant 5 studies upon which to base their assessment of causality, on which the important public health policy (i.e., vaccination) ostensibly hinged:

> *The committee reviewed 22 studies to evaluate the risk of autism after the administration of MMR vaccine. Twelve studies . . . were not considered in the weight of epidemiologic evidence because they provided data from a passive surveillance sys-*

tem lacking an unvaccinated comparison population or an ecological comparison study lacking individual-level data. Five controlled studies (DeStefano et al., 2004; Richler et al., 2006; Schultz et al., 2008; Taylor et al., 2002; Uchiyama et al., 2007) had very serious methodological limitations that precluded their inclusion in this assessment. Taylor et al. (2002) inadequately described the data analysis used to compare autism compounded by serious bowel problems or regression (cases) with autism free of such problems (controls).

DeStefano et al. (2004) and Uchiyama et al. (2007) did not provide sufficient data on whether autism onset or diagnosis preceded or followed MMR vaccination. The study by Richler et al. (2006) had the potential for recall bias since the age at autism onset was determined using parental interviews and their data analysis appeared to ignore pair-matching of cases and controls, which could have biased their findings toward the null. Schultz et al. (2008) conducted an Internet-based case-control study and excluded many participants due to missing survey data, which increased the potential for selection and information bias.

The five remaining controlled studies (Farrington et al., 2001; Madsen et al., 2002; Mrozek-Budzyn et al., 2010; Smeeth et al., 2004; Taylor et al., 1999) contributed to the weight of epidemiologic evidence and are described below.

It is amazing that five studies—and only five studies—were used in the report concluding no association between vaccines and autism. Moreover, these studies suffered serious flaws, many of which have been outlined in this chapter. Note that although subsequent NAS/IOM reports concluded no link between autism and vaccines, the proceedings were subsequently demonstrated to be influenced by directives from the CDC *to not find* an association, and are also generally considered misinformed by misleading studies currently under investigation by the CDC.

OVERCOMING DESIGN FLAWS IN VACCINE SAFETY RESEARCH STUDIES

There are three ways to study the effects of an environmental factor on molecular subtypes: massively powering a study, molecular allocation, and molecular stratification. To massively power a study, rare events can be recognized due to an immense sample size. These studies can be prospective or retrospective, with the results from prospective studies being much more legitimate. In molecular allocation studies, individuals are assigned to treatment or control groups based on genotype. These are typically prospective studies. In molecular stratification studies, study groups are enriched by molecular subtypes (subgroup analysis).

USE OF APPROPRIATE PLACEBOS

Prospective placebo-controlled clinical trials are conducted for some vaccines. However, they often use inappropriate placebos, such as adjuvant versus vaccine. Two tiers of knowledge are required to fully assess the safety and efficacy of vaccines. The first is whether a specific antigen is effective and safe. This requires the design vaccinated versus unvaccinated, with placebo adjuvant. This is useful because other antigens may be more efficacious and/or safer. This tests the combined effects of the antigen and adjuvant (and other excipients).

It is sometimes said unvaccinated versus vaccinated studies would be unethical; however, there are plenty of families who decline vaccination. If proper matching algorithms are used to minimize confounders, reasonable studies can be conducted that honor patients' rights to informed consent and the right to refuse medical procedures.

However, safety concerns—and concerns with adjuvant and additives on both health outcomes and efficacy—require additional specific comparisons. To address the safety of the vaccine, *vaccine* versus *saline* placebo comparisons are required. Patients are entitled to know overall safety profiles, not just the relative safety of specific antigens. Studies of the vaccines versus adjuvant may be conducted but do not reflect the full risk profile for a given vaccine.

Studies of combinations of vaccinations are rarely conducted, and while new schedule vs existing schedule studies have been conducted, they are inadequate because they do not address cumulative dose effects, which can have thresholds. Four years after Congressional Representative Dan Burton asked Dr. Coleen Boyle (CDC) in the House Oversight and Government Reform Committee hearings of November 2012, the safety of the full schedule versus unvaccinated has not been studied, and yet more vaccines have been added to the schedule since that testimony.

MULTICENTER INDEPENDENT TRIALS

Five research institutions should be tasked with undertaking safety trials on each vaccine individually and on each and every change to the vaccine schedule via extramural research programs. Three of these should be qualified institutions chosen at random (to reduce influence by profit interests), and two should be awarded by grant competitions. The funding to each of the five should be identical in scale; they should work and publish independently, and there should be strict ethical checks on conflicts of interest for all investigators involved. The safety trials should be randomized, prospective clinical trials of antigen, adjuvant, antigen+adjuvant, and saline control—and *all* health outcomes should be monitored, not just those for autism. The American public deserves to know the risks involved in participating in the vaccination program, and it is unethical and illegal to compel, coerce, and misinform participants by denying their informed consent. The scientific research we conduct should reflect that level of standard.

When the National Academy of Sciences, Institute of Medicine declared that 17 of 22 such studies were flawed, it did so for very good reason: those 17 studies were so fundamentally flawed that they should not be included for further consideration. The public health policy of entire nations rely on conclusions from such studies, and the CDC has not acknowledged or acted upon the limitations identified by the National Academy of Sciences.

It is time for the medical community to call for retraction of these studies; they are doing much more harm than good.

These types of fundamental flaws, so rampant in the epidemiological study of the health outcomes of vaccines, are no longer tolerable. Others types of research flaws to avoid include:

- Lack of reporting of power estimates (power to detect).
- Rejection of significant results after power to detect has been demonstrated.
- Small sample size. Results from studies with small N samples should be labeled *pilot studies,* and public health policy should not be based on their negative results.
- Failure to calculate power given incidence of disease.
- Other forms of selection bias (as noted by NAS/IOM).
- Cryptic clinical heterogeneity (mixing ASD with Rett syndrome, Fragile X syndrome, etc.).
- Cryptic genetic heterogeneity (well-known Wahlund effect).
- Cohort effects (time-related changes in incidence or covariates not accommodated by blocking). This can be avoided by matching patients by age during allocation on multivariate measurements.
- Fraud and scientific misconduct (Barr, 2015).

Statistical control of variates is the weakest and riskiest form of control. The full toolbox of study designs should instead be used (e.g., blocking, stratification, matching, and molecular allocation). The Verstraeten et al. (2003) study especially suffers from the overuse of statistical control to the point of rendering the results of little value. They removed variance in highly collinear variables, including gestational age and birth weight, age of mother, and income of mother. The published results were the final set of results after repeated rounds of analysis. This model overfitting was potentially intentional. A four-year period of time lapsed between the time when the first analysis was conducted, in which a strong finding of association between vaccination and autism was reported, and publication. The original findings of association were not disclosed in the publication. Malfeasance has been alleged.

Instead of rejecting the association of autism with vaccines, the results of the covariates should have been used to conclude that low-birth-weight babies, born to low-income mothers, may be at the highest risk of autism due to vaccines.

We need to sharpen and mature our scientific approach and rigor and enable the right questions to be asked. We can no longer rely on the past studies for a firm conclusion about the role of vaccines in autism.

The research to date on the vaccine-autism link has not been sufficiently refined, with aims too obtusely defined to detect populations of individuals made susceptible by genetics. The studies may not have had the power to detect an effect because the effect was diluted and weakened by the inclusion of people who did not have a genotype conferring risk of sensitivity to the environmental trigger. It is simply no longer acceptable to study risk of autism and ignore that some of the alleles may confer risk of sensitivity to environmental toxins. This would explain why the penetrance of autism is not 100 percent in some individuals carrying risk alleles, including parents of autistic children, who had a much milder vaccination schedule as children themselves.

Of course, an institutional review board might refuse such a randomized or molecular allocation prospective study on the basis of how unethical it would be to willfully expose people with genetic risk of autism to vaccines containing aluminum. Perhaps our only recourse is to move away from vaccines toward safer approaches to immunization and produce immunization policies that respect human dignity regardless of genotype.

Additional information and review of professional critique of many of the published epidemiological studies has been published by SafeMinds (2015).

References : see envgencauses.com

Chapter 15.

BIOLOGICAL PATHWAYS AND NETWORKS VIEWS OF AUTISM

Throughout this book, I have been critical of the Centers for Disease Control and Prevention (CDC) and various individuals for cherry-picking results from the literature in support of their policy, instead of allowing a rigorous, integrative scientific approach to inform them what their position of public health policies should be. Under testimony, officials have cited dozens of studies that failed to find an association between vaccines and autism; I have cited the National Academy of Science/Institute of Medicine (NAS/IOM) rejection of nearly all of them. These defenders of the status quo report that "vaccines do not cause autism" and also that "vaccine ingredients do not cause autism." These absolute statements are egregiously misleading and must be changed. Not only is the scientific evidence weak, flawed, and most likely fraudulent, but their statement also includes an overarching generalization to all vaccines, when not all vaccines have been studied for links to autism, individually or in combination as an entire schedule.

So how biased is my own take on the biological plausibility of the links between vaccines, glyphosate, and acetaminophen, among others? I performed a directed search studying autism, not vaccines. I have used a relatively unbiased approach. Admittedly, I tracked down further information on specific details to give the reader background as often as I could. I have surveyed more than two thousand research studies and would hope that this book provides a reflection of the full body of knowledge.

To determine whether the conclusions represented in this book are biased, I surveyed autism studies focused on biological pathways. Genes interact via proteins, and vice versa. Pathway and network analyses are used to understand the system biology of diseases. Much of the knowledge represented in the published literature reviewed thus far is confirmed by independent, more sophisticated, and less subjective views.

A variety of ingenious methods have been developed that allow researchers to summarize overall themes present in large, complex data sets into clusters, networks, and information on known pathways. This area is sometimes referred to as *systems biology*. Alternative approaches, by design, emphasize different angles on the data to shed light on related but slightly different questions; the totality of the results from these varied approaches helps to confirm the objectivity of the conclusions drawn in this book.

DISTINCTION BETWEEN NATAL AUTISM AND LATE-ONSET AUTISM VERIFIED

In an analysis relating mutations in genes to overall gene expression, Hormozdiari et al. (2014) found two primary modules enriched for mutations in autism spectrum disorder (ASD). The first was a collection of genes and proteins that are involved in early embryonic development (8 to 16 weeks post-conception). The second module included synaptic genes, calcium signaling, and long-term potentiation that are more important during postnatal development. Thus, the distinction between natal autism and late-onset autism is supported by the genetic data at the functional level.

In their study, Hormozdiari et al. (2014) compared low-IQ ASD and higher IQ ASD and found quite a large number of potentially differentiated genes. This finding implies a degree of syndromic basis for intellectual disability (ID) in autism. However, they also reported a larger proportion of de novo truncating in mutations ASD with ID vs. high-functioning ASD.

Hormozdiari et al. (2014) also studied overlap of genes with mutations in ASD, schizophrenia, and epilepsy, finding minor overlap. The genes identified are likely important in understanding the manifestation of these condition with ASD; the distinct genes may provide differentiating biomarkers.

SYNDROMIC AUTISM DISSOLVES FROM A MOLECULAR VIEWPOINT

Motivated to understand the distinctions between syndromic and non-syndromic ASD, Kelleher et al. (2012) took a pathways viewpoint on interpretation of variation in nonsyndromic ASD. In addition to finding new evidence of a risk gene (the postsynaptic density-localized scaffolding protein HOMER1), they also found evidence that genes in pathways previously implicated in syndromic ASD have functionally significant mutations in nonsyndromic ASD. Notably, these include TSC1, TSC2, and SHANK3. Of these, SHANK3 interacts with HOMER1 in the synaptic glutamate (mGluR) pathway. Copy number variations are found in excess in the mGluR pathway in autistics compared to neurotypicals (Wenger et al., 2016).

"Syndromic" autism here refers to autism that occurs *within* other syndromic conditions. The movement to turn some parts of the autism puzzle into syndromes will only progress further for subtypes that have narrow clinical variability; other types of ASD associated with specific genes and pathways will be difficult to completely tease apart clinically. A pathway-level view will likely be more productive.

EXTREMES CONFIRM DISTINCT BUT IMPORTANT PATHWAYS

In a unique approach in which they considered pathways, Campbell et al. (2013) looked at patients they considered outlier within ASD. They used a Mahalanobis distance-from-centroid method, which would effectively enrich the samples they could use to characterize ASD endophenotypes in gene expression data from blood samples in autistics. Basically, they used an enrichment study design based on multivariate gene expression phenotypes and found signatures of three impacted pathways overrepresented in the ASD cases as follows:

- Neuron development including axonogenesis and neurite development (29 percent of ASD, 3 percent of control).
- Nitric oxide signaling (29 percent, 3 percent).
- Skeletal development (27 percent, 3 percent).

They also found a hint of the *broader autism phenotype* in unaffected family members in neurogenesis.

Nitric oxide (NO) signaling has become more recognized as an important potentially reversible indicator of severity of ASD. Tetrahydrobiopterin (BH4) is a neurotransmitter precursor and is involved in the production of nitrous oxide, which is present in notably decreased amounts in some people with autism. Frye et al. (2012) found improved behavioral measures compared with baseline in NO-deficient autistics after treatment with BH4. There are likely numerous systemic effects on NO, and although the exact mechanisms of the effect of BH4 treatment may be unclear, Frye et al. (2013) also reported improved immune markers. Good (2015) provides an interesting in-depth analysis of additional, alternative, and likely effects of NO production increase in ASD. Nitric oxide has numerous, powerful effects on circulation, maintenance of healthy tissue, and destruction of damaged tissue, and may stimulate nearby blood flow during neuronal activity. The nitrate/NO balance may come to be seen as an important metabolic marker for some autistics, especially those with ID and others with ID with any condition.

SPEECH, MICROGLIA, AND NERVE CELL EXTENSION ROLES IN LOSS-OF-FUNCTION MUTATIONS

Loss-of-function (LoF) driven pathway analysis revealed three major clusters of functionally aggregate gene modules in ASD (Liu et al., 2014), reflecting functional groups involved in the following:

- Speech and language, clustering around the gene FOXP2.
- Microglial activation, clustering around the gene PTEN.
- Microtubule-processes in nerve cell function, clustering around the gene SPAST.

The importance of FOXP2 and PTEN in ASD has been discussed previously in this book. The SPAST cluster found by Liu et al. (2014) may indicate the importance of a microtubule reorganization, which is important for both cell shape development (neurite extension and neuronal arborization) and microglial and astrocyte functioning. Another effect could be disruption of the modulation of the endoplasmic reticulum, important for cellular waste transport and detoxification. Mutations in genes in this cluster could lead to sequestration of toxins in cells such as astrocytes (disrupting glutamate uptake) and microglia, which hinder proper mediation of synapses and autophagy.

CONFIRMATION OF PATHWAY CLUSTERS BY RISK TYPE CLASS AND MULTIPLE-HIT HYPOTHESIS

In an astonishing contribution, including an analysis of genetic variation in ASD and neurotypical controls, Pinto et al. (2014) identified three large clusters of pathways:

- Neuronal development and axon guidance (reflecting autism risk genes).

- Chromatic modification and transcription regulation (mixed autism risk genes + environmental susceptibility genes).
- MAPK and other molecular signaling pathways reflecting risk, environmentally susceptible genes, and modifier genes.

Although a thorough accounting of how the genes fall into risk categories is needed, many autism risk genes are found in the neuronal development and axon guidance cluster reported by Pinto et al. (2014). Similarly, genes with large environmental influences predominate in the chromatic modification and transcription regulation cluster, suggesting that many are environmental susceptibility genes. Chromatin remodeling pathways, important in methylation-mediated control of gene expression, were also detected by the analysis (O'Roak et al., 2012).

An example of environmental effectors of chromatin remodeling effects includes increasing H3K9 acetylation disruption by acetate treatment, with consequences for microglia activation (Soliman et al., 2013). Similarly, it is well known that p38 MAPK will reflect the innate autoimmune processes in ASD leading to microglial activation. See Grayson and Guidott (2016) for a review of additional environmental factors that impact the expression of sets of genes by altering methylation-hydroxymethylation patterns, local histone modification patterns, and chromatin remodeling in autism.

One of most exciting demonstrations of translational potential of the multiple-hit hypothesis for ASD, and strong evidence for use of risk assessment by counting risk genes with variations of all types, is the estimation of odds ratios by numbers of insertions and deletions by the Pinto et al. (2014) study. Their figure, presented as Figure 4 (page 77), provides a clear model how the genetic information may be useful for risk assessment. They used a model in which the patient's group label (ASD or control) was studied and found that the best models fit CNV status, the number of genes covered by each CNV, and their average brain expression levels. Thus, de novo CNVs that influence gene expression in the brain are very important in the etiology of autism.

CLASSIFICATION INFORMATION CONTENT ACROSS PATHWAYS INDICATES INDEPENDENCE OF MULTIPLE FACTORS

A clever study by Skafidas et al. (2014) confirmed that pathway views can lead to useful knowledge, not only for etiologies of ASD, but also on the potential clinical utility of the information. It is reasonable to expect that patients with mutations in different genes in the same pathways likely carry similar risks and clinical presentation. They found evidence of independent classification utility in a large number of canonical KEGG database pathways, noting especially calcium signaling, gap junction, long-term potentiation, and purine metabolism for potential utility across ethnic groups. Others such as axon guidance may have ethnic-group specific utility; therefore, population substructure and ancestry is important to consider for clinical translation.

Clustering of approval of clinical utility of specific function-altering mutations using pathways knowledge may yield a faster route to routine and automated use of genetic data for assessing ASD risk. They also identified a list of single nucleotide variations that appear to confer risk and others that may confer protection. One of these, GRM5, was found in both lists. GRM5 is expressed in microglia and plays an important role synaptic plasticity, modulation of synaptic excitation, innate immune function, and microglial activation (Skafidas et al., 2014).

THREE SUBNETWORKS OF COEXPRESSED GENES

Another important and brilliant analysis (Ben-David and Shifman, 2012) used weighted coexpression network analysis to examine coexpression subnetworks of genes involved in ASD. Ben-David and Shifman found three clustered networks:

- General neuronal biology
- Astrocytes
- Oligodendrocytes

Each of these three clustered networks provides insights into shifts in the processes involved in the autistic brain. Again, we see shifts in the biology of astrocytes, which regulate microglia and also oligodendrocytes, which are active in the maintenance of myelin in the CNS. Oligodendroglial precursors are highly susceptible to oxidative stress and excitotoxic insult (Zeidán-Chuliá et al., 2015).

Ben-David and Shifman (2012) then also analyzed autism spectrum disorders (ASD) genome-wide association studies GWAS data and found two major signatures: the first reflects synaptic and neuronal plasticity via genes expressed in areas associated with learning and memory, and the second involves sensory perception genes.

Zeidán-Chuliá et al.'s (2015) closer look at networks specifically involving oligodendrocytes in autism is revealing as well. Alterations in demyelination in the autistic brain appear to change long-range interconnectivity among brain regions with tissue differentiation and functional specialization, which may help explain some stereotyped ASD behaviors involving attention and focus shifting dynamics (Zikopoulos and Barbas, 2010).

IMPACT OF MUTATIONS IN GENES BY BRAIN REGION WITH SIGNIFICANT OVERLAP

As various brain regions exhibit developmentally derived tissue specialization and functions, it seems sensible to surmise that autism risk and modifier genes may exhibit varying degree of importance for different brain region phenotypes. This is indeed what is reflected by a shrewd analysis by Kumar et al. (2011), who studied the likely regions in which various ASD-related genes might have the largest impact on phenotypes. First, they conducted a gene ontology (GO) analysis and found signatures of neurogenesis and projection, cell adhesion, and ion channel activity.

Then, using the NCBI DAVID resource, Kumar et al. found differences in localization of function (expression) in ASD genes, specifically enrichment in brain regions critical for sensory information processing (olfactory bulb, occipital lobe), executive function (prefrontal cortex), and hormone secretion (pituitary). From a neurobiology perspective, this all makes sense. However, their analysis further highlights genes expression across four, three, and two regions. Those expressed in all four regions include A2BP1, APC, CNTNAP2, DPP6, FABP7, IL1RAPL1, NBEA, NF1, NLGN3, NLGN4X, NRXN1, PCDH9, RAPGEF4, RIMS3, SCN2A, and SEZ6L2. This highlights the importance of the fact that single LoF mutations or methylation repatterning can have profound brain-wide effects. These are especially likely to be penetrant ASD genes. Those reachable by environmental-induced methylation repatterning are likely candidates for direct environmental susceptibility genes, with or without mutations.

These pathway and network studies confirm much of the knowledge base and conclusions I have gleaned during my research for the prior chapters. Clearly, some of the studies are based on data from some of the same literature I have reviewed in previous chapters. However, the objectivity reflected in discovery of emergent clusters and networks, as well as the robustness of the conclusions under objective analysis, provides welcome reassurance that the knowledge base and conclusions I independently derived is sufficiently objective to be considered robust knowledge.

References : see envgencauses.com

Chapter 16.

TOWARD A MULTIDIMENSIONAL MATRIX RISK MODEL FOR AUTISM

It is clear there are risks due to both environmental exposure and genetics. Measures of lifetime exposure to environmental factors may be difficult; however, the cumulative exposure of specific additives in vaccines are reasonably estimable. Knowing which genes confer risk of occurrence of autism helps, and while the knowledge base is not yet complete, it appears that not only do only a subset of genes confer risk, but particular mutations may prove more useful than others in predicting risk. Uddin et al. (2014) found that mutations in brain-expressed exons have an excess of de novo mutations in ASD compared to neurotypical siblings.

A promising gene–single nucleotide polymorphism (SNP)-based diagnosis developed and proposed by Skafidas et al. (2014) showed reasonably high accuracy; however, follow-up analysis revealed that it likely confounded population substructure by using cases and controls with different ancestry (Belgard et al., 2014; Robinson et al., 2014). Also, the analysis setup appears to have used the entire data set for the feature selection set (identifying the set of potentially informative SNPs), which should be done on the training set only. Random resampling validation can allow for external generalizability as well, but a truly independent test set should be used in the construction of machine-learning optimized prediction models.

Three of the genes found by Skafidas et al. (2014) have potential for use in diagnostics based on biological plausibility, along with the others outlined in this book. One gene, GRM5, is a glutamate receptor and is among the glutamate receptors found by other studies to be associated with autism (Strom et al., 2010). Now that the story on the causes, processes, and manifestations of autism is clarified, their finding looks more interesting. Mutations in GNAO1 has been found in patients with epileptic encephalopathy (Talkvik et al., 2015), which is often an alternative diagnosis to autism. KCNMB4 is a potassium calcium-activated challenge gene associated with ASD and schizophrenia (Glessner et al., 2010).

Variation (LoF and CNV) in these genes should cause concern for increased risk of autism.

DIVERGENT WORLD VIEWS ON G, E, AND G × E

The overview of the literature I conducted for this book suggests three types of causes of autism: *endogenous autism*, caused purely by genetics; *environmentally induced autism*, caused purely by environmental toxins; and *mixed-cause autism*, caused by a combination of genetic and environmental factors. Conceptually, these ideas help organize our thinking about cause and effect, prevention, liability, and ultimately about what clinically actionable knowledge is available to help patients. Thus, with respect to the causes of autism, the three divergent views on the relative important of genetic and environmental causes have emerged. In the following section, I summarize the three views as a step toward model-based risk assessment, diagnosis, and treatment. The three models are presented graphically in Figure 7.

GENOCENTRIC VIEW OF G, E AND G × E RISK OF ASD

In the genocentric view, a simple risk model counts the number of ASD-associated genes in which an LoF score might be useful, or perhaps one weighted on functional categories such as synaptic genes, neurotransmitter genes, mitochondrial genes, neuronal migration-axon guidance genes, and glutamate pathway genes. Independent hits in three or more of genes in these categories likely confers increased risk (Figure 7A). A simple or weighted diagnostic nomogram based on gene counting may apply in such cases. The number of hits and the number of functional categories represented both likely provide key information. This view emphasizes the role of mutations in genes, with environmental toxins considered passively, something that we must all live with; and while it would be a good idea to minimize risk of exposure, the main focus is on neurological genes. Generalization of this view tends to lead to the incorrect position that autism is primarily a genetic disorder. Such a geocentric risk model downplays environmental exposures.

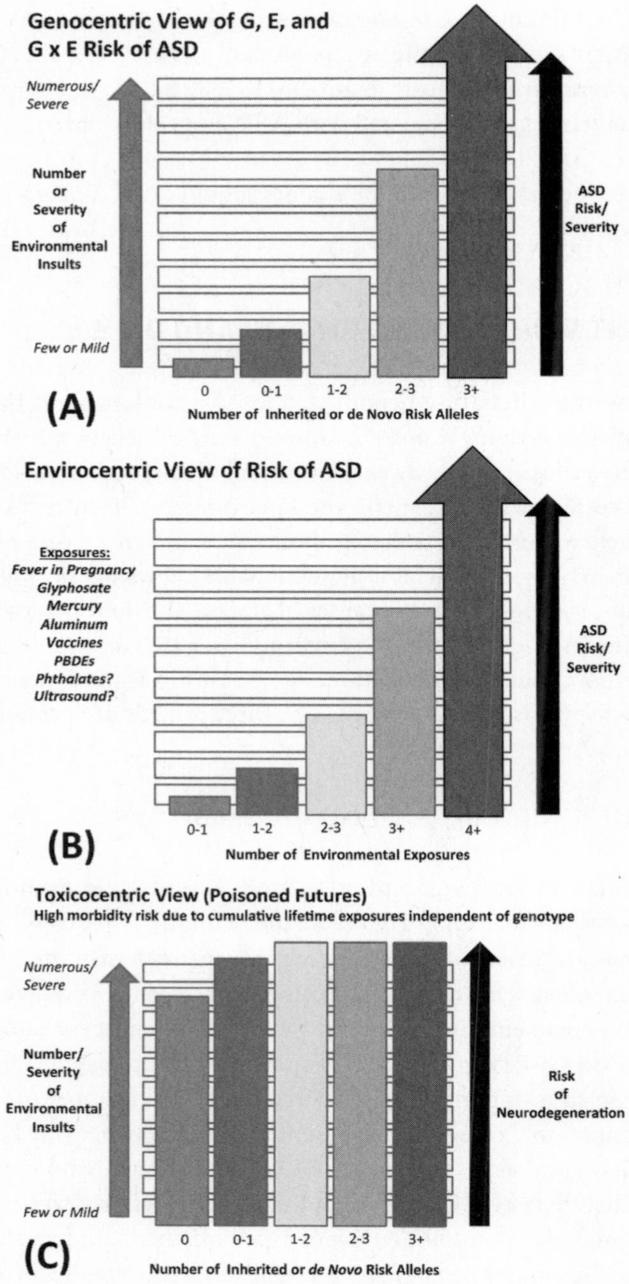

Figure 7. Three views on the relationships among genetic risk (G), environmental risk (E), and G × E interactions in terms of risk of ASD (A, B) and lifetime risk of neurodegeneration (C).

ENVIROCENTRIC VIEW OF RISK OF ASD

Mutations in environmental susceptibility genes would include genes that influence the uptake, sequestration, and detoxification of neurotoxins. These could add an additional likelihood of chronic microglial activation, and it is possible that a single LoF mutation could greatly increase the risk of ASD due to cumulative exposure (Figure 7B). Such mutations would likely amplify the risk of ASD incurred by mutations in other neurological genes, which are also included in the count.

This view more correctly places the responsibility and liability on environmental factors and is the most likely general case. It also is the model we can control more easily than our genetics. The genetic variation that we carry is either ancient (common alleles) or new (rare and de novo alleles). The increase in the concentration of environmental toxins that could trigger CMA is recent (see Nevison et al., 2014). When mutations exist in this class of genes, reductions in exposures to toxins could prevent or minimize autism symptoms.

TOXICOCENTRIC VIEW (POISONED FUTURES)

Valproic acid can induce autism in wild-type mice. Autism risk due to gestational thalidomide or valproic acid exposure leads to high morbidity risk without requiring any genetic risk. The same concern exists for lifetime risk of neurodegenerative diseases (Alzheimer's disease, Parkinson's disease, multiple sclerosis, etc.) due to multiple environmental exposures and cumulative lifetime exposures independent of genotype (Figure 7C). This is the *Poisoned Futures* model of autism risk with which society must grapple, because it is the fact-based reality for an increasing number of families. Sufficient evidence now exists to condemn an increasing number of toxins in our environment as causal factors in autism. Exposure to each of them independently may be controllable to a certain degree, and those that can be minimized must be minimized. This view minimizes the role of genetic variation, and it likely to apply to more individuals as the diversity and amount of toxins in our environment increase.

FORMALIZING A MULTIVARIATE RISK MATRIX MODEL

Multivariate thinking takes a bit of doing. It simplifies the process if we agree at the beginning with the assumption of additivity. This assumption, however, is merely for the sake of convenience, and when used in the practice of discovery of relationships among variables of interest, it can restrict our discovery of important knowledge. We saw this with the multicollinearity among closely related variables like birth weight, gestational age, age of mother, and income of mother, which destroyed and finally buried an initially strong association between autism and vaccines in the Verstraeten et al. (2003) study.

In the discussion that follows, I will explore the concepts of risk prediction modeling in autism from the perspective of a multidimensional matrix risk model. The goal is to foster development of robust, real-time actionable models that can be used with each pregnancy, each child, in real-time in the clinic and to inform parents on the need to reduce risk via reduction of exposures.

MAJOR CAUSAL DIMENSION 1: CUMULATIVE ENVIRONMENTAL NEUROTOXIN DOSE

A list of common environmental toxic compounds include aluminum, mercury, acetaminophen, monosodium glutamate, thalidomide, valproic acid, PBDE (flame retardant), air pollution, pthalates, ultrasound exposure, and parents who work with solvents, among many others. These are all measurable elements, both in their sources and in human tissue, as elements and compounds. While they are measureable with available analytical techniques, knowledge of meaningful metabolic fates, localization, and tissue concentration of these toxins through biological processes is not sufficiently worked out. Thus, compartments such as macrophages and cerebral spinal fluid may be more reliable than serum or urine levels, especially if tissue-specific sequestration can be related to neurotoxicity. Environmental factors have four dimensions: dose, duration, frequency, and nature of action. Ignorance of tissue sequestration can prolong duration and determine the sometimes cryptic natures of a toxin's action.

Just like chemicals, stress can be an important part of an individual's environment. Autism has been seen as a psychological condition resulting from severe abuse and neglect. Remarkably, stress causes corticotropin-releasing hormone to be secreted, which, acting with neurotensin, stimulates microglia, resulting in focal brain inflammation and neurotoxicity—so environmental stress could be included in this group of predictive factors.

MAJOR CAUSAL DIMENSION 2: ENVIRONMENTAL GENETIC SUSCEPTIBILITY

Absolute genetic susceptibility acts independently of environment. Environmental genetic susceptibility variants make specific compounds in the child's environment hazardous to them. When those toxins can be removed from the environment, they clearly should be. Mutations in genes that encode glutamate receptors (e.g., GluR6, GluR8, GRM5, GRIN2A, GRIN2C, GRM7, and NMDAR) and anything that would make a person more susceptible to factors such as aluminum neurotoxicity (e.g., mutations in endoplasmic reticulum genes) could lead to ASD and would thus belong in this category. Synaptic structural genes and regulatory developmental genes do not.

MAJOR CAUSAL DIMENSION 3: ABSOLUTE ASD GENETIC RISK

Add to the genetic risk factors enumerated in the previous section, tiered by expected degree of risk, as presented in the following:

- **First tier:** For example, neuronal development regulatory genes, such as RBFOX1, Reelin, AUTS2, and genes that regulate glutamate receptors). These genes will have a large phenotype effect and will not likely require much of an environmental injury.
- **Second tier:** Synaptic genes (e.g., CASK/VELI/MINT/CAMK, GUK/GKAP/SHANK, CTNND2, CNTN4, NRXN1, PARK2, MDGAs). Variation in these genes may cause minor symptoms, excitability, ADHD, some repetitive motions, tics, stutters, Tourette's syndrome, and other motor behavioral differences, but rarely full-blown autism without environmental injury.
- **General:** Number of CNVs of biological and clinical significance will depend on the precise copy variations, genes involved, etc. The correlation between increased numbers of CNVs and ASD is likely often due to satisfaction of the multiple-hit hypothesis, predisposition to environmental toxins, or both.

The number of dimensions here in terms of inputs to risk is a function of the number of tiers multiplied by number of genes and multiplied by the severity of mutation. That is, given that a person has one mutation in a glutamate receptor, the risk due to mutations in the second glutamate receptor—or in the glutamate pathway—is not likely to be as high as the increase in risk added due to mutations in genes that encode for other synaptic proteins. The greatest increase in risk is likely derived from variation in those genes that are demonstrated to direct neurological development.

We can add additional genetic dimensions, which are equal to the number of clinical and subclinial indicators that inform a pediatrician on a patient's diagnosis.

MINOR CAUSAL DIMENSION 1: AUTISM PHENOTYPE MODIFIER GENES

Autism phenotype modifier genes are likely to include genes that influence secondary causes and processes that may be largely independent of autism per se. They likely include common, high-frequency variations that are individually not at all pathogenic but instead influence phenotypes in both the unaffected and affected population. Their influence in the affected population may appear to be exaggerated by autism, but this reflects interaction between autism genes and modifier genes. They will be found to be otherwise independent of core autism phenotypes, and are therefore not likely to contribute to risk of autism. This distinction is important because not all genetic variation found to influence the degree or severity of autism reveal "autism genes." Although they are not primary causes, and do not contribute to risk, they can have surprisingly large phenotypic effects. Genes that influence intellectual ability may be an example.

Other clinical diagnostic risk markers reflecting the degree of severity of individual phenotypes represent additional minor secondary causal markers, as they may represent intermediate endpoints. They may also represent environment × gene or gene × gene interactions, but do not provide the necessary nor sufficient conditions for autism to occur.

MINOR CAUSAL DIMENSION 2: DEMOGRAPHIC AND CLINICAL FACTORS

Demographic and clinical factors include possible predictive factors, such as *parental age*, *complicated birth*, *blood relative with autism*, *birth weight*, *age of gestation*, and *family income*. Each of these factors have at least one dimension and some may prove more important individually than others. For example, Shelton et al. (2010) reminded us that "older women have a dramatically small chance of having a child with autism." A goal would be to see if they are useful in constructing an translationally informative risk prediction model.

However, most risk factors are not independent of each other or other factors. For example, *blood relative with autism* reflects genetic risk; *birth weight* and *complicated birth* must be examined for intercausality. That is, birth weight may have a genetic component, which may or may not be related to autism risk, and *parental age* could be due to nationwide cohort effects (autism increase). There are techniques in risk prediction modeling to assess these relationships and accommodate them, such as covariance analysis, feature selection, and principle components analysis.

With those variables arranged thusly, it seems imperative to develop a confluence between conceptual models of autism, genetic data and observations, and environmental data and observations, for comprehensive ASD risk prediction model. From a population standpoint, risk models and outcome models in autism resemble a tesseract. From the individual standpoint, the relevant markers are likely few, but important.

A multivariate-risk-matrix model cross-validated for prediction accuracy, sensitivity, specificity (ASD-neurotypical), and disease specificity (ASD, other neurological conditions, or disorders) would be important to have. Use of multiple research centers and performance sites that allow independent development and multiple instance of cross-validation will help assess generalizability. Awareness of the population structure would be important if "discovery" genetics were conducted, but it would be fruitful to pursue targeted genetic assays that focus on genes in the pathways of interest in ASD: synaptic genes, glutamate, serotonin, microglial signaling, and function. Prediction models explored should include those that do not assume that all biomarkers are relevant for all patients (such as linear models and logistic regression); *k* of *m* prediction modeling, for example, counts the number of aberrant markers and uses machine learning to optimize a cutoff on *w*, a threshold for optimal generalized accuracy for diagnosis. It could be useful to explore models in which markers are weighted for risk by functional class. Random Forest by Breiman and Culter (Breiman, 2001) could be valuable in this arena as well. Models such as the Pramparo et al. (2015) may be made more accurate by counting number of indicators, weighted by a function of the frequency of the markers in the affected and unaffected, and could, like *k* of *m* models, transcend the limits of additive regression models. Machine-learning techniques could be used to optimize either a cutoff in the critical number of markers between cases and controls, or made to learn and recognize specific constellations of mutations that might signify high risk for particular exposures.

Such models would be useful for more than diagnosis. And the confluence possible is beautiful: the point of diagnostic modeling here would be tailored prevention and treatment, indicated by the markers used for risk assessment, etiology, and diagnosis.

HISTORICAL CONCEPTUAL MODELS OF AUTISM

In this confusing context, differential diagnosis and disease classification of autism, the diseases in the ASD, and related conditions have been approached by various thinkers and remain controversial due to overlapping phenotypes and genetic etiologies. A number of conceptual models have been presented to comprehend autism, ASD, and comorbid conditions as categories (Table 3).

TABLE 3. CONCEPTUAL MODELS OF AUTISM

Theory of mind	Baron-Cohen et al., 1985
Global coherence	Frith, 1989
Deficient eye tracking	Leekam, 2007; Baron-Cohen et al., 1997
Deficient attention switching mechanism	Courchesne et al., 1994
Executive function deficit	Ozonoff et al. 1991; Russell, 1996
Deficient imitation mechanism	Meltzoff & Gopnik, 1993
Paused contingency detection module	Gergely & Watson, 1999 (focus on self)

These category-based models may all dissolve, as the reductionism made possible by molecular biology could, if taken to an extreme, call for reclassification of individual syndromes. I believe while in most cases this ability will illuminate causes and targets for individuals, it could also lead to a rigid, inflexible view of conditions and diseases and to a loss of something that is also essential to progressive biomedical research: our ability to communicate clearly and to generalize.

Each of the models discussed in this chapter has a basis that makes sense in light of the genetic variation contributing to autism risk and the variation that modulates autism phenotypes. That is, each has a molecular basis. Each of these phenomenological models focuses on and emphasizes one or more phenotypes present in autism that may or may not be present in a given patient and represent endpoints. Endpoints are descriptions, not causal explanations.

The paused contingency module (Gergely and Watson, 1999) is set apart in that it invokes a failure of a genetically encoded development program by which autistics fail to progress to (or regress back to) a mental state focused on learning elementary basics of their environment, which involves primarily their own body and the movement of others. This would place the model closer to a causal explanation, but these are also secondary causes.

Vision processing in the primate brain is well characterized. Complex visual messages have many features, including shape, color, speed, or direction of a moving object. All of these pieces of information are processed in dedicated visual areas of the brain. Proceeding as a stepwise process, vision processing begins with inputs relayed from the thalamus to the primary visual area. The messages are then dispatched to extrastriate areas, which are usually organized in a hierarchical manner, involving reciprocal connections (Felleman and Van Essen, 1991). Refined messages are received, and high-order complex integrative and associative processing takes place (Mountcastle, 1997).

In neurotypical development, the contingency module is set to preferentially explore perfect response-contingent stimulation, switching at approximately three months of age to a preference for less-than-perfect contingent actions of others, such as reciprocal imitation. In ASD, children fail to switch preference from perfect to less-than-perfect contingency. This effect has been shown to have a neurobiological basis.

Milne (2009) and Okamoto et al. (2014) found difference in brain activity in an extrastriate body area (EBA), which, with the right temporoparietal junction (TPJ), have been found to be critical for the sense of embodiment (the feeling of being located within one's body; Abraham et al., 2008). Okamoto et al. (2014) found these differences to be responsible for why autistics seem to be unaware that they are being imitated. In neurotypical adults, the extrastriate body area region is decoupled from motor systems. The "cross-wiring" found repeatedly throughout the literature may be at play, as different developmental programs may link motor circuits with the EBA (Kontaris et al., 2009). Although it is generally recognized the EBA region highly overlaps with the human motion–selective complex, the EBA region itself has been shown to be more complex, with functional differentiation of separate areas for specific body part and movement recognition (Weiner et al., 2011).

CALL FOR ANIMAL STUDIES INFORMED BY GENETICS

Animal studies, when conducted in a manner that ignores the wealth of knowledge about the environmental and genetic causes of autism, are essentially pointless. Animal models could be created that reflect the mutational profile of an individual child; animal siblings could be challenged with various environmental toxins to determine if the mutations alone were sufficient to cause autism, or if a specific environmental challenge caused autism in those animals. Although mice are not humans, this would be very useful for causal determination. A number of initiatives have born fruit (e.g., Schroeder et al. 2015).

References : see envgencauses.com

Chapter 17.

THE LOGIC OF PREVENTION IN AUTISM AND GENE-INFORMED TREATMENT

Too much time, energy, and expense has been spent in the back-and-forth between those who would like the public to continue to believe there are no links between vaccines and autism, and those who acknowledge vaccine-induced immunoneurotoxicity and mitochondrial dysfunction. It is time to move on. The mechanisms are established and the scientific evidence is clear: aluminum and mercury can cause autism in some people.

The question is, what are we going to do about it? There is much work to be done.

We need to build reliable risk prediction models that can inform doctors which patients should forgo exposure. These models need to be researched using state-of-the-art practices for phased risk and biomarker development. We need to work out rational medical exemptions. I believe parents concerned about vaccine-induced immunoneurotoxicity should be granted exemptions, without conflict from their pediatricians. Pediatricians are sometime reluctant to issue medical exemptions for vaccines for fear of sanctions. I do not see why doctors are not pushing hard for autism risk models that include vaccines. Perhaps most do not have time to do their homework on the issue and rely on the position of the Centers for Disease Control and Prevention (CDC) and the American Academy of Pediatrics. I hope that at least one position can be changed. I am calling on these and other organizations to change their position ever so slightly to simply inform the public that some people may be susceptible to autism from vaccines. And I urge them to join the growing number of doctors and scientists who are demanding reform in vaccine science. This would be the most significant step toward prevention of vaccine-induced autism.

For those who remain skeptical that vaccines play a role in the increasing numbers of autism, population-based retrospective studies showing no association do not meet the standards required, nor the level of evidence needed, to enact public health policies. The vaccine schedule itself is untested for safety; no vaccinated versus unvaccinated study has been conducted. Genetic-informed and risk-informed association studies would be a massive improvement. Rather than use genetic and demographic factors as confounders and removing patients in an ad-hoc, semiblock design that uses some variables as covariates and others as exclusion criteria, we should undertake studies that seek to determine whether biomarkers and other risk factors exist that could have predicted which patients would have developed autism from vaccines. Let us enrich samples for people with mutations in specific genes, to see if their groupwise risk of ASD in a genetically at-risk minority is increased by vaccines. Let us conduct total health outcome awareness studies in which all health outcomes, not just autism, are examined. And most of all, we should stop pretending that we are conducting scientifically rigorous analysis when we use proxy measures of total exposure, rather than cumulative dose. Finally, let us allow lifetime exposure measures to be an independent variable in both association studies and in outcome studies.

PREVENTION

First, we need to freeze the number of vaccines in the schedule and remove aluminum. Animal safety studies of the entire pediatric schedule should be conducted with animals with various combinations of genetic predisposition alleles. We need to reduce exposure to glyphosate, to the flame retardant polybrominated diphenyl ethers (PDBEs), and to other environmental toxins, and we may need to consider familial risk factors during prenatal care (e.g., ultrasound) and perinatal care (e.g., extended umbilical cord blocking).

Until we can determine the safe numbers and frequencies of vaccines in terms of antigenic-induced immunoneurotoxicity, leading to CMA, it is unconscionable to add more vaccines to the schedule. Removal of aluminum would, I think, be the more responsible of the two options. However, there should not be an unending number of vaccines added to the schedule. Mandatory vaccine laws should require renewal when vaccine schedules changes and should require the highest possible level of clinical evidence of long-term safety. That means randomized prospective clinical trials with proper controls. We should not pass laws that give governments the power to dose the population with ever-increasing numbers of vaccines, antigens, adjuvants, or additives; such laws essentially facilitate an uncontrolled experiment run amuck.

There is also good reason to remove specific vaccines from the schedule, and for certain people to reduce their personal risk of chronic microglial activation. Pragmatic policies and practices are needed that reduce total lifetime exposure. This would include genetic screening using a panel of validated risk markers, even if they only confer risk to a small percentage of people.

Some actions can be taken to reduce autism risk in spite of exposure. Expectant and breastfeeding mothers with MTHFR and COMT variants should avoid folic acid, a synthetic form of folate. Such mothers can reduce autism risk by avoiding folic acid–containing prenatal vitamins (Schmidt et al., 2011). This is only necessary for mothers with most MTHFR mutations. Carriers of some mutations, however, appear to require extra folate. Choline supplementation may help individuals with MeCP LoF mutations or deletion (Ricceri et al., 2011).

Individuals (autistics and neurotypicals) with specific variants of the HLA-DQA1 and HLA-DQB1 genes have celiac disease; their mutations cause a sensitivity to gluten and gluten-induced enteropathy (aka celiac disease). The frequency of these mutations is roughly the same across populations, and therefore the occurrence of gluten sensitivity might be thought of as being independent of ASD. However, observations of improvement in symptoms after moving to a gluten- and dairy-free diet are widespread.

Reducing exposure to environmental sources of excitoxic chemicals is a reasonable step for high-risk individuals as well. Faber et al. (2015) studied the effect of clean room sleeping environments on markers of oxidative stress, immune regulation, and behavior in children with ASD and found that younger children showed decreased immune dysregulation (decreased CD3 and CD4) and improved behavior. Older children displayed a worsening in behavior, which the authors surmised may have been to effects of a higher load of toxins released. Five children showed decreased concentrations of oxidized glutathione.

While this was a small, uncontrolled study, it shows the potential of reducing chronic and cumulative exposure. Anecdotally, one set of twins showed divergent patterns of behavior improvement that tracked their differences in four of five markers of oxidative stress.

In the meantime, a number of compounds and foods may prevent the onset of microglial activation. First, intrinsic glutathione production is essential. Well-meaning parents and doctors, who in the past wished to use acetaminophen to reduce risk of fever after vaccination, may have done more harm than good because acetaminophen depletes glutathione. The risk of autism due to gestational acetaminophen exposure seems to have been confirmed (Avella-Garcia et al., 2016).

AVOIDING FEVERS IN PREGNANCY

As we have seen, autism involves immune system activation. Fevers during pregnancy should be avoided. Interactions between acetaminophen use and vaccines have not been fully studied. To protect pregnant women from influenza, a virus-like particle vaccine screened for unsafe epitopes that mimic human peptides is needed that does not require preservatives or adjuvants such as thimerosal and aluminum.

RISK PREDICTION MODELING

A by-product of understanding the etiology of a disease is generating routes to prevention. However, the etiology of autism is complicated, which requires clever and sophisticated approaches in its prevention. Tests are needed that can score infants, perhaps in the preterm, for risk of developing ASD.

The ability to perform rapid risk modeling would be valuable to determine which patients are in high-risk categories and should consider prevention programs. Such individuals should be monitored for elevated glutamate in their CNS and perhaps scanned for chronic microglial activation. Both conditions should be treated in as tailored a manner as genetic testing allows.

KNOWN RISK FACTORS

Many etiological factors of autism are known, and some are reflected in the specific manifestations of ASD and in some of the common comorbid conditions. Bradstreet et al. (2010) stated:

> *Newer evidence, however, reveals that ASDs are associated with: oxidative stress; decreased methylation capacity; limited production of glutathione; mitochondrial dysfunction; intestinal dysbiosis; increased toxic metal burden; immune dysregulation, characterized by a unique inflammatory bowel disease and immune activation of neuroglial cells; and ongoing brain hypoperfusion.*

Each of these conditions, or processes, have a root cause; identifying the root cause will alleviate the condition and its role in ASD. Sometimes targeted treatments will be aligned with the root cause; those treatments will be called cures. Other treatments that do not address root causes will be considered palliative and, in the long run, will be ineffective. Bradstreet et al. (2010) provide a comprehensive report on which individual biomarkers reflect physiological conditions in ASD and ADHD and how they can be corrected medically.

We can also systematically organize the information from all of the disparate sources and derive risk models that will help parents at once reduce risk and improve the symptoms of ASD in their children.

FAMILIAL RISK MARKERS

Recurrence (familial risk) is between 4 and 13 percent if the first child affected is female and approximately 7 to 20 percent if a male. The recurrence rate increases to 25 to 30 percent if a second child is also diagnosed with ASD. Studies have shown that among identical twins, if one child has ASD, then the other has a 60 to 95 percent chance of being affected (Dhillon et al., 2011).

PARENTAL AGE MARKERS

A meta-analysis by Hultmann (2011) found that men aged forty to forty-nine were 1.4 times more likely to have children with a diagnosis of autism than a comparison group (fifteen- to twenty-nine-year-old males). Risk of autism increased with father's age: fifty- to fifty-four-year-old men were 2.2 times more likely to have autistic children; for men older than fifty-five years, the risk is 4.4 times the comparison group.

One of the potential confounders for this finding is that men who tend to have children at an older age may take longer to adjust socially to adulthood, and then pass those genes forward to their children at an advanced age. Here again, we see the limits of retrospective epidemiological studies. This could be an example in which the group of interest (older men who have children later) represent a cryptic genetic subgroup.

Even so, advanced parental age could be a proxy variable for a specific causal factor. Copy number variations (CNVs) may be higher in older parents. One would have to study whether parental age adds additional, independent information to a prediction model beyond other variables, such as genetics and cumulative environmental exposures.

Other studies have shown that young fathers have similar risks to older fathers. Is this methylation in action? Or shared environment? It could possibly be a cohort effect. Or is there a genetic variation (e.g., for risk taking) that can lead to teen fathers that is also associated with ASD risk? Excellent research is needed to tease these factors apart.

GENETIC VARIATION MARKERS

In addition to the number of CNVs in general, a condensed panel of genetic markers might be one route to assaying autism risk. However, this could miss important de novo variations. A specific approach to autism risk using whole genome sequencing is needed, one that guarantees clinical-level accuracy of all types of genetic variation without bias and with extremely low false-positive rates.

BIOMARKERS OF AND HISTORY OF EXPOSURES

A checklist of known exposures now exists, and it includes cumulative doses of mercury and aluminum in vaccines and acetaminophen exposure in pregnancy or at an early age as risk factors. Some of these will be difficult to assess and thorough environmental exposure surveys can be expensive. Development opportunities and needs exist for standard assays for macrophage measures of aluminum, mercury, and other toxins, which may be most informative in general and should be given highest priority, as high measures would indicate course corrections to reduce exposures.

METABOLIC, PHYSIOLOGIC, CELLULAR BIOMARKERS THAT INDICATE RISK

Compared with the markers described in the previous sections, readily available markers exist within patients themselves. Primary markers include antibrain and specific immunoglobulin (Ig) antibodies in the mother and child. Additional markers that are potential candidates to be used in screening programs include glutathione levels, glutamate levels in the central nervous system (CNS), glial fibrillary acid protein (GFAP) measures of microglial activity, blood cytokine levels, oxidative stress and mitochondrial dysfunction biomarkers, metabolic markers of detoxification pathways, neurotropic markers, vasopressin, serotonin level, skin conductance measures, and measures of brain levels of connectivity. These latter markers could potentially be used to inform parents on specific treatment routes and course corrections such as dietary changes and addressing vitamin D_3 deficiency. Serotonin has been studied in detail as a biomarker and shows promise owing to its known causal contribution (Pagan et al., 2014). The expression of the genes neurotrophin 3 and 4 and a neurotrophin receptor (P75) was found to be potential biomarkers of ASD in the blood (Segura et al., 2015). Nelson et al. (2001) also reported finding neuropeptides and neurotrophins in neonatal blood of children with autism and mental retardation.

Many conditions share symptoms with autism, and many appear to share molecular etiologies. As we will see, the rich information available to patients via genetics is likely much more important to individual patients and families in defining road maps for specific action in terms of prevention, therapy, and treatment. A lifelong neurological disorder screen given at annual checkups is therefore much more likely to prove cost-effective than merely a screen for autism.

VACCINE RISK AND MEDICAL RIGHTS TO EXEMPTIONS FROM VACCINES

Prevention includes medical exemptions from vaccines for those concerned. The primary side effect of vaccines is fever. Children with autism are likely to experience recurrent immunological hyperactivation. Siblings of children with autism may be at more risk than siblings of neurotypicals, due to the familial risk and to birth order. Thus, it is reasonable to propose medical exemption in light of proven risk of adverse events related to vaccines, especially if the parents report temporal association. Women with antibrain antibodies in their blood should certainly avoid having their immune systems activated intentionally during pregnancy. And genetic testing is available to assess biologically informed risk.

If a woman does decide to get a flu shot while pregnant, she should wait until the last trimester, and she should request a vaccine without thimerosal (contra CDC recommendations).

Medical exemptions have been in place with vaccines for years; in fact, the CDC does not recommend vaccination for anyone with any serious medical condition. Classically, the wisdom was to never vaccinate the sick. This wisdom appears not to be no longer commonly applied in the clinical setting.

Human beings already have medical rights, under US and international law, that protect them from being experimented on, or from having medical procedures conducted upon them, without informed consent.

It is illegal to use force or coercion to cause a person to submit to a medical procedure. The medical profession must be forthright in revealing specific risks to patients. To do otherwise is to deny patients of their right to informed consent. Doctors who threaten patients with sanctions of refused health care could in principle lose their licenses for coerced medical practice, and civil suits could be filed against them for physical harm and denial of rights to informed consent. Of course, any medical practice conducted on any patient without consent should be considered assault and battery and should be reported to the local police.

SUPPLEMENTS DURING PREGNANCY

A number of supplements, if taken by women during pregnancy, have shown promise at reducing the risk of autism. For example, folic acid supplementation during pregnancy reduces incidence of autism (Surén et al., 2013) and has been observed to alter gene expression in genes involved in autism (Barus et al., 2015). Folic acid, a synthetic form of folate, cannot be metabolized by individuals with specific mutations in the gene MTHFR. Also, iron supplements taken during pregnancy also appear to reduce risk of ASD diagnosis (Schmidt et al., 2014).

TREATMENTS

There are autism advocacy groups who bristle at the idea that autism is a disease. They are sensitive to word use, and do not like the notion that autistics have a disease, or have something that needs to be cured. It is their position that autism and ASD is part of what makes them who they are. They do not want to be labeled *disabled*; they want to labeled *differently abled* and want people see them just like other people: *perfectly imperfect* (see, for example, Richard Âû's blog, 2015). And I understand why. This world can be cruel. There are mean-spirited people who will look down on those with autism or Asperger syndrome. And we should certainly respect the rights of people on the spectrum to have and express their (varied) opinions.

However, some autistics cannot write blogs. They cannot speak. They cannot walk well. They cannot learn language, math, or music. Other autistics are particularly gifted in some domains. They are, like all people, beautiful. And what the findings from scientific and biomedical research has done for some of them is to enable their immune system to stop consuming their neural precursor cells and dendrites. Parents of autistic children and autistic individuals themselves simply want to enable and empower the autistic mind to grow; they want an end to the physical pain and suffering.

As recently as 2014, it was generally perceived that although comorbid conditions that co-occur with autism may respond to treatment, the core components of ASD did not respond to treatment (Lai et al., 2014). That may no longer be the case.

As treatments come forward for specific domains of expression of autism, no one will force anyone to take the treatments. It will be up to the parent or the autistic adult himself to make decisions. Patients have a right to informed consent both for vaccination risks and for treatments of any kind. If an autistic person cannot provide his own consent, it is up to his legal guardian to do so.

For this book, I interviewed an autistic fellow, Mr. Jonathan Mitchell, who would really like to have new, effective treatments for autism. His call for cures has made national news, as they were interpreted to be insulting by people in the neurodiversity movement. Jonathan thinks autism should be curable. He told me: "Sure, I'd like to have less executive function problems and sure, I'd like to have my hand flapping to stop, after it starts. I'd like to be more approachable, socially, you know and maybe have a date. You know, I've never even had a date."

Given that environment toxicity is preventable, but perhaps not reversible, *cures* might not be the best terms for the possible goal. The difference between treating and curing autism is clear. Treatments are aimed at specific phenotypes; cures would undo the damage caused by the toxins. The best and most effective doctors see the patient, not the disease.

TREATMENT OF AUTISM WITH PHARMACEUTICAL PRODUCTS

Very few medicines have been developed specifically to treat AD and ASD overall. Antipsychotic medications may be useful to modulate behavior problems such as aggressiveness, and can appear to ameliorate repetitive behavior patterns. Seizures are managed with anticonvulsant medications, and bipolar symptoms are approached with typical treatments for those symptoms.

However, to date population-based medicine has for the most part failed to render significant success in the treatment of autism and ASD. The routes that biomedical science could travel to help shut down brain inflammation are clear. In this chapter, I review past, current, and future treatments of autism and ASD. I do this with respect for people on all sides of the "curing autism" issue, including those who feel there is no need for a cure.

Promising treatments for autism are summarized in Table 4.

TABLE 4. EXAMPLES OF POSSIBLE FUTURE TREATMENTS OF AUTISM BY PHENOTYPE

Phenotype	Treatment
Aggression	Aripiprazole
Gastrointestinal	Fecal matter transplants, vancomycin
Language delay/loss	Adenosine receptor agonists
Microglial activation	Amantadine, luteolin, cannabinoids, many others
Renal peptiduria	Vitamin E, selenium
Repetitive Motor	Fluoxetine,[a] risperidone,[b] adenosine receptor agonists[c]
Seizures	Carbamazepine, ketogenic diet
Social	Oxytocin, tetrahydrobiopterin (cofactor BH4)

Gene-Directed Treatment Examples	
Mitochondrial dysfunction	Carnitine, various drugs
SCN1A (serotonin)	Clonazepam (microdoses)

[a]Hollander E et al. A double-blind placebo-controlled trial of fluoxetine for repetitive behaviors and global severity in adult autism spectrum disorders. *Am J Psychiatry.* 2012;169(3):292–299. doi:10.1176/appi.ajp.2011.10050764.

[b]McDougle CJ et al. Risperidone for the core symptom domains of autism: results from the study by the autism network of the research units on pediatric psychopharmacology. Am J Psychiatry. 2005;162(6):1142–1148.

[c]Tanimura Y et al. Indirect basal ganglia pathway mediation of repetitive behavior: attenuation by adenosine receptor agonists. Behav Brain Res. 2010;210(1):116–122. doi:10.1016/j.bbr.2010.02.030.

AGGRESSION

The US Food and Drug Administration (FDA) has approved the atypical antipsychotic drugs risperidone and aripiprazole for treatment of aggression and irritability in autistics ages five to sixteen. Risperidone can reduce aggression in mice with an R451C (arginine to cysteine residue 451 substitution) mutation in neuroligin-3 (NL3). This mutation is found in some cases of ASD (Burrows et al., 2015). The basis of approval for use in ASD is in part that it is used for the treatment of schizophrenia, which shares clinical features with ASD, such as social deficits and shifts in the *N*-methyl-D-aspartic acid (NMDA), gamma-aminobutyric acid (GABA), and dopamine receptors. Risperidone has been shown to alleviate repetitive behaviors in mice, but to date has not shown to impact social deficits (Jeste and Geschwind, 2014).

ACETYLCYSTEINE

Stutzman and Dopheide (2015) concluded that treatment with acetylcysteine improved ASD symptoms, including irritability and aggression, in their teenage patient. They wrote:

> *A 17-year-old Hispanic male with ASD and intellectual disability was hospitalized for inpatient psychiatric treatment due to impulsive and violent behavior. Despite receiving various medications in the initial weeks of hospitalization, including intramuscular lorazepam and diphenhydramine injections (four days a week on average), the patient continued to exhibit aggressive and unpredictable behaviors. Treatment with 20% acetylcysteine oral solution was initiated at a dosage of 600 mg twice daily as an adjunct to quetiapine therapy. Over the next six weeks, reductions in the patient's aggressive behavior, tantrums and irritability were noted. The use of as-needed medications to control aggression was decreased and the dosage of quetiapine was lowered from 700 to 400 mg daily over the course of the hospitalization. Acetylcysteine was well tolerated, with no observed or reported adverse effects. Unlike clonidine or guanfacine (other medications used for ASD-related behavioral symptoms), acetylcysteine is not sedating; moreover, it lacks the metabolic, extrapyramidal and endocrine adverse effects of atypical antipsychotics. Published data from small controlled trials and case reports suggest that acetylcysteine use is associated with improvements in irritability and aggression in prepubertal children with ASD; these therapeutic benefits may be associated with acetylcysteine's glutamatergic, dopaminergic, antioxidant and anti-inflammatory properties.*

TREATMENT OF SPEECH AND LANGUAGE PROCESSING DISORDER IN AUTISM

Intranasal delivery of davunetide (NAP), a neuroprotective octapeptide NAPVSPIQ, from the ADNP protein, has been reported to alleviate cognitive abnormalities observed in a knockout mouse model (Vulih-Shultzman et al., 2007; Gozes et al., 2011).

The mechanism of action of NAP has been elucidated and involves interaction of ADNP with the MAP1LC3 protein (autophagy regulating microtubule-associated protein 1 light chain 3) with microtubule end binding proteins (Gozes, 2015). MAP1LC3 is one of the genes in the chromosome 16 region 16q24.2 found to be association with autism (Handrigan et al., 2013). The ability of macrophages to function properly is highly dependent on microtubules.

A number of drugs approved for the treatment of Alzheimer disease are under exploration for use in ASD. Some target specific phenotypes, whereas many others target microglial activation.

TREATMENTS TO ENHANCE SOCIAL SKILLS

Tetrahydrobiopterin is a naturally occurring substance (essential cofactor) that targets L-dopamine production pathways. Administration of 20 mg/kg of BH4 per day led to significant improvements in social awareness, autism mannerisms, hyperactivity, and inappropriate speech (Frye et al., 2010). Placebo-controlled studies in Japan showed long-term efficacy and minor side effects (Takesada et al., 1990)

Treatment of autistic disorder (AD) with inhaled oxytocin has been observed to increase the frequency and duration of eye contact and improvement in social skills in autistic children. Auyeung et al. (2015) found in a randomized, placebo-controlled clinical trial that doses of 24 international units of oxytocin, administered to adult males with an AD diagnosis and control males, enhanced gaze to the eyes in both the autism and control groups. Within the autism group, oxytocin had the largest effect on fixation duration in individuals with impaired levels of eye contact at baseline.

This was not the first study of the potential utility of oxytocin to improve social skills in autism. It had already been shown to increase retention of social cognition (Hollander et al., 2007), and clinical trials point to improvements in emotion recognition and eye gaze (Preti et al., 2014; Guastella et al., 2010). In Asperger syndrome, oxytocin improves emotion recognition and social skills including turn taking and a decrease in social anxiety (Andari et al., 2010). A more recent study by Yatawara (2015) also showed that oxytocin treatment improved social interaction deficits in young children with autism. Domes et al. (2013) found that right amygdala activity to facial stimuli increased in ASD in response to treatment with oxytocin. Randomized placebo-controlled functional magnetic resonance imaging (fMRI) studies have shown that oxytocin restores activity in the ventromedial prefrontal cortex (vmPFC) in a friend-foe recognition task-dependent manner (Aoki et al., 2015). It is generally recognized that oxytocin mutations may not represent important variants in all, or even most, cases of autism. Tansey et al. (2010) found no OXTR single nucleotide variant alleles to be significantly associated with autism in Irish, Portuguese, and British cases, after correction for multiple comparisons. However, the lack of a strong association of genomic variants (single nucleotide variations, CNVs, etc.) is due to the heterogeneous nature of autism and ASD, and the finding does not mean that oxytocin receptor mutations are not important in a subset of cases.

VITAMIN D_3

Vitamin D deficiency exists in autistics. Feng et al. (2016) found that serum levels of vitamin D_3 were significantly lower in autistic children compared to neurotypicals. They found that serum levels were also negatively correlated with ABC total scores (a behavior analysis) and language subscale scores. After supplementation with vitamin D_3, autism symptom scores were significantly improved, and improvement seemed more significant in younger children.

ALLEVIATING MITOCHONDRIAL DYSFUNCTION

Studies have shown some promise for mutation-based and nonmutation-based mitochondrial dysfunction, notably carnitine, coenzyme Q10, ubiquinol, and B vitamins (Rossignol and Frye, 2012). Multiple molecular dysfunctions exist, however, and specific targeted treatments may be possible for each.

SEROTONIN PATHWAY DYSFUNCTION

Serotonin reuptake inhibitors are used for depression and obsessive-compulsive disorder in children seven years and older. Divalproex sodium is used to treat manic symptoms and epilepsy, and the psychostimulant drug methylphenidate is used to treat attention deficit hyperactivity disorder (ADHD). Targeted therapy is now possible given that whole genome and whole exome sequencing is possible; mutations in the relevant genes and pathways may indicate likely efficacy, lack of efficacy, and/or safety issues with these drugs.

The outcomes of the use of these drugs in autism and ASD have been mixed at best, and in general prescriptions are still hit-or-miss for any individual patient. Gene-guided treatments are needed so patients and parents can avoid the disappointment, stress, discouragement, and attrition of will that can result from ineffectual treatments. The negative experiences can be replaced with experiences of joy and celebration at young patients' renewed progress in development and learning.

REDOX METABOLISM

Frye and Rossignal (2014) discussed the use of methylcobalamin with and without folinic acid and vitamin C and *N*-acetyl-L-cysteine in other studies, with improved core and associated ASD symptoms.

CHRONIC MICROGLIAL ACTIVATION

A great number of opportunities exist to reduce microglial activation, a root cause of many cases of autism. Immunoneuroexcitotoxicity via chronic microglial cell activation is a prevalent, lifelong cause of autism, and microglia activation can be prevented in a myriad of ways. Therefore, rational design of a study that complements treatment with drugs—and supplements—with those that shut down microglial activation via different routes should be high priority. Otherwise, autistics will be treated for symptoms, not reversal of causes, of their condition.

Chronic microglial activation is a positive feedback loop, which, if short-circuited, could alleviate symptoms in numerous domains of AD and ASD. People with ASD should understand that no one wants to take away what makes them special. The type of damage that can be stopped ranges from simple migraines and allergies to severe intellectual disability, lack of speech and language, and death.

Given the central role of microglial hyperactivation, tiered treatment strategies might be worth exploring. Assessment of symptoms after each tier might indicate rationale, or obviation, of treatment of further symptoms. Not all of these drugs are approved on-label for treatment of autism or autism symptoms.

Anti-inflammatory therapy designed to reduce microglial activation to non-deleterious levels holds the promise of slowing and perhaps halting progressive brain injury.

Luteolin, for example, is a bioflavinoid antioxidant that reduces microglia activation. Treatment of activated microglia with luteolin blocked proinflammatory and proapoptotic gene expression. Ramification of microglia (return to resting state) was significantly increased. Activated microglia showed reduced nitrous oxide secretion (Dirscherl et al., 2010). Chamomile tea is one good source of luteolin. Theorhides et al. (2015) found that "brain fog" and inflammation were both reduced by luteolin, and Tsilioni et al. (2015) found that autistics with luteolin in their diet showed reductions in markers of microglial activation (tumor necrosis factor [TNF] and interleukin [IL]-6 levels) in their serum.

Sulforaphane attenuates the lipopolysaccharide (LPS)-induced increase of IL-1β, IL-6, and TNF-α expression in microglia (Brandenburg et al., 2010). Sulfoaphane also dramatically improved social skills in two-thirds of patients in a prospective, placebo-controlled clinical trial (Singh et al., 2014). Forty-six percent of patients treated with sulfoaphane exhibited noticeable improvement in social interaction, fifty-four percent improved in aberrant behaviors, and forty-two percent improved in verbal communication.

A large number of microglial suppressors is reviewed in Appendix A, online at http://envgencauses.com. Clinical studies are needed.

THE PARADOX OF VALPROATE

Valproic acid has been shown to reduce inflammation from postinjury-induced brain damage (Suda et al., 2013). It is ironic, then, that autism is clearly a condition with chronic microglial activation and innate immunity-induced inflammation. How can we resolve that valproic acid can induce autism and reduce brainwide inflammation with measureably improved outcomes? How can it have both neuroprotective and neurotrophic effects?

If we keep in mind that ischemia-reperfusion of the type induced in animal studies leads to massive numbers of damaged brain cells, it would appear that when environmental inducement of microglial activation has no damaged cells as targets, activated cells go after healthy cells. Signals from damaged cells also include a set of cytokines and signals that activate microglia (IL-1, TNF-α, and granulocyte-macrophage colony-stimulating factor, also known as colony stimulating factor [GM-CSF]), whereas most other interleukins deactivate microglia and return them to their ramified state. In the absence of the turnoff signals, the microglia are free to cause damage unchecked and can induce apoptosis in nearby neurons.

This idea is bolstered by the observation that valproic acid injected in the spines of mice after spinal injury caused improved conservation of hind limb function (Lu et al., 2013), accompanied by a reduction in the accumulation of microglia-macrophages and astrocytes in the spinal fluid. Similarly, microglial activation after global cerebral schemia was *reduced* by valproic acid (Xuan et al., 2012).

The mechanism of autism via gestational valproic acid exposure may have an intermediate step: exposure, microglial apoptosis (Chen et al., 2007), cytokine release, microglial activation, and dendritic extension and neural precursor death. It induces the upregulation of the expression of neurotrophic factors, including glial cell line-derived neurotrophic factor (GDNF) and brain-derived neurotrophic factor (BDNF) from astrocytes (Chen et al., 2006). Valproic acid is thought to be effective in neurodegenerative diseases such as Alzheimer's disease, Parkinson's disease, and human immunodeficiency virus (HIV) dementia by "selectively killing microglia" (Dragunow et al., 2006).

Naturally, autistics who plan on having children should avoid using valproic acid, given the increased combined genetic × exposure risk.

TREATMENT OF COMORBID CONDITIONS

Physicians who attempt to treat comorbid conditions may find treating some with autism and ASD challenging. At times, a diagnosis of autism and ASD is given to enable a family to access resources they would not qualify for without the diagnosis.

For accuracy in any diagnosis, the symptoms must not be explicable by other diagnoses. This ambiguous nature of symptoms is also a concern for this book, as many of the autism phenotypes may be shared with other conditions due to the same underlying genetic pathways and environmental causes. However, the *Diagnostic and Statistical Manual of Mental Disorders, Fifth Edition* (DSM-5) allows an autism diagnosis with or without specification of "association with" a known medical or genetic condition or environmental factor. This frame of reference neither commits one to think of autism as a subset of other conditions nor to consider all co-occurring symptoms as being part of autism. There are important medical and legal implications for one's view on such exercises in classification. This classification exercise is dealt with in Chapter 13, which deals with concepts of comorbidity, as comorbidities are critically important to the definition of populations for clinical studies.

Other specifications include whether the symptoms appear with or without accompanying intellectual impairment and also with or without accompanying language impairment. These allowances are useful in that they may help refine clinical populations that can be compared for discovery of differentiating molecular etiologies. The DSM-5 also prescribes levels of severity related to level of care needed.

All of these conditions, including Asperger syndrome, fall under the umbrella of autism spectrum disorders in the DSM-5. This lumping of conditions into ASD can lead to placing groups of individuals into clinical categories replete with heterogeneity, making the use of ASD as a well-defined comparator group problematic. Each study of autism and ASD, for example, risks missing more refined important findings. The most reasonable approach for research studies is the focus on association of genes and environmental factors with phenotypes, not heterogeneous populations. The basis of categories and subcategories is not questioned; however, the utility of subsuming these subcategories into "ASD" again begs the question of shared versus unique molecular and environmental etiologies.

SCN1A MUTATIONS: FROM ASSOCIATION TO ANIMAL MODELS TO TARGETED TREATMENT OF SEIZURES

In a study of Chinese children with SCN1A mutations, Wong et al. (2012) detected a high frequency of ASD (79 percent) and vaccination-induced encephalopathy (57 percent) in those with Dravet syndrome with SCN1A mutation. The authors concluded that it would be wise to evaluate further relationships between SCN1A mutations and ASD with epilepsy or vaccination-induced encephalopathy. A study of a patient with intractable myoclonic epilepsy and familial migraines revealed a potential role of SCN1A mutation (Frosk et al., 2013).

Note especially the observations by Huynh et al. (2008) that ". . . a large percentage of children who suffered vaccination-induced encephalopathy exhibited clinical progression similar to severe myoclonic epilepsy in infancy (SMEI), which is an epileptic encephalopathy with long seizures accompanied by fever, intractable myoclonic seizure (muscle jerking) and psychomotor decline."

Huynh et al. also noted that more than 50 percent of severe myoclonic epilepsy in infancy patients experienced their first seizure after diphtheria, pertussis, and tetanus (DPT) vaccination.

In studying this population, Huynh et al. (2008) identified mutations in the SCN1A gene in 11 of 14 patients with suspected vaccine encephalopathy. The SCN1A gene encodes a voltage-gated sodium channel protein. It has been hypothesized that SCN1A mutations are predisposing factors "waiting to be triggered by fever or other stresses" (Huynh et al., 2008). A mouse strain with a defective copy of SCN1A (Scn1a+/- mice) was found to exhibit autism-like behavior, including hyperactivity, stereotyped behaviors, social interaction deficits, impaired context-dependent spatial memory, aversion to novel food, and social odors. The authors also found that a low dose of clonazepam "completely reversed" the phenotypes, indicating that mutational screening in autistic children for SCN1A mutations may aid in alleviating some of the most important types of impairments due to those mutations. The result has been replicated (Han et al., 2012).

This has implications for the treatment of autistic patients with SCN1A mutations. Very low doses may be effective in these cases. A search at clinicaltrials.gov (Jan 2016) found no prospective studies are underway.

KETOGENIC DIET, SOCIAL BEHAVIOR, AND SEIZURES

Seizures are examples of a condition that is considered comorbid but that also appears to share major etiologic pathways with core ASD symptoms. A high-fat, low-carbohydrate ketogenic diet improves social behavior and metabolism in one ASD model mouse (Ahn at al., 2014) and reduced seizures in another (Rushkin et al., 2013). Results in human studies are early but promising, showing improved learning abilities and social skills in a handful of studies (Napoli et al., 2014).

BEHAVIORAL THERAPIES

Behaviorial therapies are used to help children learn or relearn language, self-care, and social skills, but are typically only moderately successful for severe AD. The focus is primarily on the use of rewards to reinforce desirable behavior.

Lee and Tomblin (2012) showed that the ability for reinforcement learning is retained in ASD and provides a neurobiological basis for such programs. Other studies have shown that autistics retain a great deal more information than many give them credit for. It is easy to underestimate someone on the basis of stereotyped behaviors that may not reflect at all on whether a person is paying attention. The sensory input overload, along with the excitatory-inhibitive overdrive, perhaps leading to input signals traveling into the motor cortex as signals for motor movement, may be present, but until an autistic is given the opportunity to demonstrate their knowledge retention, it is best to presume that all types of learning are occurring.

ANTAGONISTIC TREATMENT AND NEGLECT

Studies have shown neglect along with stressful, antagonizing treatment by others can lead to microglial activation. How the brain is treated by others influences not only its immediate chemistry, but stress also alters gene expression, inducing activation of microglia. Reduction of microglial activation should reduce long-term damage to dendrites, stripping inhibitory synapses and devouring neural precursor cells.

Being good to children can help, and it does not cost anything.

GENE-INFORMED TREATMENTS

It is now known that autism is a medical condition. The bewildering possible combinations of symptoms and severity levels can be clarified greatly via whole genome or whole exome sequencing.

One of the most exciting developments for autism and ASD in a long time is the advent of whole genome sequencing. When clinicians are informed by molecular mechanisms, the knowledge can then be useful for defining routes to effective therapies and treatments. High resolution, personalized medicine focuses on the link between genotype and phenotypes in the individual patient, not necessarily clinical subtypes (domains).

Genetics lends itself well to fine-resolution diagnostics driven by a desire to provide best treatment for individual phenotypes (i.e., *medical phenostics*). When chromosomal (karyotypic) molecular etiologies of multiple phenotypes are suspected, *medical syndromics* may be a better term. Neither syndromics nor phenostics is mutually exclusive because individuals with a syndrome may also have a constellation of inherited or de novo mutations that lead to any of the phenotypes associated with ASD.

When the focus of research involves the study of genetic or genomic modification, the term *medical genomics* seems more appropriate than other terms. However, such study groups should be defined by phenotype and informed by genotype and environmental exposure. The practice of naming syndromes after molecular aberrations in the genome may be convenient, but it may lead to *reductio ad absurdum.* Each person's unique constellation of inherited and de novo risk and modifier mutations could lead to a constellation of unique names and a proliferations of syndromes, many of which are nearly identical.

Some, but not all, information is available in genomic assays. In breast cancer, the disease is not defined away by the additional information provided by knowledge of the hormone (estrogen and progesterone) receptor status. Instead, the cancer is referred to, for example, as "ER+" or "ER–", or "triple negative" (ER–, PR–, and HER2Neu–). This knowledge helps oncologists direct the treatment, and I have listed the use of breast cancer receptor status as one of the greatest translational successes in medical history (Lyons-Weiler, 2016).

Similar molecular characteristic designations can be envisioned for autism—MeCP2+ autism, for example, would inform clinicians of a function-altering mutation in the MeCP2 gene. *MeCP2–* could refer to the outright loss (knock-out) of that gene for a patient (MeCP2 is X-linked). Copy number variations could be referred to as MeCP2+N, where *N* is the number of copies. The dosage effect of CNV variation is thus communicated as well, without demoting every case of autism to its own developmental or regressive molecular disorder. The combinatoric number of possible mutational and molecular "types" of autism is nearly infinite.

A survey of parents of autistics and parents of children with no diagnosed disability revealed that parents of autistic children were more likely to use and pay for genetic testing than neurotypical parents. (May 2012). Parents of autistics also reported being more willing to pay for genetic testing out of pocket if it was a test for aggression or if the test could help develop a tool for early diagnosis. Two genes in particular have polymorphisms in the general population that are associated with proactive aggression (monoamine oxidase A gene and CD13). Although IQ is related to use of adaptive behaviors (Kanne et al., 2011), alleles can occur in individuals with and without ASD, and signs of aggression in ASD are independent of most ASD phenotypes with the exception of repetitive behaviors (Kanne et al., 2011).

Although interest is high, parents of autistics in the United States are less likely to add a genetic test to their toolbox than those in France (Amiet et al., 2014). It makes little sense to study environmental risk factors independent of genetic factors, and vice versa. Environmental risks can be aggregated by families just like genetic factors. Studies are needed that examine independent and combined risk of genes and environment through interactions.

The environment is heterogeneous in space and time. Certainly, population-level associations may miss some very important environmental factors; however, variation across conditions within ASD could be an important study for specific (narrow) age groups. Lumping variously manifested phenotypes into a broad spectrum may be useful for expediting current diagnostic purposes (e.g., family member with partial autism-like [clinical] or autism-associated [subclinical] features as a risk factor). When genetic researchers study molecular etiologies by focusing on individual phenotypes and sets of phenotypes, a much better resolved picture of disease etiology is seen. Use of unaffected sibs can weaken the association if any of the siblings fall into broader autism phenotype. The focus of some studies should be on phenotypes, not necessarily on diagnosis; these issues need to be consider in the design of future studies.

Therefore, to eliminate the guesswork, patients could be matched to particular combinations of treatments that are likely to be effective, given the specific mutations they carry that might be related to their autism symptoms. Enrolled patient information could be added to a large study that afforded treatment options based on their specific profile—a process called molecular allocation. This would involve whole genome sequencing in case they have other candidate LoF mutations or deletions. This would allow an overall test of all available treatments to molecular subgroups as indicated by their disabled pathways and also allow for the use of a standardized set of outcome measurements for each phenotype.

References : see envgencauses.com

Chapter 18.

INJECTING OBJECTIVE ASSOCIATION AND CAUSAL INFERENCE INTO CLINICAL TRIALS, PREVENTION, DIAGNOSIS, AND TREATMENT OF ASD

The *Diagnostic and Statistical Manual of Mental Disorders, Fifth Edition* (DSM-5) brought autistic disorder (AD), Asperger disorder, childhood disintegrative disorder (CDD), and pervasive developmental disorder not otherwise specified (PDD-NOS) under one umbrella of *autism spectrum disorder* (ASD). The categories attempt to address variation in severity levels of some of the clinical features, and diagnosis is largely driven by anticipated degree of need for services.

The rates of autism and ASD have increased in recent years and have now reached almost 1 in 50 births in the United States. That is a remarkable increase from 2003, when autism rates were 1 in 250 births. Some have argued that the increase in autism and ASD is due to the most recent and more inclusive classification of ASD; however, the increase in autism was well underway before 2013. Others have implied that the increase is due to improved diagnosis, contagion of self-diagnosis, and other factors. Although each of these other explanations is worthy of further consideration, they can also detract from focus on a search for environmental factors. These nonepidemiological factors do not account for the significant increase in the diagnosis of autism. Something biological is amiss. Genes cannot explain the increase because gene frequencies do not change that rapidly overnight.

Autism spectrum disorder clinical diagnostic categories are moving targets designed for clinical utility and may not reflect the optimal set of categories for research on association, definitions of biomarker, and risk factors. Also, ASD is diagnosed based on behavioral characteristics presented in a clinical setting. Various instruments exist for use in formal diagnosis, including checklists and questionnaires (e.g., Social Responsiveness Scale and Social Communication Questionnaire), diaries (observational schedules), and structured interviews. The Autism Diagnostic Observation Schedule–Generic is used in combination with the Autism Diagnostic Interview–Revised (ADI-R). Together, these tests assess social and communication impairments (Autism Diagnostic Observation Schedule–Generic) and restricted, repetitive, and stereotyped behaviors. Such tools may be efficient but are not specific. Risi et al. (2006) found that individually, these two tools had specificity below 50 percent, both finding 29 percent of non-ASD children as false positives. Used in combination, there were fewer false positives, but they disagreed in approximately 15 percent of cases. Thus, they are used in combination with clinical observation. Due to the lack of specificity of such instruments, they should not be used to define clinical populations for research studies, as they will add non-ASD individuals to a case-control or cohort study.

More problematic than the two tests described in the previous paragraph, the clinical categories themselves presume common etiology within any defined category. Therefore, a phenotypic approach to autism and ASD is proposed. It requires focus both on the timing of events leading to the condition and the presence or absence of a role of environmental factors. These disease phenotypic categories reflect manifestation of processes that cause ASD and will be critical for defining useful clinical populations for studying the functional role(s) of specific mutations and genes, involvement of brain regions, as well as for attributing causality. The phenotypic categories of ASD are:

1. **Prenatal, congenital autism and ASD.** Persons born with autism or ASD purely as a result of their genotype. They usually have one very serious developmental abnormality due to a loss-of-function (LoF) mutation in a regulatory gene, or they may have two or three mutations (inherited or germline) that disrupt normal development. These individuals are destined, regardless of environmental factors, to fail to develop typically.
2. **Prenatal, induced autism and ASD.** Persons born with autism or ASD as a combined result of zero, one, or two mutations plus an environmental insult in the womb. Candidates include fever, maternal measles, mumps, and rubella (MMR) infection, maternal immunity against fetal

brain proteins, and neurotoxin exposure (e.g., metals such mercury and aluminum, pesticides, valproic acid, thalidomide).

3. **Perinatal, induced autism, and ASD.** Induced autism or ASD may result as a consequence of injuries such as hypoxia due to labor difficulties or physician error. Immediate reactions have been observed due to hepatitis B vaccination shortly after birth. The hepatitis B vaccine exceeds the Food and Drug Administration (FDA) limit for aluminum exposure for typical birth weights. The early vaccine schedule to two months also includes aluminum quantities that exceed the recommended exposure. Neurotoxicity of aluminum is extremely well established in the literature, as is described in Chapter 11.
4. **Regressive, congenital autism and ASD.** Autism that was predestined to occur at a later stage, due to one to three or (rarely) more mutations, with or without an environmental trigger. This type of autism includes Rett syndrome if there is a confirmed genetic basis, and childhood disintegrative disorder if the mutations are known to lead to specific late-onset brain development abnormalities. This is likely to be the rarest type of autism.
5. **Regressive, induced autism, and ASD.** Autism that is triggered by listed environmental factors, but at a later age (two to three years). There are instances of very late onset of autism after exposure (such as those caused in adults by *Herpes simplex* infection). In ages two to three, these cases likely involve zero to three mutations; therefore, genetics is a cofactor, and the trigger is a definite causal factor.
6. **Gender bias.** It may be useful to distinguish clinically, for research purposes, between male autism or ASD and female autism or ASD as another dimension in the tesseract. Males have nearly a fivefold greater risk of autism and ASD relative to females. This greater risk probably has multiple factors, which likely reflect risk, but also etiology, specific constellation of symptoms, progression, and outcome.

Combining these various phenotypic classes of autism and ASD into one overall population for cohort and case-control studies will confound attempts to attribute cause to either genetics or environment. Without a clear demarcation of these "onset" categories, large-scale studies of association to rule in or rule out causal factors will likely prove to be completely fruitless, with negative results of finding associations due to high heterogeneity in a sample. One of the most fundamental assumptions of statistical hypothesis testing is that measurements from a variable being studied are randomly sampled from a homogeneous population. Negative results from poorly designed studies may thus be utterly misleading.

HOW DOES ASD FALL INTO THE SUBTYPES?

A *Mortality and Morbidity Weekly Report* (MMWR) study of ASD children aged eight years at 14 monitoring sites in 2008 found 44 percent autistic disorder, 46 percent ASD or PDD, and 9 percent Asperger disorder (CDC, 2014). The same study from data in 2010 using 15 monitor sites found the following percentages for 2010: autistic disorder (43 percent), ASD or PDD (46 percent), or Asperger disorder (11 percent). These percentages reflect "of those with ASD of these three types" to make the percentages comparable among reports.

The proposed disease phenotypic classes are not intended to supplant DSM-5 clinical categories; rather, they provide focus on timing of onset, which is critical to causal inference, and are designed to empower the community to study autism and ASD in a manner more likely to objectively enrich clinical populations with individuals of common etiologies. Studies of any one subcategory should include proper (i.e., clinically relevant) control groups, whereas studies across these groups (comparisons) may provide key information useful for identifying specific associations, risk factors, and causal factors.

CDD AND PPD-NOS

The MMWR reports do not summarizes percentage of PPD-NOS or childhood disintegrative disorder as percentages. Childhood disintegrative disorder occurs in approximately two per 100,000 children (Fombonne, 2009), approximately 60 times less prevalent than autistic disorder. It is described as a "relentlessly progressive neurologic disorder" (Rosman et al., 2013) and is characterized as having an onset later in life than autism, with more complete and severe symptoms than autism, with more frequent seizures, with much worse long-term prognosis, especially for cases with seizures.

Pervasive developmental disorder not otherwise specified includes three recognized groups, most likely reflecting differences in underlying etiology or severity of injury to specific brain functions. The three groups of PPD-NOS are:

1. A high-functioning group with symptoms similar to those in Asperger syndrome, but with the addition of a delay in language development and mild cognitive impairment (25 percent).
2. Autistic disorder-like, but with missing key criteria for a full autistic disorder diagnosis (25 percent).
3. Autistic disorder-like, but missing or mild stereotypical and repetitive behaviors (50 percent).

Depending on the specific hypothesis at hand, these clinical subcategories may need to be studied separately from the other three (AD, Asperger syndrome, and ASD-PDD) for association studies. The full complement of possible combination of symptoms and their relative severity in individuals makes combining individuals into clinical groups risky without prior molecular knowledge.

I have spoken with many pediatricians who work with families with autistic members, and they are, by and large, not concerned about an exacting classification. They prefer to identify clinically actionable information about a patient or a family that at least appears to inform on a given autism or ASD phenotype. Some report amelioration of severity; others report a complete turnaround (nonverbal to approaching normal in communication skills).

SUMMARY

The concepts of co-occurrence, comorbidity, and syndromic occurrence of specific phenotypes are difficult to study without a full delineation of molecular etiologies. Current categories of autism and related conditions do not comprehensively reflect aggregated phenotypes that are well-enough defined for definitive studies of association of ASD with genetic variation, nor of ASD with environmental causal factors. A time-of-onset focused pathway for future studies is presented with the definition of at least five distinct phenotypic classes of autism and ASD, defined so as to provide a clearer definition of useful clinical populations geared for causal analysis, and much more likely to reveal both distinct etiologies and risk factors for the identification of clinically actionable knowledge for bona fide subtypes of autism and ASD. Many of the autism and ASD phenotypes are not permanent in their severity, and some can be remarkably responsive to treatment. Thus, an individual could float among the existing categories on the spectrum on any given day, depending on their health. In short, the current clinical designations are hypotheses based in part on constellation of symptoms and severity, but are hypotheses, nevertheless.

References : see envgencauses.com